NUR
POC
DRU
2005

EDITOR

Judith Barberio Pollachek, PhD, APRN,

BC, ANPC, GNPC
Assistant Professor
Rutgers, The State University of New Jersey
College of Nursing
Newark, New Jersey

CONSULTING EDITOR

Leonard G. Gomella, MD, FACS
The Bernard W. Godwin, Jr., Professor
Chairman, Department of Urology
Jefferson Medical College
Thomas Jefferson University
Philadelphia, Pennsylvania

McGraw-Hill
MEDICAL PUBLISHING DIVISION
New York Chicago San Francisco Lisbon
London Madrid Mexico City Milan New Delhi
San Juan Seoul Singapore Sydney Toronto

The McGraw·Hill Companies

Nurse's Pocket Drug Guide 2005

Copyright © 2004 by Judith Barberio Pollachek. Based on CLINICIAN'S POCKET DRUG REFERENCE 2004 Copyright © 2004 by Leonard G. Gomella. Published by **The McGraw-Hill Companies, Inc.** All rights reserved. Printed in Canada. Except as permitted under the United States copyright Act of 1976, no part of this publication may be reproduced or distributed in any form or by any means, or stored in a data base or retrieval system, without the prior written permission of the publisher.

1 2 3 4 5 6 7 8 9 0   WBCWBC   0 9 8 7 6 5 4

ISBN 0-07-144056-9
ISSN 1550-2554

This book was set in Times Roman by Pine Tree Composition, Inc.
The editors were Janet Foltin, Harriet Lebowitz, and Karen Davis.
The production supervisor was Richard C. Ruzycka.
The cover designer was Mary McKeon.
The text designer was Marsha Cohen/Parallelogram Graphics.
The index was prepared by Pat Perrier.
Webcom Limited was printer and binder.

This book is printed on acid-free paper.

CONTENTS

PREFACE

On behalf of the entire editorial board, we are pleased to present the first edition of the *Nurse's Pocket Drug Guide*. This book is based on the basic drug presentation style used since 1983 in the *Clinician's Pocket Reference*.

Our goal is to identify the most frequently used and clinically important medications based on input from our readers and editorial board. The book includes more than 1000 generic medications and is designed to represent a cross section of those used in health care practices across the country.

The style of drug presentation includes key elements of commonly used medications that are essential information for the student, practicing nurse, and health care provider. Key medication elements include generic and selected brand names; common uses; mechanisms of action; adult and pediatric dosages with key dosing modifiers (elderly, renal/hepatic disease); major cautions and contraindications (pregnancy, breast-feeding, and others); available dosing formulations; key notes; common side effects for the medication; common drug-drug, drug-herb, and drug-lab interactions; common laboratory test results; and nursing indications and patient education highlights. A unique feature is the inclusion of common uses of medications rather than just the official labeled indications. These recommendations are based on the actual uses of the medication supported by publications and community standards of care. All common uses have been reviewed by our editorial board.

It is essential that students, registered nurses, and advanced-practice nurses learn more than the name and dose of the medications they prescribe and administer. Certain common side effects and significant contraindications are associated with most prescription medications. Although a nurse or other health care practitioner should ideally be completely familiar with the entire package insert of any medication being prescribed, such a requirement is unreasonable. References such as the *Physician's Desk Reference* and in many cases the drug manufacturer's Web site make package inserts readily available for many medications, but they may not provide key data for generic and over-the-counter drugs. The limitations of difficult-to-read package inserts were acknowledged by the Food and Drug Administration in early 2001, when it noted that health care providers do not have time to read the many pages of small print in the typical package insert. In the future, package inserts will be redesigned to ensure that important drug interactions, contraindications, and common side effects are highlighted for easier practitioner reference. We have made this key prescribing information available to you now in this pocket-sized book. Information in this book is meant for use by health care professionals who order and administer commonly prescribed medications.

The 2005 edition has been completely reviewed by our editorial board. New FDA drug approvals of more than two dozen key medications have been included. Recent changes in indications and available forms of other drugs have been added based on new FDA approvals.

We express special thanks to our families for their support of this book and the entire project. The contributions of the members of the editorial board are deeply appreciated. Janet Foltin and the team at McGraw-Hill have been supportive in our goal of creating a pocket drug reference for nursing professionals.

Your comments and suggestions are always welcome and encouraged because improvements to this and all our books would be impossible without the interest and feedback of our readers. We hope this book will help you learn some of the key elements in prescribing medications and allow you to care for your patients in the best way possible.

Judith Barberio Pollachek, PhD, APRN, BC, ANPC, GNPC
Newark, New Jersey
pollachek@nursetech.rutgers.edu

Leonard G. Gomella, MD
Philadelphia, PA
Leonard.Gomella@jefferson.edu

Medications are listed by prescribing class, and the individual medications are then listed in alphabetical order by generic name. Some of the more commonly recognized trade names are listed for each medication (in parentheses after the generic name).

Generic Drug Name (Selected Common Brand Names [Controlled Substance]) WARNING: Summary of the "Black Box" precautions that are deemed necessary by the FDA. These are significant precautions and contraindications concerning the individual medication. **Uses:** This includes both FDA labeled indications and other "off label" uses of the medication. Because many medications are used to treat various conditions based on the medical literature and not listed in their package insert, we list common uses of the medication rather than the official "labeled indications" (FDA approved) based on input from our editorial board **Action:** How the drug works. This information is helpful in comparing classes of drugs and understanding side effects and contraindications **Dose:** *Adults.* Where no specific pediatric dose is given, the implication is that this drug is not commonly used or indicated in that age group. At the end of the dosing line, important dosing modifications may be noted (ie, take with food, avoid antacids, etc) **Caution/Contra:** [pregnancy/fetal risk categories, breast-feeding] Other common contraindications or cautions **Supplied:** Common dosing forms **Notes/SE:** Lists other key information about the drug as well as the more common or significant side effects. **Interactions:** Common drug-drug, drug-herb, and drug-food interactions that may change the drug response **Labs:** Common laboratory test results that are changed by the drug and/or significant lab monitoring requirements **NIPE:** (Nursing Indications and/or Patient Education) Significant information that the nurse must be aware of with administration of the drug and/or information that should be given to any patient taking the drug.

CONTROLLED SUBSTANCE CLASSIFICATION

Medications under the control of the U.S. Drug Enforcement Agency (Schedule I–V controlled substances) are indicated by the symbol [C]. Most medications are "uncontrolled" and do not require a DEA prescriber number on the prescription. The following is a general description for the schedules of DEA controlled substances:

Schedule (C–I) I: All nonresearch use forbidden (eg, heroin, LSD, mescaline, etc).

Schedule (C–II) II: High addictive potential; medical use accepted. No telephone call-in prescriptions; no refills. Some states require special prescription form (eg, cocaine, morphine, methadone).

Schedule (C–III) III: Low to moderate risk of physical dependence, high risk of psychologic dependence; prescription must be rewritten after 6 months or five refills (eg, acetaminophen plus codeine).

Schedule (C–IV) IV: Limited potential for dependence; prescription rules same as for schedule III (eg, benzodiazepines, propoxyphene).

Schedule (C–V) V: Very limited abuse potential; prescribing regulations often same as for uncontrolled medications; some states have additional restrictions.

FDA FETAL RISK CATEGORIES

Category A: Adequate studies in pregnant women have not demonstrated a risk to the fetus in the first trimester of pregnancy; there is no evidence of risk in the last two trimesters.

Category B: Animal studies have not demonstrated a risk to the fetus, but no adequate studies have been done in pregnant women.

or

Animal studies have shown an adverse effect, but adequate studies in pregnant women have not demonstrated a risk to the fetus during the first trimester of pregnancy and there is no evidence of risk in the last two trimesters.

Category C: Animal studies have shown an adverse effect on the fetus, but no adequate studies have been done in humans. The benefits from the use of the drug in pregnant women may be acceptable despite its potential risks.

or

No animal reproduction studies and no adequate studies in humans have been done.

Category D: There is evidence of human fetal risk, but the potential benefits from the use of the drug in pregnant women may be acceptable despite its potential risks.

Category X: Studies in animals or humans or adverse reaction reports, or both, have demonstrated fetal abnormalities. The risk of use in pregnant women clearly outweighs any possible benefit.

Category ?: No data available (not a formal FDA classification; included to provide complete data set).

BREAST-FEEDING

No formally recognized classification exists for drugs and breast-feeding. This shorthand was developed for the *Nurse's Pocket Drug Guide*.

+	Compatible with breast-feeding
M	Monitor patient or use with caution
+/–	Excreted, or likely excreted, with unknown effects or at unknown concentrations
?/–	Unknown excretion, but effects likely to be of concern
–	Contraindicated in breast-feeding
?	No data available

ABBREVIATIONS

AAA: abdominal aortic aneurysm
AB: antibody, abortion, antibiotic
ABG: arterial blood gases
ABL: African Burkitt lymphoma
ABMT: autologous bone marrow transplantation
ACE: angiotensin-converting enzyme
ACEIs: angiotensin-converting enzyme inhibitors
ACLS: advanced cardiac life support
ACP: American College of Physicians
ACS: Acute coronary syndrome, American Cancer Society, American College of Surgeons
ad lib: as much as needed (*ad libitum*, OR as desired)
ADH: antidiuretic hormone
ADHD: attention-deficit hyperactivity disorder
AF: atrial fibrillation
AHF: antihemophilic factor
ALL: acute lymphocytic leukemia
ALT: alanine aminotransferase
AMI: acute myocardial infarction
AML: acute myelogenous leukemia
AMP: ampule
ANA: antinuclear antibody
ANC: absolute neutrophil count
AODM: adult-onset diabetes mellitus
aPTT: activated partial thromboplastin time

APAP: acetaminophen [*N*-acetyl-*p*-aminophenol]
ARA-C: cytarabine
ARB: angiotensin II receptor blocker
ARDS: adult respiratory distress syndrome
ARF: acute renal failure
AS: aortic stenosis
ASA: aspirin (acetylsalicylic acid)
AST: aspartate aminotransferase
AUB: abnormal uterine bleeding
AUC: area under the curve
AV: atrioventricular
AVM: arterio-venous malformation
BBs: beta blockers
BCL: B-cell lymphoma
BMT: bone marrow transplantation
BP: blood pressure
BRM: biologic response modifiers
BSA: body surface area
BUN: blood urea nitrogen
BW: body weight
C&S: culture and sensitivity
c: with (*cum*)
Ca: calcium
CA: cancer
CAD: coronary artery disease
CAP: cancer of prostate
CBC: complete blood count
CCBs: calcium channel blockers
CF: cystic fibrosis
CHF: congestive heart failure

CK: creatinine kinase
CLL: chronic lymphocytic leukemia
CML: chronic myelogenous leukemia
CMV: cytomegalovirus
CNS: central nervous system
COAD: chronic obstructive airway disease
COMT: catechol-*O*-methyl-transferase
Contra: contraindicated
COPD: chronic obstructive pulmonary disease
CP: chest pain
CPK: creatinine phosphokinase
CPP: central precocious puberty
CR: controlled release
CrCl: creatinine clearance
CRF: chronic renal failure
CRP: C-reactive protein
CVA: cerebrovascular accident, costovertebral angle
CVH: common variable hypergammaglobulinemia
CVP: central venous pressure
D5LR: 5% dextrose in lactated Ringer's solution
D5NS: 5% dextrose in normal saline
D5W: 5% dextrose in water
DC: discontinue, discharge, direct current
d/c: discontinue
DEA: Drug Enforcement Administration
DI: diabetes insipidus
DIC: disseminated intravascular coagulation
DJD: degenerative joint disease
DKA: diabetic ketoacidosis
dL: deciliter
DM: diabetes mellitus
DN: diabetic nephropathy
dT: diphtheria-tetanus toxoid
DTs: delirium tremens

DVT: deep venous thrombosis
EC: enteric-coated
ECC: emergency cardiac care
ECG: electrocardiogram
ELISA: enzyme-linked immunosorbent assay
ENT: ear, nose, and throat
eod: every other day
EPS: extrapyramidal symptoms
ESR: erythrocyte sedimentation rate
ESRD: end-stage renal disease
ET: endotracheal
ETOH: ethanol
ETT: endotracheal tube
Fab: antigen-binding fragment
FBS: fasting blood sugar
FSH: follicle-stimulating hormone
5-FU: fluorouracil
FU: follow-up
GC: gonorrhea (gonococcus)
G-CSF: granulocyte colony-stimulating factor
GDP: guanosine diphosphate
GERD: gastroesophageal reflux disease
GF: growth factor
GFR: glomerular filtration rate
GI: gastrointestinal
GM-CSF: granulocyte-macrophage colony-stimulating factor
GnRH: gonadotropin-releasing hormone
gr: grain
gt, gtt: drop, drops (*gutta*)
HA: headache
HBP: high blood pressure
HCL: hairy cell leukemia
HCT: hematocrit
HCTZ: hydrochlorothiazide
Hgb: hemoglobin
HIT: heparin-induced thrombocytopenia

HIV: human immunodeficiency virus

HMG-CoA: hydroxymethylglutaryl coenzyme A

hs: at bedtime (*hora somni*)

HSV: herpes simplex virus

5-HT: 5-hydroxytryptamine

HTLV-III: human T-lymphotropic virus, type III (HIV)

HTN: hypertension

HUS: hemolytic uremic syndrome

Hx: history

IBD: irritable bowel disease

IBS: irritable bowel syndrome

ICP: intracranial pressure

IDDM: insulin-dependent diabetes mellitus

Ig: immunoglobulin

IHSS: idiopathic hypertrophic subaortic stenosis

IM: intramuscular

INH: isoniazid

INR: international normalized ratio

ISA: intrinsic sympathomimetic activity

IT: intrathecal

ITP: idiopathic thrombocytopenic purpura

IV: intravenous

K: potassium

L/day: liters per day

LDL: low-density lipoprotein

LFT: liver function test

LH: luteinizing hormone

LHRH: luteinizing hormone-releasing hormone

lln: lower limits of normal

LMW: low molecular weight

LR: lactated Ringer's solution

LVD: left ventricular dysfunction

LVH: left ventricular hypertrophy

MAC: *Mycobacterium avium* complex

MAI: *Mycobacterium avium-intracellulare*

MAO/MAOI: monoamine oxidase/inhibitor

MAT: multifocal atrial tachycardia

mEq: milliequivalent

MI: myocardial infarction, mitral insufficiency

mL: milliliter

6-MP: mercaptopurine

MRSA: methicillin-resistant *Staphylococcus aureus*

MS: mitral stenosis, morphine sulfate, multiple sclerosis

MSSA: methicillin-sensitive *Staphylococcus aureus*

MTT: monotetrazolium

MTX: methotrexate

MyG: myasthenia gravis

ng: nanogram

NG: nasogastric

NHL: non-Hodgkin's lymphoma

NIDDM: non-insulin-dependent diabetes mellitus

NIPE: nursing implications/ patient education

NPO: nothing by mouth (*nil per os*)

NS: normal saline

NSAID: nonsteroidal antiinflammatory drug

NSR: normal sinus rhythm

NT: nasotracheal

NTG: nitroglycerin

N/V: nausea and vomiting

N/V/D: nausea, vomiting, diarrhea

OCP: oral contraceptive pill

OD: overdose, right eye (*oculus dexter*)

OS: opening snap, left eye (*oculus sinister*)

OTC: over the counter

OU: both eyes

PAC: premature atrial contraction

PAT: paroxysmal atrial tachycardia

pc: after eating (*post cibum*)

PCP: *Pneumocystis carinii* pneumonia, phencyclidine

PCWP: pulmonary capillary wedge pressure

PDGF: platelet-derived growth factor

PE: pulmonary embolus, physical examination, pleural effusion

PEA: pulseless electrical activity

PFT: pulmonary function test

pg: picogram

PI: pulmonic insufficiency

PID: pelvic inflammatory disease

PMDD: premenstrual dysphoric disorder

PO: by mouth (*per os*)

PPD: purified protein derivative

PPN: peripheral parenteral nutrition

PR: by rectum

PRG: pregnancy

PRN: as often as needed (*pro re nata*)

PS: pulmonic stenosis, partial saturation

PSVT: paroxysmal supraventricular tachycardia

pt: patient

PT: prothrombin time, physical therapy, posterior tibial

PTCA: percutaneous transluminal coronary angioplasty

PTH: parathyroid hormone

PTT: partial thromboplastin time

PTU: propylthiouracil

PUD: peptic ulcer disease

PV: polycythemia vera

PVC: premature ventricular contraction

PWP: pulmonary wedge pressure

PZI: protamine zinc insulin

q: every (*quaque*)

q_h: every _ hours

qd: every day

qh: every hour

qhs: every hour of sleep (before bedtime)

qid: four times a day (*quater in die*)

QNS: quantity not sufficient

qod: every other day

QS: quantity sufficient

QT: in an electrocardiogram, the refractory period of the ventricles when they depolarize and repolarize.

RA: rheumatoid arthritis

RCC: renal cell carcinoma

RDA: recommended dietary allowance

RDS: respiratory distress syndrome

RSV: respiratory syncytial virus

RT: rubella titer, respiratory therapy, radiation therapy

RTA: renal tubular acidosis

Rx: treatment

s: without (*sine*)

SC: subcutaneous

SCr: serum creatinine

SIADH: syndrome of inappropriate antidiuretic hormone

sig: write on label (*signa*)

SL: sublingual

SLE: systemic lupus erythematosus

soln: solution

SPAG: small particle aerosol generator

s/s: signs and symptoms

SSRI: selective serotonin reuptake inhibitor

SSS: sick sinus syndrome

stat: immediately (*statim*)

STD: sexually transmitted disease

supp: suppository

SVT: supraventricular tachycardia

Sx: symptoms
Tab/Tabs: tablet/tablets
TB: tuberculosis
T&C: type and crossmatch
TCA: tricyclic antidepressant
TCC: transitional cell carcinoma
TCP: transcutaneous pacer
Td: tetanus-diphtheria toxoid
TFT: thyroid function test
6-TG: 6-thioguanine
T&H: type and hold
TIA: transient ischemic attack
TIBC: total iron-binding capacity
tid: three times a day (*ter in die*)
TIG: tetanus immune globulin
TKO: to keep open
TMP: trimethoprim
TMP-SMX: trimethoprim-sulfamethoxazole
TPA: tissue plasminogen activator
TPN: total parenteral nutrition
TPR: total peripheral resistance
T&S: type and screen
TURBT: transurethral bladder tumor

TT: thrombin time
TTP: thrombotic thrombocytopenic purpura
TU: tuberculin units
tw: twice a week
U Cr: urine creatinine
ud: as directed (*ut dictum*)
uln: upper limits of normal
URI: upper respiratory infection
UTI: urinary tract infection
VF: ventricular fibrillation
VT: ventricular tachycardia
WHI: Women's Health Initiative
w/n: within
wnl: within normal limits
w/o: without
WPW: Wolff–Parkinson–White syndrome
wt(s): weight(s)
ZE: Zollinger–Ellison (syndrome)
⊘: avoid or not recommended
< (less than): before
> (greater than): after

CLASSIFICATION (Generic and common brand names)

ALLERGY

Antihistamines

Cetirizine (Zyrtec)
Chlorpheniramine
(Chlor-Trimeton)
Clemastine fumarate
(Tavist)

Cyproheptadine
(Periactin)
Desloratadine (Clarinex)
Diphenhydramine
(Benadryl)

Fexofenadine (Allegra)
Hydroxyzine (Atarax,
Vistaril)
Loratadine (Claritin)

Miscellaneous Antiallergenic Agents

Budesonide (Pulmicort)

Cromolyn (Cromolyn
sodium)

Montelukast (Singulair)

ANTIDOTES

Acetylcysteine
(Mucomyst)
Amifostine (Ethyol)
Charcoal (Activated
Charcoal, Actidose-
Aqua, CharcoAid,
Charcodote)

Dexrazoxane (Zinecard)
Digoxin Immune FAB
(Digibind)
Flumazenil (Romazicon)
Ipecac Syrup (OTC
Syrup)

Mesna (Mesnex)
Naloxone (Narcan)
Physostigmine (Antilir-
ium, Isopto, Eserine)
Succimer (Chemet)

ANTIMICROBIAL AGENTS

Antibiotics

AMINOGLYCOSIDES
Amikacin (Amikin)
Gentamicin (Garamycin)

Neomycin (Mycifradin)
Streptomycin

Tobramycin (Nebcin)

CARBAPENEMS
Ertapenem (Invanz)

Imipenem-Cilastatin
(Primaxin)

Meropenem (Merrem)

CEPHALOSPORINS, FIRST GENERATION

Cefadroxil (Duricef)
Cefazolin (Ancef, Kefzol)
Cephalexin (Keflex, Keftab)
Cephalothin (Keflin)
Cephradine (Velosef)

CEPHALOSPORINS, SECOND GENERATION

Cefaclor (Ceclor)
Cefmetazole (Zefazone)
Cefonicid (Monocid)
Cefotetan (Cefotan)
Cefoxitin (Mefoxin)
Cefprozil (Cefzil)
Cefuroxime (Ceftin [oral], Zinacef [parenteral])
Loracarbef (Lorabid)

CEPHALOSPORINS, THIRD GENERATION

Cefdinir (Omnicef)
Cefditoren (Spectracef)
Cefixime (Suprax)
Cefoperazone (Cefobid)
Cefotaxime (Claforan)
Cefpodoxime (Vantin)
Ceftazidime (Fortaz, Ceptaz, Tazidime, Tazicef)
Ceftizoxime (Cefizox)
Ceftriaxone (Rocephin)

CEPHALOSPORINS, FOURTH GENERATION

Cefepime (Maxipime)

FLUOROQUINOLONES

Ciprofloxacin (Cipro)
Gatifloxacin (Tequin)
Levofloxacin (Levaquin)
Lomefloxacin (Maxaquin)
Moxifloxacin (Avelox)
Norfloxacin (Noroxin)
Ofloxacin (Floxin, Ocuflox Ophthalmic)
Sparfloxacin (Zagam)

MACROLIDES

Azithromycin (Zithromax)
Clarithromycin (Biaxin)
Dirithromycin (Dynabac)
Erythromycin (E-Mycin, Ilosone, Erythrocin)
Erythromycin and Sulfisoxazole (Eryzole, Pediazole)

PENICILLINS

Amoxicillin (Amoxil, Polymox)
Amoxicillin-Clavulanate (Augmentin)
Ampicillin (Amcill, Omnipen)
Ampicillin-Sulbactam (Unasyn)
Dicloxacillin (Dynapen, Dycill)
Mezlocillin (Mezlin)
Nafcillin (Nallpen)
Oxacillin (Bactocill, Prostaphlin)
Penicillin G Aqueous (potassium or sodium) (Pfizerpen, Pentids)
Penicillin G Benzathine (Bicillin)
Penicillin G Procaine (Wycillin)
Penicillin V (Pen-Vee K, Veetids)
Piperacillin (Pipracil)
Piperacillin-Tazobactam (Zosyn)
Ticarcillin (Ticar)
Ticarcillin-Clavulanate (Timentin)

TETRACYCLINES

Doxycycline (Vibramycin)

Tetracycline (Achromycin V, Sumycin)

MISCELLANEOUS ANTIBACTERIAL AGENTS

Aztreonam (Azactam)
Clindamycin (Cleocin, Cleocin-T)
Fosfomycin (Monurol)
Linezolid (Zyvox)
Metronidazole (Flagyl, MetroGel)

Quinupristin-Dalfopristin (Synercid)
Trimethoprim-Sulfamethoxazole [Co-trimoxazole] (Bactrim, Septra)

Vancomycin (Vancocin, Vancoled)

Antifungals

Amphotericin B (Fungizone)
Amphotericin B Cholesteryl (Amphotec)
Amphotericin B Lipid Complex (Abelcet)
Amphotericin B Liposomal (AmBisome)
Caspofungin (Cancidas)

Clotrimazole (Lotrimin, Mycelex)
Clotrimazole and Betamethasone (Lotrisone)
Econazole (Spectazole)
Fluconazole (Diflucan)
Itraconazole (Sporanox)
Ketoconazole (Nizoral)

Miconazole (Monistat)
Nystatin (Mycostatin)
Oxiconazole (Oxistat)
Terbinafine (Lamisil)
Triamcinolone and Nystatin (Mycolog-II)
Voriconazole (VFEND)

Antimycobacterials

Clofazimine (Lamprene)
Dapsone (Avlosulfon)
Ethambutol (Myambutol)

Isoniazid (INH)
Pyrazinamide
Rifabutin (Mycobutin)

Rifampin (Rifadin)
Rifapentine (Priftin)
Streptomycin

Antiprotozoals

Nitazoxanide (Alinia)

Antiretrovirals

Abacavir (Ziagen)
Amprenavir (Agenerase)
Atazanavir (Reyataz)
Bortezomib (Velcade)
Delavirdine (Rescriptor)
Didanosine [ddI] (Videx)
Efavirenz (Sustiva)
Emtricitabine (Emtriva)

Enfuvirtide (Fuzeon)
Indinavir (Crixivan)
Lamivudine (Epivir, Epivir-HBV)
Lopinavir/Ritonavir (Kaletra)
Nelfinavir (Viracept)
Nevirapine (Viramune)

Ritonavir (Norvir)
Saquinavir (Fortovase)
Stavudine (Zerit)
Tenofovir (Viread)
Zalcitabine (Hivid)
Zidovudine (Retrovir)
Zidovudine and Lamivudine (Combivir)

Antivirals

Acyclovir (Zovirax)
Adefovir (Hepsera)
Amantadine (Symmetrel)
Cidofovir (Vistide)
Famciclovir (Famvir)
Foscarnet (Foscavir)
Ganciclovir (Cytovene, Vitrasert)

Interferon Alfa-2b and Ribavirin Combination (Rebetron)
Oseltamivir (Tamiflu)
Palivizumab (Synagis)
Peg interferon alfa 2 a (Pegasys)
Penciclovir (Denavir)

Ribavirin (Virazole)
Rimantadine (Flumadine)
Valacyclovir (Valtrex)
Valganciclovir (Valcyte)
Zanamivir (Relenza)

Miscellaneous Antimicrobial Agents

Atovaquone (Mepron)
Atovaquone/Proguanil (Malarone)

Pentamidine (Pentam 300, NebuPent)

Trimetrexate (Neutrexin)

ANTINEOPLASTIC AGENTS

Alkylating Agents

Altretamine (Hexalen)
Busulfan (Myleran)
Carboplatin (Paraplatin)

Cisplatin (Platinol AQ)
Procarbazine (Matulane)

Triethylene-triphosphamide (Thio-Tepa, TESPA, TSPA)

NITROGEN MUSTARDS

Chlorambucil (Leukeran)
Cyclophosphamide (Cytoxan, Neosar)

Ifosfamide (Ifex, Holoxan)
Mechlorethamine (Mustargen)

Melphalan [l-PAM] (Alkeran)

NITROSOUREAS

Carmustine [BCNU] (BiCNU)

Streptozocin (Zanosar)

Antibiotics

Bleomycin sulfate (Blenoxane)
Dactinomycin (Cosmegen)

Daunorubicin (Daunomycin, Cerubidine)
Doxorubicin (Adriamycin, Rubex)

Idarubicin (Idamycin)
Mitomycin (Mutamycin)
Pentostatin (Nipent)
Plicamycin (Mithracin)

Antimetabolites

Cytarabine [ARA-C] (Cytosar-U)
Cytarabine Liposomal (DepoCyt)
Floxuridine (FUDR)

Fludarabine (Fludara)
Fluorouracil [5-FU] (Adrucil)
Gemcitabine (Gemzar)

Mercaptopurine [6-MP] (Purinethol)
Methotrexate (Folex, Rheumatrex)
6-Thioguanine (Tabloid)

Hormones

Anastrozole (Arimidex)
Bicalutamide (Casodex)
Estramustine phosphate (Estracyt, Emcyt)
Fluoxymesterone (Halotestin)
Flutamide (Eulexin)

Fulvestrant (Faslodex)
Goserelin (Zoladex)
Leuprolide acetate (Lupron, Viadur)
Levamisole (Ergamisol)
Megestrol acetate (Megace)

Nilutamide (Nilandron)
Tamoxifen acetate (Nolvadex)
Triptorelin (Trelstar Depot, Trelstar LA)

Mitotic Inhibitors

Etoposide [VP-16] (VePesid)
Vinblastine (Velban, Velbe)

Vincristine (Oncovin, Vincasar PFS)

Vinorelbine (Navelbine)

Miscellaneous Antineoplastic Agents

Aldesleukin [Interleukin-2, IL-2] (Proleukin)
Aminoglutethimide (Cytadren)
L-Asparaginase (Elspar, Oncaspar)
BCG (TheraCys, Tice BCG)
Cladribine (Leustatin)
Dacarbazine (DTIC)

Docetaxel (Taxotere)
Gefitinib (Iressa)
Hydroxyurea (Hydrea, Droxia)
Imatinib mesylate (Gleevec)
Irinotecan (Camptosar)
Letrozole (Femara)
Leucovorin (Wellcovorin)

Mitotane (Lysodren)
Mitoxantrone (Novantrone)
Paclitaxel (Taxol)
Pentostatin (Nipent)
Rasburicase (Elitek)
Topotecan (Hycamtin)
Tretinoin [Retinoic acid] (Vesanoid)

CARDIOVASCULAR AGENTS

Aldosterone Antagonist

Eplerenone (Inspra)

Alpha1-Adrenergic Blockers

Alfuzosin (Uroxatral)
Doxazosin (Cardura)

Prazosin (Minipress)

Terazosin (Hytrin)

Angiotensin-Converting Enzyme Inhibitors

Benazepril (Lotensin)
Captopril (Capoten)
Enalapril and Enalaprilat
    (Vasotec)

Fosinopril (Monopril)
Lisinopril (Prinivil,
    Zestril)
Moexipril (Univasc)

Perindopril (Aceon)
Quinapril (Accupril)
Ramipril (Altace)
Trandolapril (Mavik)

Angiotensin II Receptor Antagonists

Candesartan (Atacand)
Eprosartan (Teveten)
Irbesartan (Avapro)

Losartan (Cozaar)
Olmesartan (Benicar)

Telmisartan (Micardis)
Valsartan (Diovan)

Antiarrhythmic Agents

Adenosine (Adenocard)
Amiodarone (Cordarone,
    Pacerone)
Atropine
Digoxin (Lanoxin,
    Lanoxicaps)
Disopyramide (Norpace,
    NAPAmide)

Dofetilide (Tikosyn)
Esmolol (Brevibloc)
Flecainide (Tambocor)
Ibutilide (Corvert)
Lidocaine (Anestacon
    Topical, Xylocaine)
Methoxamine (Vasoxyl)
Mexiletine (Mexitil)

Moricizine (Ethmozine)
Procainamide (Pronestyl,
    Procan)
Propafenone (Rythmol)
Quinidine
Sotalol (Betapace,
    Betapace AF)
Tocainide (Tonocard)

Beta-Adrenergic Blockers

Acebutolol (Sectral)
Atenolol (Tenormin)
Atenolol and Chlorthali-
    done (Tenoretic)
Betaxolol (Kerlone)
Bisoprolol (Zebeta)
Carteolol (Cartrol,
    Ocupress Ophthalmic)

Carvedilol (Coreg)
Labetalol (Trandate,
    Normodyne)
Metoprolol (Lopressor,
    Toprol XL)
Nadolol (Corgard)

Penbutolol (Levatol)
Pindolol (Visken)
Propranolol (Inderal)
Timolol (Blocadren)

Calcium Channel Antagonists

Amlodipine (Norvasc)
Bepridil (Vascor)
Diltiazem (Cardizem,
    Dilacor, Tiazac)
Felodipine (Plendil)

Isradipine (DynaCirc)
Nicardipine (Cardene)
Nifedipine (Procardia,
    Procardia XL, Adalat,
    Adalat CC)

Nimodipine (Nimotop)
Nisoldipine (Sular)
Verapamil (Calan,
    Isoptin)

Centrally Acting Antihypertensive Agents

Clonidine (Catapres)   Methyldopa (Aldomet)

Diuretics

Acetazolamide (Diamox)
Amiloride (Midamor)
Bumetanide (Bumex)
Chlorothiazide (Diuril)
Chlorthalidone
  (Hygroton)
Furosemide (Lasix)
Hydrochlorothiazide
  (HydroDIURIL,
  Esidrix)

Hydrochlorothiazide and
  Amiloride (Moduretic)
Hydrochlorothiazide and
  Spironolactone
  (Aldactazide)
Hydrochlorothiazide and
  Triamterene (Dyazide,
  Maxzide)

Indapamide (Lozol)
Mannitol
Metolazone (Zaroxolyn)
Spironolactone
  (Aldactone)
Torsemide (Demadex)
Triamterene (Dyrenium)

Inotropic/Pressor Agents

Amrinone (Inocor)
Digoxin (Lanoxin,
  Lanoxicaps)
Dobutamine
  (Dobutrex)
Dopamine (Intropin)

Epinephrine (Adrenalin,
  Sus-Phrine)
Isoproterenol (Isuprel,
  Medihaler-Iso)
Methoxamine (Vasoxyl)
Milrinone (Primacor)

Nesiritide (Natrecor)
Norepinephrine
  (Levophed)
Phenylephrine (Neo-
  Synephrine)

Lipid-Lowering Agents

Atorvastatin (Lipitor)
Cholestyramine (Ques-
  tran)
Colesevelam (Welchol)
Colestipol (Colestid)

Ezetimibe (Zetia)
Fenofibrate (Tricor)
Fluvastatin (Lescol)
Gemfibrozil (Lopid)
Lovastatin (Mevacor)

Niacin (Nicolar)
Pravastatin (Pravachol)
Rosuvastatin (Crestor)
Simvastatin (Zocor)

Vasodilators

Alprostadil
  [Prostaglandin E_1]
  (Prostin VR)
Epoprostenol (Flolan)
Fenoldopam (Corlopam)
Hydralazine
  (Apresoline)
Isosorbide Dinitrate
  (Isordil, Sorbitrate)

Isosorbide Mononitrate
  (Ismo, Imdur)
Minoxidil (Loniten,
  Rogaine)
Nitroglycerin (Nitrostat,
  Nitrolingual, Nitro-
  Bid Ointment, Nitro-
  Bid IV, Nitrodisc,
  Transderm-Nitro)

Nitroprusside (Nipride,
  Nitropress)
Tolazoline (Priscoline)
Treprostinil sodium
  (Remodulin)

CENTRAL NERVOUS SYSTEM AGENTS

Antianxiety Agents

Alprazolam (Xanax)
Buspirone (BuSpar)
Chlordiazepoxide (Librium)
Clorazepate (Tranxene)
Diazepam (Valium)
Doxepin (Sinequan, Adapin)
Hydroxyzine (Atarax, Vistaril)
Lorazepam (Ativan, others)
Meprobamate (Equanil, Miltown)
Oxazepam (Serax)

Anticonvulsants

Carbamazepine (Tegretol)
Clonazepam (Klonopin)
Diazepam (Valium)
Ethosuximide (Zarontin)
Fosphenytoin (Cerebyx)
Gabapentin (Neurontin)
Lamotrigine (Lamictal)
Levetiracetam (Keppra)
Lorazepam (Ativan, others)
Oxcarbazepine (Trileptal)
Pentobarbital (Nembutal)
Phenobarbital
Phenytoin (Dilantin)
Tiagabine (Gabitril)
Topiramate (Topamax)
Valproic acid (Depakene, Depakote)
Zonisamide (Zonegran)

Antidepressants

Amitriptyline (Elavil)
Bupropion (Wellbutrin, Zyban)
Citalopram (Celexa)
Desipramine (Norpramin)
Doxepin (Sinequan, Adapin)
Escitalopram (Lexapro)
Fluoxetine (Prozac, Sarafem)
Fluvoxamine (Luvox)
Imipramine (Tofranil)
Maprotiline (Ludiomil)
Mirtazapine (Remeron)
Nefazodone (Serzone)
Nortriptyline (Aventyl, Pamelor)
Paroxetine (Paxil)
Phenelzine (Nardil)
Sertraline (Zoloft)
Trazodone (Desyrel)
Trimipramine (Surmontil)
Venlafaxine (Effexor)

Antiparkinson Agents

Amantadine (Symmetrel)
Benztropine (Cogentin)
Bromocriptine (Parlodel)
Carbidopa/Levodopa (Sinemet)
Entacapone (Comtan)
Pergolide (Permax)
Pramipexole (Mirapex)
Procyclidine (Kemadrin)
Selegiline (Eldepryl)
Trihexyphenidyl (Artane)

Antipsychotics

Aripiprazole (Abilify)
Chlorpromazine (Thorazine)
Clozapine (Clozaril)
Fluphenazine (Prolixin, Permitil)
Haloperidol (Haldol)
Lithium carbonate (Eskalith)
Mesoridazine (Serentil)

Molindone (Moban)
Olanzapine (Zyprexa)
Perphenazine (Trilafon)
Prochlorperazine
(Compazine)
Quetiapine (Seroquel)
Risperidone (Risperdal)
Thioridazine (Mellaril)
Thiothixene (Navane)
Trifluoperazine
(Stelazine)
Ziprasidone (Geodon)

Sedative Hypnotics

Chloral hydrate
Diphenhydramine
(Benadryl)
Estazolam (ProSom)
Flurazepam (Dalmane)
Hydroxyzine (Atarax,
Vistaril)
Midazolam (Versed)
Pentobarbital (Nembutal)
Phenobarbital
Propofol (Diprivan)
Quazepam (Doral)
Secobarbital (Seconal)
Temazepam (Restoril)
Triazolam (Halcion)
Zaleplon (Sonata)
Zolpidem (Ambien)

Miscellaneous CNS Agents

Atomoxetine (Strattera)
Galantamine (Reminyl)
Nimodipine (Nimotop)
Rivastigmine (Exelon)
Sodium oxybate
(Xyrem)
Tacrine (Cognex)

DERMATOLOGIC AGENTS

Acitretin (Soriatane)
Acyclovir (Zovirax)
Alefacept (Amevive)
Anthralin (Anthra-Derm)
Amphotericin B
(Fungizone)
Bacitracin (Baci-IM)
Bacitracin, Topical
(Baciguent)
Bacitracin and Polymyxin
B, Topical (Polysporin)
Bacitracin, Neomycin
and Polymyxin B,
Topical (Neosporin
Ointment)
Bacitracin, Neomycin,
Polymyxin B and Hy-
drocortisone, Topical
(Cortisporin)
Bacitracin, Neomycin,
Polymyxin B and Li-
docaine, Topical
(Clomycin)
Calcipotriene (Dovonex)
Capsaicin (Capsin,
Zostrix)
Ciclopirox (Loprox)
Ciprofloxacin (Cipro)
Clindamycin, Topical
(Cleocin-T)
Clotrimazole and Be-
tamethasone
(Lotrisone)
Dibucaine (Nupercainal)
Doxepin, Topical
(Zonalon)
Econazole (Spectazole)
Erythromycin, Topical
Gentamicin, Topical
Haloprogin (Halotex)
Imiquimod (Aldara)
Isotretinoin [13-*cis*
Retinoic acid]
(Accutane)
Ketoconazole
(Nizoral)
Lactic Acid and Ammo-
nium Hydroxide
(Lac-Hydrin)
Lindane (Kwell)
Metronidazole
(MetroGel)
Miconazole (Monistat)
Minoxidil (Loniten,
Rogaine)
Mupirocin (Bactroban)
Naftifine (Naftin)

Nystatin (Mycostatin, Nilstat)
Nystatin and Triamcinolone
Oxiconazole (Oxistat)
Penciclovir (Denavir)
Permethrin (Nix, Elimite)
Pimecrolimus (Elidel)
Pramoxine (Anusol Ointment, Proctofoam-NS)
Pramoxine and Hydrocortisone (Enzone, Proctofoam-HC)
Podophyllin (Podocon-25, Condylox Gel 0.5%, Condylox)
Tretinoin, Topical [Retinoic Acid] (Retin-A, Avita)
Selenium Sulfide (Exsel Shampoo, Selsun Blue Shampoo, Selsun Shampoo)
Silver Sulfadiazine (Silvadene)
Steroids, Topical (Table 5, page 249–252)
Tacrolimus (Prograf)
Tazarotene (Tazorac)
Terbinafine (Lamisil)
Tolnaftate (Tinactin)
Witch Hazel

DIETARY SUPPLEMENTS

Calcium acetate (Calphron, Phos-Ex, PhosLo)
Calcium Glubionate (Neo-Calglucon [OTC])
Calcium Gluceptate
Calcium salts [calcium chloride and gluconate]
Cholecalciferol [Vitamin D_3] (Delta D)
Cyanocobalamin [Vitamin B_{12}]
Ferric gluconate Complex (Ferrlecit)
Ferrous gluconate (Fergon)
Ferrous sulfate
Folic acid
Iron Dextran (DexFerrum, InFeD)
Magnesium Oxide (Mag-Ox 400)
Magnesium sulfate
Phytonadione [Vitamin K] (Aqua-MEPHYTON)
Potassium Supplements (Kaon, Kaochlor, K-Lor, Slow-K, Micro-K, Klorvess)
Pyridoxine [Vitamin B_6]
Sodium bicarbonate [Bicarbonate]
Thiamine [Vitamin B_1]

EAR (OTIC) AGENTS

Acetic acid and Aluminum acetate (Otic Domeboro)
Benzocaine and Antipyrine (Auralgan)
Ciprofloxacin and Hydrocortisone (Cipro HC Otic)
Neomycin, Colistin and Hydrocortisone (Cortisporin-TC Otic Drops)
Neomycin, Colistin, Hydrocortisone and Thonzonium (Cortisporin-TC Otic Suspension)
Neomycin, Polymyxin and Hydrocortisone (Cortisporin Ophthalmic and Otic)
Polymyxin B and Hydrocortisone (Otobiotic Otic)
Sulfacetamide and Prednisolone (Blephamide)
Triethanolamine (Cerumenex)

ENDOCRINE SYSTEM AGENTS

Antidiabetic Agents

Acarbose (Precose)
Chlorpropamide
  (Diabinese)
Glimepiride (Amaryl)
Glipizide (Glucotrol)
Glyburide (DiaBeta,
  Micronase)

Glyburide/Metformin
  (Glucovance)
Insulins (Table 6,
  page 252)
Metformin (Glucophage)
Miglitol (Glyset)
Nateglinide (Starlix)

Pioglitazone (Actos)
Repaglinide (Prandin)
Rosiglitazone
  (Avandia)
Tolazamide (Tolinase)
Tolbutamide (Orinase)

Hormone and Synthetic Substitutes

Calcitonin (Cibacalcin,
  Miacalcin)
Calcitriol (Rocaltrol)
Cortisone
Desmopressin (DDAVP,
  Stimate)
Dexamethasone
  (Decadron)

Fludrocortisone acetate
  (Florinef)
Glucagon
Hydrocortisone (Cortef,
  Solu-Cortef)
Methylprednisolone
  (Solu-Medrol)

Metyrapone
  (Metopirone)
Prednisolone (Delta-
  Cortef, others)
Prednisone (Deltasone,
  others)
Vasopressin (Pitressin)

Hypercalcemia Agents

Etidronate (Didronel)
Gallium nitrate (Ganite)

Pamidronate (Aredia)
Plicamycin (Mithracin)

Zoledronic acid
  (Zometa)

Obesity

Sibutramine (Meridia)

Osteoporosis Agents

Alendronate (Fosamax)
Raloxifene (Evista)

Risedronate (Actonel)
Teriparatide (Forteo)

Zoledronic acid
  (Zometa)

Thyroid/Antithyroid

Levothyroxine
  (Synthroid)

Liothyronine (Cytomel)
Methimazole (Tapazole)

Potassium iodide (SSKI)
Propylthiouracil [PTU]

Miscellaneous Endocrine Agents

Demeclocycline
  (Declomycin)

Diazoxide (Hyperstat,
  Proglycem)

Metyrosine (Demser)

EYE (OPHTHALMIC) AGENTS

Glaucoma Agents

Acetazolamide (Diamox)
Apraclonidine (Iopidine)
Betaxolol (Kerlone)
Brimonidine (Alphagan)
Brinzolamide (Azopt)
Carteolol (Cartrol, Ocupress Ophthalmic)
Dipivefrin (Propine)
Dorzolamide (Trusopt)
Dorzolamide and Timolol (Cosopt)
Echothiophate Iodine (Phospholine Ophthalmic)
Latanoprost (Xalatan)
Levobunolol (A-K Beta, Betagan)
Levocabastine (Livostin)
Lodoxamide (Alomide Ophthalmic)
Timolol (Blocadren)

Ophthalmic Antibiotics

Bacitracin (AK-Tracin Ophthalmic)
Bacitracin and Polymyxin B (AK-Poly-Bac Ophthalmic, Polysporin Ophthalmic)
Bacitracin, Neomycin and Polymyxin B (AK Spore Ophthalmic, Neosporin Ophthalmic)
Bacitracin, Neomycin, Polymyxin B and Hydrocortisone (AK Spore HC Ophthalmic, Cortisporin Ophthalmic)
Ciprofloxacin (Ciloxan)
Erythromycin (Ilotycin Ophthalmic)
Gentamicin (Garamycin, Genoptic, Gentacidin, Gentak)
Neomycin and Dexamethasone (AK-Neo-Dex Ophthalmic, NeoDecadron Ophthalmic)
Neomycin, Polymyxin-B and Dexamethasone (Maxitrol)
Neomycin, Polymyxin-B and Prednisolone (Poly-Pred Ophthalmic)
Ofloxacin (Ocuflox Ophthalmic)
Silver Nitrate (Dey-Drop)
Sulfacetamide (Bleph-10, Cetamide, Sodium Sulamyd)
Sulfacetamide and Prednisolone (Blephamide)
Tobramycin (AKTob, Tobrex)
Tobramycin and Dexamethasone (TobraDex)
Trifluridine (Viroptic)

Other Ophthalmic Agents

Artificial Tears (Tears Naturale)
Cromolyn (Opticrom)
Cyclopentolate (Cyclogyl)
Dexamethasone, Ophthalmic (AK-Dex Ophthalmic, Decadron Ophthalmic)
Emedastine (Emadine)
Ketorolac (Acular)
Ketotifen (Zaditor)
Lodoxamide (Alomide)
Naphazoline and Antazoline (Albalon-A Ophthalmic)
Naphazoline and Pheniramine (Naphcon A)
Olopatadine (Patanol)

GASTROINTESTINAL AGENTS

Antacids

Alginic acid (Gaviscon)
Aluminum carbonate (Basaljel)
Aluminum hydroxide (Amphojel, Alter-naGEL)
Aluminum hydroxide with Magnesium carbonate (Gaviscon)

Aluminum hydroxide with Magnesium hydroxide (Maalox)
Aluminum hydroxide with Magnesium hydroxide and Simethicone (Mylanta, Mylanta II, Maalox Plus)

Aluminum hydroxide with Magnesium Trisilicate (Gaviscon, Gaviscon-2)
Calcium carbonate (Tums, Alka-Mints)
Magaldrate (Riopan, Lowsium)
Simethicone (Mylicon)

Antidiarrheals

Bismuth Subsalicylate (Pepto-Bismol)
Diphenoxylate with Atropine (Lomotil)

Kaolin/Pectin (Kaodene, Kao-Spen, Kapectolin, Parepectolin)
Lactobacillus (Lactinex Granules)

Loperamide (Imodium)
Octreotide (Sandostatin, Sandostatin LAR)
Paregoric [Camphorated Tincture of Opium]

Antiemetics

Aprepitant (Emend)
Chlorpromazine (Thorazine)
Dimenhydrinate (Dramamine, others)
Dolasetron (Anzemet)
Dronabinol (Marinol)
Droperidol (Inapsine)

Granisetron (Kytril)
Meclizine (Antivert)
Metoclopramide (Reglan, Octamide)
Ondansetron (Zofran)
Palonosetron (Aloxi)
Prochlorperazine (Compazine)

Promethazine (Phenergan)
Scopolamine (Transderm-Scop)
Thiethylperazine (Torecan)
Trimethobenzamide (Tigan)

Antiulcer Agents

Cimetidine (Tagamet)
Esomeprazole (Nexium)
Famotidine (Pepcid)
Lansoprazole (Prevacid)

Nizatidine (Axid)
Omeprazole (Prilosec)
Pantoprazole (Protonix)

Rabeprazole (Aciphex)
Ranitidine (Zantac)
Sucralfate (Carafate)

Cathartics/Laxatives

Bisacodyl (Dulcolax)
Docusate calcium (Surfak)

Docusate potassium (Dialose)

Docusate sodium (Doss, Colace)

Glycerin Suppositories
Lactulose (Chronulac, Cephulac)
Magnesium citrate
Magnesium hydroxide (Milk of Magnesia)

Mineral Oil
Polyethylene Glycol-Electrolyte Solution (GoLYTELY, CoLyte)
Sorbitol

Psyllium (Metamucil, Serutan, Effer-Syllium)

Enzymes

Pancreatin (Creon)

Pancrelipase [Lipase, Protease, Amylase] (Pancrease, others)

Miscellaneous GI Agents

Alosetron (Lotronex)
Balsalazide (Colazal)
Dexpanthenol (Ilopan-Choline Oral, Ilopan)
Dibucaine (Nupercainal)
Dicyclomine (Bentyl)
Hydrocortisone, Rectal (Anusol-HC Suppository, Cortifoam Rectal, Proctocort)
Hyoscyamine (Anaspaz, Cystospaz, Levsin)

Hyoscyamine, Atropine, Scopolamine and Phenobarbital (Donnatal)
Infliximab (Remicade)
Mesalamine (Rowasa, Asacol, Pentasa)
Metoclopramide (Reglan, Clopra, Octamide)
Misoprostol (Cytotec)
Olsalazine (Dipentum)

Pramoxine (Anusol Ointment, Procto-foam-NS)
Pramoxine with Hydro-cortisone (Enzone, Proctofoam-HC)
Propantheline (Pro-Banthine)
Sulfasalazine (Azulfidine)
Tegaserod maleate (Zelnorm)
Vasopressin (Pitressin)

HEMATOLOGIC AGENTS

Anticoagulants

Ardeparin (Normiflo)
Argatroban (Acova)
Bivalirudin (Angiomax)
Dalteparin (Fragmin)

Enoxaparin (Lovenox)
Fondaparinux (Arixtra)
Heparin
Lepirudin (Refludan)

Protamine
Tinzaparin (Innohep)
Warfarin (Coumadin)

Antiplatelet Agents

Abciximab (ReoPro)
Aspirin (Bayer, St. Joseph)
Clopidogrel (Plavix)

Dipyridamole (Persantine)
Dipyridamole and Aspirin (Aggrenox)

Eptifibatide (Integrilin)
Reteplase (Retavase)
Ticlopidine (Ticlid)
Tirofiban (Aggrastat)

Antithrombotic Agents

Alteplase, Recombinant
[TPA] (Activase)
Aminocaproic acid
(Amicar)
Anistreplase (Eminase)

Aprotinin (Trasylol)
Dextran 40
(Rheomacrodex)
Reteplase (Retavase)

Streptokinase (Streptase,
Kabikinase)
Tenecteplase (TNKase)
Urokinase (Abbokinase)

Hematopoietic Stimulants

Darbepoetin alfa
(Aranesp)
Epoetin Alfa [Erythro-
poietin, EPO]
(Epogen, Procrit)

Filgrastim [G-CSF] (Neu-
pogen)
Oprelvekin (Neumega)
Pegfilgrastim (Neulasta)

Sargramostim [GM-
CSF] (Prokine,
Leukine)

Volume Expanders

Albumin (Albuminar,
Buminate,
Albutein)

Dextran 40 (Rheo-
macrodex)
Hetastarch (Hespan)

Plasma Protein Fraction
(Plasmanate)

Miscellaneous Hematologic Agents

Antihemophilic Factor
VIII (Monoclate)

Desmopressin (DDAVP,
Stimate)

Pentoxifylline (Trental)

IMMUNE SYSTEM AGENTS

Immunomodulators

Adalimumab (Humira)
Anakinra (Kineret)
Etanercept (Enbrel)
Interferon Alfa (Roferon-
A, Intron A)

Interferon Alfacon-1
(Infergen)
Interferon Beta-1b
(Betaseron)

Interferon Gamma-1b
(Actimmune)
Peg interferon alfa 2b
(PEG-Intron)

Immunosuppressive Agents

Azathioprine (Imuran)
Basiliximab
(Simulect)
Cyclosporine (Sandim-
mune, Neoral)
Daclizumab
(Zenapax)

Lymphocyte Immune
Globulin [Antithymo-
cyte Globulin, ATG]
(Atgam)
Muromonab-CD3
(Orthoclone
OKT3)

Mycophenolate Mofetil
(CellCept)
Sirolimus (Rapamune)
Steroids, Systemic
(Table 4, page 248)
Tacrolimus (Prograf,
Protopic)

Vaccines/Serums/Toxoids

CMV Immune Globulin
[CMV-IG IV]
(CytoGam)

Diphtheria and Tetanus
Toxoids

Diphtheria, Tetanus
Toxoids, and Acellular
Pertussis Adsorbed

Diphtheria, Tetanus
Toxoids, and Acellular
Pertussis Adsorbed,
Hepatitis B (recombi-
nant), and Inactivated
Poliovirus Vaccine
(IPV) Combined
(Pediarix)

Haemophilus B Conju-
gate Vaccine (ActHIB,
HibTITER, Pedvax-
HIB, Prohibit,
Comvax)

Hepatitis A Vaccine
(Havrix, Vaqta)

Hepatitis A (inactivated)
and Hepatitis B Re-
combinant Vaccine
(Twinrix)

Hepatitis B Immune
Globulin (HyperHep,
H-BIG)

Hepatitis B Vaccine
(Engerix-B, Recom-
bivax HB)

Immune Globulin, Intra-
venous (Gamimune N,
Sandoglobulin,
Gammar IV)

Influenza (Fluzone,
FluShield, Fluvirin)

Meningococcal Polysac-
charide Vaccine
(Menomune)

Pneumococcal Vaccine,
Polyvalent (Pneu-
movax-23)

Pneumococcal 7-Valent
Conjugate
(Prevnar)

Tetanus Immune
Globulin

Tetanus Toxoid

Varicella Virus Vaccine
(Varivax)

MUSCULOSKELETAL AGENTS

Antigout Agents

Allopurinol (Zyloprim,
Lopurin, Alloprim)

Colchicine
Probenecid (Benemid)

Sulfinpyrazone
(Anturane)

Muscle Relaxants

Baclofen (Lioresal)
Carisoprodol (Soma)
Chlorzoxazone
(Paraflex, Parafon
Forte DSC)

Cyclobenzaprine
(Flexeril)
Dantrolene (Dantrium)
Diazepam (Valium)

Metaxalone (Skelaxin)
Methocarbamol
(Robaxin)
Orphenadrine (Norflex)

Neuromuscular Blockers

Atracurium (Tracrium)
Mivacurium (Mivacron)
Pancuronium
(Pavulon)

Pipecuronium (Arduan)
Succinylcholine (Anec-
tine, Quelicin,
Sucostrin)

Vecuronium (Norcuron)

Miscellaneous Musculoskeletal Agents

Edrophonium (Tensilon)
Leflunomide (Arava)

Methotrexate (Folex, Rheumatrex)

OB/GYN AGENTS

Contraceptives

Estradiol Cypionate and Medroxyprogesterone acetate (Lunelle)
Etonogestrel/Ethinyl Estradiol (NuvaRing)
Levonorgestrel Implants (Norplant)
Medro...

Norgestrel (Ovrette)
Norelgestromin and Ethinyl Estradiol, Ortho Evra (Ortho)
Oral Contraceptives, Monophasic (Table 7, page...

Oral Contraceptives, Triphasic (Table 7, page 253)
Oral Contraceptives, Progestin Only (Table 7...

...ep-
...ge 259)
...trex)
...ptan (Imitrex)
...ptan (Zomig)

Meperidine (Demerol)
Methadone (Dolophine)
Morphine (Roxanol, MS Contin)
Duramorph, MS Contin)
Nalbuphine (Nubain)
Oxycodone (OxyContin, OxyIR, Roxicodone)
Oxycodone and Aceta- minophen (Percocet, Tylox)
Oxycodone and Aspirin (Percodan, Percodan-Demi)

...osal
...nyl

...done and Aceta- ...ophen (Lorcet, Vi- ...codin)
Hydrocodone and As- pirin (Lortab ASA)
Hydrocodone and Ibupro- fen (Vicoprofen)
Hydromorphone (Dilaudid)
Levorphanol (Levo- Dromoran)

...an)

...oblimaze)
...Transdermal

...ragesic)

Miscellaneous Ob/Gyn Agents

Dinoprostone (Cervidil
Vaginal Insert,
Prepidil Vaginal Gel)
Gonadorelin (Lutrepulse)
Leuprolide (Lupron)
Magnesium Sulfate

Medroxyprogesterone
(Provera,
Depo-Provera)
Methylergonovine
(Methergine)

Mifepristone [RU486]
(Mifeprex)
Oxytocin (Pitocin)
Terbutaline (Brethine,
Bricanyl)

PAIN MEDICATIONS

Local Anesthetics

Benzocaine and An-
tipyrine (Auralgan)
Bupivacaine (Marcaine)
Capsaicin (Capsin,
Zostrix)

Cocaine
Dibucaine (Nupercainal)
Lidocaine (Anestacon
Topical, Xylocaine)

Lidocaine (ELA-Max)
Lidocaine and Prilocaine
(EMLA)
Pramoxine

Migraine Headache Medications

Acetaminophen with Bu-
talbital w/wo Caffeine
(Fioricet, Medigesic,
Repan, Sedapap-10
Two-Dyne, Triapin,
Axocet, Phrenilin
Forte)

Almotriptan (Axert)
Aspirin with Butalbital
and Caffeine (Fiorinal
with Codeine)
Eletriptan (Relpax)
Naratriptan (Amerge)
Rizatriptan (Maxalt)

Serotonin 5-HT$_1$ Re
tor Agonists (
Table 11, p
Sumatript
Zolmit

Narcotics

Acetaminophen with
Codeine (Tylenol No.
1, 2, 3, 4)
Alfentanil (Alfenta)
Aspirin with Codeine
(Empirin No. 2, 3, 4)
Buprenorphine
(Buprenex)
Butorphanol (Stadol)
Codeine
Dezocine (Dal
Fentanyl (S
Fentanyl
(D

Fentanyl Transmu
(Actiq, Fenta
Oralet)
Hydroco
mi

Oxymorphone (Numorphan)
Pentazocine (Talwin)
Propoxyphene (Darvon)
Propoxyphene and Acetaminophen (Darvocet)

Propoxyphene and Aspirin (Darvon Compound-65, Darvon-N with Aspirin)

Sufentanil (Sufenta)

Nonnarcotic Agents

Acetaminophen [APAP] (Tylenol)
Aspirin (Bayer, St. Joseph)

Tramadol (Ultram)
Tramadol/Acetaminophen (Ultracet)

Nonsteroidal Antiinflammatory Agents

Celecoxib (Celebrex)
Diclofenac (Cataflam, Voltaren)
Diflunisal (Dolobid)
Etodolac (Lodine)
Fenoprofen (Nalfon)
Flurbiprofen (Ansaid)

Ibuprofen (Motrin, Rufen, Advil)
Indomethacin (Indocin)
Ketoprofen (Orudis, Oruvail)
Ketorolac (Toradol)
Meloxicam (Mobic)
Nabumetone (Relafen)

Naproxen (Aleve, Naprosyn, Anaprox)
Oxaprozin (Daypro)
Piroxicam (Feldene)
Rofecoxib (Vioxx)
Sulindac (Clinoril)
Tolmetin (Tolectin)
Valdecoxib (Bextra)

Miscellaneous Pain Medications

Amitriptyline (Elavil)

Imipramine (Tofranil)

Tramadol (Ultram)

RESPIRATORY AGENTS

Antitussives, Decongestants and Expectorants

Acetylcysteine (Mucomyst)
Benzonatate (Tessalon Perles)
Codeine
Dextromethorphan (Mediquell, Benylin DM, PediaCare 1)
Guaifenesin (Robitussin)
Guaifenesin and Codeine (Robitussin AC, Brontex)

Guaifenesin and Dextromethorphan (Many OTC Brands)
Hydrocodone and Guaifenesin (Hycotuss Expectorant, others)
Hydrocodone and Homatropine (Hycodan)
Hydrocodone and Pseudoephedrine (Entuss-D, Histussin-D, others)

Hydrocodone, Chlorpheniramine, Phenylephrine, Acetaminophen and Caffeine (Hycomine)
Potassium Iodide
Pseudoephedrine (Sudafed, Novafed, Afrinol)

Bronchodilators

Albuterol (Proventil, Ventolin)
Albuterol and Ipratropium (Combivent)
Aminophylline
Bitolterol (Tornalate)
Ephedrine
Epinephrine (Adrenalin, Sus-Phrine)

Formoterol (Foradil Aerolizer)
Isoetharine (generic)
Isoproterenol (Isuprel)
Levalbuterol (Xopenex)
Metaproterenol (Alupent, Metaprel)

Pirbuterol (Maxair)
Salmeterol (Serevent)
Terbutaline (Brethine, Bricanyl)
Theophylline (Theolair, Somophyllin-CRT)

Respiratory Inhalants

Acetylcysteine (Mucomyst, Mucosil)
Beclomethasone (Beconase, Vancenase Nasal Inhaler)
Beractant (Survanta)
Budesonide (Pulmicort)
Calfactant (Infasurf)
Colfosceril Palmitate (Exosurf Neonatal)

Cromolyn sodium (Intal, Nasalcrom, Opticrom)
Dexamethasone, Nasal (Dexacort Phosphate Turbinaire)
Flunisolide (AeroBid, Nasalide)
Fluticasone, Oral, Nasal (Flonase, Flovent)

Fluticasone Propionate and Salmeterol Xinafoate (Advair Diskus)
Ipratropium (Atrovent)
Nedocromil (Tilade)
Triamcinolone (Aristocort, Kenalog)

Miscellaneous Respiratory Agents

Alpha$_1$-Protease Inhibitor (Prolastin)
Dornase Alfa (Pulmozyme)

Montelukast (Singulair)
Omalizumab (Xolair)

Zafirlukast (Accolate)
Zileuton (Zyflo)

URINARY/GENITOURINARY AGENTS

Alprostadil (Caverject, Edex)
Alprostadil Urethral Suppository (Muse)
Ammonium Aluminum Sulfate [Alum]
Belladonna and Opium Suppositories (B & O Supprettes)
Bethanechol (Urecholine, others)

Dimethyl Sulfoxide [DMSO] (Rimso-50)
Flavoxate (Urispas)
Hyoscyamine (Anaspaz, Cystospaz, Levsin)
Methenamine (Hiprex, Urex)
Nalidixic acid (NegGram)
Neomycin-Polymyxin Bladder Irrigant [GU Irrigant]

Nitrofurantoin (Macrodantin, Furadantin, Macrobid)
Oxybutynin (Ditropan, Ditropan XL, Oxytrol)
Pentosan polysulfate (Elmiron)
Phenazopyridine (Pyridium)
Potassium citrate (Urocit-K)

Potassium citrate and
Citric acid
(Polycitra-K)
Sildenafil (Viagra)

Sodium citrate (Bicitra)
Tolterodine (Detrol,
Detrol LA)
Tadalafil (Cialis)

Trimethoprim (Trimpex,
Proloprim)
Vardenafil (Levitra)

Benign Prostatic Hyperplasia Medications

Doxazosin (Cardura)
Dutasteride (Avodart)

Finasteride (Proscar,
Propecia)

Tamsulosin (Flomax)
Terazosin (Hytrin)

WOUND CARE

Becaplermin (Regranex
Gel)

Silver nitrate (Dey-Drop)

MISCELLANEOUS THERAPEUTIC AGENTS

Drotrecogin alfa (Xigris)
Megestrol Acetate
(Megace)
Metaraminol (Aramine)
Naltrexone (ReVia)
Nicotine Gum (Nicorette,
Nicorette DS)

Nicotine Nasal Spray
(Nicotrol NS)
Nicotine Transdermal
(Habitrol, Nicoderm,
Nicotrol, ProStep)
Potassium iodide

Sodium Polystyrene sul-
fonate (Kayexalate)
Triethanolamine
(Cerumenex)

GENERIC DRUG DATA

Abacavir (Ziagen) **WARNING:** Hypersensitivity manifested as fever, rash, fatigue, GI, and respiratory reported; stop drug immediately and do not rechallenge; lactic acidosis and hepatomegaly/steatosis reported **Uses:** HIV infection **Action:** Nucleoside reverse transcriptase inhibitor **Dose:** *Adults.* 300 mg PO bid. *Peds.* 8 mg/kg bid **Caution/Contra:** [C, –] CDC recommends HIV-infected mothers not breast-feed due to risk of infant HIV transmission **Supplied:** Tabs 300 mg; soln 20 mg/mL **Notes/SE:** Numerous drug interactions **Interactions:** Alcohol ↓ drug elimination and ↑ drug exposure **Labs:** Monitor LFTs, FBS, CBC & differential, BUN & creatinine, triglycerides **NIPE:** ⊘ alcohol; monitor & teach pt about hypersensitivity reactions; d/c drug immediately if hypersensitivity reaction and DO NOT rechallenge; take with or w/o food

Abciximab (ReoPro) **Uses:** Prevents acute ischemic complications in PTCA **Action:** Inhibits platelet aggregation (glycoprotein IIb/IIIa inhibitor) **Dose:** 0.25 mg/kg bolus 10–60 min prior to PTCA, then 0.125 μg/kg/min (max = 10 μg/min) cont inf for 12 h **Caution/Contra:** [C, ?/–] Contra if active or recent (w/n 6 wk) internal hemorrhage, CVA w/n 2 y or CVA with significant neurologic deficit, bleeding diathesis or administration of oral anticoagulants w/n 7 d (unless PT = 2 × control), thrombocytopenia (<100,000 cells/μL), recent trauma or major surgery (w/n 6 wk), CNS tumor, AVM, aneurysm, severe uncontrolled HTN, vasculitis, use of dextran prior to or during PTCA, hypersensitivity to murine proteins **Supplied:** Inj 2 mg/mL **Notes/SE:** Use with heparin; allergic reactions, bleeding, thrombocytopenia possible **Interactions:** May ↑ bleeding with anticoagulants, antiplatelets, NSAIDs, thrombolytics **Labs:** Monitor CBC, PT, PTT, INR, guaiac stools, urine for blood **NIPE:** Monitor for ↑ bleeding & bruising; do not shake vial or mix with another drug, avoid contact sports.

Acarbose (Precose) **Uses:** Type 2 DM **Action:** α-Glucosidase inhibitor; delays digestion of carbohydrates, thus ↓ glucose levels **Dose:** 25–100 mg PO tid with 1st bite each meal; avoid if CrCl <25 mL/min **Caution/Contra:** [B, ?] Contra in IBD **Supplied:** Tabs 25, 50, 100 mg **Notes/SE:** May take with sulfonylureas; can affect digoxin levels; abdominal pain, diarrhea, flatulence, ↑ LFTs; check LFTs q3mo for 1st year of therapy. **Interactions:** ↑ hypoglycemic effect with sulfonylureas, juniper berries, ginseng, garlic, coriander, celery; ↓ effects with intestinal absorbents, digestive enzyme preparations, diuretics, corticosteroids, phenothizides, estrogens, phenytoin, isoniazid, sympathomimetics, calcium channel blockers, thyroid hormones; ↓ concentrations of digoxin **Labs:** LFTs, FBS,

HbA1c, LFTs, HGB & HCT **NIPE:** Take drug tid with first bite of food, ↓ GI side effects by ↓ dietary starch, treat hypoglycemia with dextrose instead of sucrose, continue diet & exercise program

Acebutolol (Sectral) **Uses:** HTN **Action:** Competitively blocks β-adrenergic receptors, β₁, and ISA **Dose:** 200–800 mg/d, ↓ if CrCl <50 mL/min **Caution/Contra:** [B, D in 2nd and 3rd trimesters, +] Contra in 2nd- and 3rd-degree heart block; can exacerbate ischemic heart disease, do not DC abruptly **Supplied:** Caps 200, 400 mg **Notes/SE:** Fatigue, HA, dizziness, bradycardia **Interactions:** ↓ antihypertensive effect with NSAIDS, salicylates, thyroid preparations, anesthetics, antacids, α-adrenergic stimulants, ma-huang, ephedra, licorice; ↓ hypoglycemic effect of glyburide; ↑ hypotensive response with other antihypertensives, nitrates, alcohol, diuretics, black cohash, hawthorn, goldenseal, parsley; ↑ bradycardia with digoxin, amiodarone; ↑ hypoglycemic effect of insulin **Labs:** Monitor lipids, uric acid, K⁺, FBS, LFTs, thyroxin, ECG **NIPE:** Teach pt to monitor BP, pulse, s/s CHF

Acetaminophen [APAP, N-acetyl-p-aminophenol] (Tylenol) **Uses:** Mild pain, HA, and fever **Action:** Nonnarcotic analgesic; inhibits synthesis of prostaglandins in the CNS; inhibits hypothalamic heat-regulating center **Dose:** *Adults.* 650 mg PO or PR q4–6h or 1000 mg PO q6h; max 4 g/24 h. *Peds. <12 y.* 10–15 mg/kg/dose PO or PR q4–6h; max 2.6 g/24 h. See Quick Dosing Table 1 (page 240). Administer q6h if CrCl 10–50 mL/min and q8h if CrCl <10 mL/min; avoid alcohol intake **Caution/Contra:** [B, +]. G6PD deficiency; alcoholic liver disease; hepatotoxicity reported in elderly and with alcohol use at doses >4 g/day **Supplied:** Tabs 160, 325, 500, 650 mg; chew tabs 80, 160 mg; liq 100 mg/mL, 120 mg/2.5 mL, 120 mg/5 mL, 160 mg/5 mL, 167 mg/5 mL, 325 mg/5 mL, 500 mg/5 mL; gtt 48 mg/mL, 60 mg/0.6 mL; supp 80, 120, 125, 300, 325, 650 mg **Notes/SE:** No antiinflammatory or platelet-inhibiting action; overdose causes hepatotoxicity, which is treated with *N*-acetylcysteine **Interactions:** ↑ hepatotoxicity with alcohol, barbiturates, carbamazepine, isoniazid, rifampin, phenytoin; ↑ risk of bleeding with NSAIDS, salicylates, warfarin, feverfew, ginkgo biloba, red clover; ↓ absorption with antacids, cholestyramine, colestipol. **Labs:** Monitor LFTs, CBC, BUN, creatinine, PT, INR; false ↑ urine 5-HIAA, urine glucose, serum uric acid; false ↓ serum glucose, amylase **NIPE:** Delayed absorption if given with food, ⊘ alcohol, teach s/s hepatotoxicity, consult health provider if temp.↑103° F/>3 d

Acetaminophen + Butalbital +/– Caffeine (Fioricet, Medigesic, Repan, Sedapap-10, Two-Dyne, Triapin, Axocet, Phrenilin Forte) [C-III] **Uses:** Mild pain; HA, especially associated with stress **Action:** Nonnarcotic analgesic with barbiturate **Dose:** 1–2 tabs or caps PO q4/6h PRN; ↓ in renal/hepatic impairment; 4 g/24 h APAP max; avoid alcohol intake **Caution/Contra:** [D, +] G6PD deficiency; alcoholic liver disease **Supplied:** Caps *Medigesic, Repan, Two-Dyne:* Butalbital 50 mg, caffeine 40 mg, + APAP 325 mg. Caps *Axocet, Phrenilin Forte:* Butalbital 50 mg + APAP 650 mg; *Triapin:* Butalbital 50 mg + APAP 325 mg. Tabs *Medigesic, Fioricet, Repan:* Butalbital 50 mg, caffeine 40 mg, + APAP 325 mg; *Phrenilin:* Butalbital 50 mg + APAP 325 mg; *Sedapap-10:* Butalbital 50 mg + APAP 650 mg **Notes/SE:** Butalbital habit-forming; drowsiness, dizziness, "hangover" effect **Interactions:** ↑ effects of benzodiazepines, opioid analgesics, sedatives/hypnotics, alcohol, methylphenidate hydrochloride; ↓ effects of MAO inhibitors, tricyclic antidepressants, corticosteroids, theophylline, oral contraceptives, BBs, doxycycline **NIPE:** ⊘ alcohol & CNS depressants, may impair coordination, monitor for depression, use barrier protection contraception

Acetaminophen + Codeine (Tylenol No. 1, No. 2, No. 3, No. 4) [C-III, C-V]
Uses: No. 1, No. 2, and No. 3 for mild–moderate pain; No. 4 for moderate–severe pain **Action:** Combined effects of APAP and a narcotic analgesic **Dose: Adults.** 1–2 tabs q3–4h PRN (max dose APAP = 4 g/d). **Peds.** APAP 10–15 mg/kg/dose; codeine 0.5–1.0 mg/kg dose q4–6h (useful dosing guide: 3–6 y, 5 mL/dose; 7–12 y, 10 mL/dose); ↓ in renal/hepatic impairment; do not exceed 4 g/24 h of APAP in adults **Caution/Contra:** [C, +] G6PD deficiency; alcoholic liver disease **Supplied:** Tabs 300 mg of APAP + codeine; caps 325 mg of APAP + codeine; helix, susp (C-V) APAP 120 mg + codeine 12 mg/5 mL **Notes/SE:** Codeine in No. 1 = 7.5 mg, No. 2 = 15 mg, No. 3 = 30 mg, No. 4 = 60 mg; drowsiness, dizziness, N/V **Interactions:** ↑ respiratory &/or CNS depression with alcohol, antihistamines, barbiturates, cimetidine, benzodiazepines, MAO inhibitors, tricyclic antidepressants, sedatives/hypnotics, muscle relaxants; ↑ effects of digoxin, phenytoin, rifampin; **Labs:** ↑ urine morphine, serum amylase, and lipase **NIPE:** Monitor respiratory rate & for constipation, may cause physical dependency, take with milk to ↓ GI distress

Acetazolamide (Diamox)
Uses: Diuresis, glaucoma, prevent high-altitude sickness, and refractory epilepsy **Action:** Carbonic anhydrase inhibitor; ↓ renal excretion of hydrogen and ↑ renal excretion of Na, K, bicarbonate, and water **Dose: Adults.** *Diuretic:* 250–375 mg IV or PO q24h. *Glaucoma:* 250–1000 mg PO q24h in ÷doses. *Epilepsy:* 8–30 mg/kg/d PO in ÷ doses. *Altitude sickness:* 125–250 mg PO q8–12h or SR 500 mg PO q12–24h start 24 h before ascent. **Peds.** *Epilepsy:* 8–30 mg/kg/24 h PO in (÷) doses; max 1 g/d. *Diuretic:* 5 mg/kg/24 h PO or IV. *Alkalinization of urine:* 5 mg/kg/dose PO bid–tid. *Glaucoma:* 5–15 mg/kg/24 h PO in ÷ doses; max 1 g/d; adjust in renal impairment (avoid if CrCl <10 mL/min) **Caution/Contra:** [C, +] Renal/hepatic failure, sulfa hypersensitivity **Supplied:** Tabs 125, 250 mg; SR caps 500 mg; inj 500 mg/vial **Notes/SE:** Follow Na⁺ and K⁺; watch for metabolic acidosis; SR dosage forms not recommended for use in epilepsy; malaise, metallic taste, drowsiness, photosensitivity, hyperglycemia **Interactions:** Causes ↑ effects of amphetamines, quinidine, procainamide, tricyclic antidepressants, ephedrine; ↓ effects of lithium, phenobarbital, salicylates, barbiturates; ↑ K⁺ loss with corticosteroids and amphotericin B **Labs:** Monitor serum electrolytes, FBS, CBC, creatinine, intraocular pressure; false positives for urinary protein, urinary urobilinogen; ↓ iodine uptake; ↑ serum and urine glucose, uric

acid, calcium, serum ammonia **NIPE:** ↓ GI distress with food, monitor for s/s metabolic acidosis, ↑ fluid to ↓ risk of kidney stones

Acetic Acid and Aluminum Acetate (Otic Domeboro)   Uses:
Otitis externa **Action:** Antiinfective **Dose:** 4–6 gtt in ear(s) q2–3h **Caution/Contra:** [C, ?] **Supplied:** Otic soln **NIPE:** Burning with instillation or irrigation

Acetylcysteine (Mucomyst)   Uses: Mucolytic agent as adjuvant Rx for
chronic bronchopulmonary diseases and CF; antidote to APAP hepatotoxicity, best results used w/n 24 h **Action:** Splits disulfide linkages between mucoprotein molecular complexes; protects liver by restoring glutathione levels in APAP overdose **Dose:** *Adults & Peds. Neb:* 3–5 mL of 20% soln diluted with an equal vol of water or NS tid–qid. *Antidote:* PO or NG: 140 mg/kg loading dose, then 70 mg/kg q4h for 17 doses. Dilute 1:3 in carbonated beverage or orange juice **Caution/Contra:** [C, ?] **Supplied:** Soln 10%, 20% **Notes/SE:** Bronchospasm when used by inhalation in asthmatics; N/V, drowsiness; activated charcoal adsorbs acetylcysteine when given PO for acute APAP ingestion **Interactions:** Discolors rubber, iron, copper, silver; incompatible with multiple antibiotics – administer drugs separately **Labs:** Monitor ABGs & pulse oximetry with bronchospasm **NIPE:** Inform pt of ↑ productive cough, clear airway before aerosol administration, ↑ fluids to liquefy secretions, unpleasant odor will disappear & may cause N/V

Acitretin (Soriatane)   Uses: Severe psoriasis and other keratinization dis-
orders (lichen planus, etc) **Action:** Retinoid-like activity **Dose:** 25–50 mg/d PO, with main meal; can ↑ if no response by 4 wk to 75 mg/d **Caution/Contra:** [X, –] Caution in renal/hepatic impairment; caution in women of reproductive potential **Supplied:** Caps 10, 25 mg **Notes/SE:** Teratogenic, contra in PRG; follow LFTs; response often takes 2–3 mon; cheilitis, skin peeling, alopecia, pruritus, rash, arthralgia, GI upset, photosensitivity, thrombocytosis, hypertriglyceridemia **Interactions:** ↑ ½ life with alcohol use, ↑ hepatotoxicity with methotrexate, ↓ effects of progestin-only contraceptives **Labs:** Monitor LFTs, lipids, FBS, HbA1c **NIPE:** Use effective contraception; ⊘ donate blood for 3 y after treatment, teach pt s/s pancreatitis

Acyclovir (Zovirax)   Uses: Herpes simplex and herpes zoster viral infec-
tions **Action:** Interferes with viral DNA synthesis **Dose:** *Adults. Oral: Initial genital herpes:* 200 mg PO q4h while awake, total of 5 caps/d for 10 d or 400 mg PO tid for 7–10 d. *Chronic suppression:* 400 mg PO bid. *Intermittent Rx:* As for initial treatment, except treat for 5 d, or 800 mg PO bid, initiate at earliest prodrome. *Herpes zoster:* 800 mg PO 5×/d for 7–10 d. *IV:* 5–10 mg/kg/dose IV q8h. *Topical initial herpes genitalis:* Apply q3h (6×/d) for 7 d. *Peds.* Herpes simplex or PO q8h or 750 mg/m²/24 h ÷ q8h. *Chickenpox:* 20 mg/kg/dose PO qid; ↓ for CrCl <50 mL/min **Caution/Contra:** [C, +] **Supplied:** Caps 200 mg; tabs 400, 800 mg; susp 200 mg/5 mL; inj 500 mg/vial; oint 5% **Notes/SE:** PO better than topical for herpes genitalis; dizziness, lethargy, confusion, rash, inflammation at IV inj site **Interactions:** ↑ CNS SE with methotrexate & zidovudine, ↑ blood levels with

probenecid **Labs:** monitor BUN, serum creatinine, LFTs, CBC **NIPE:** start immediately with symptoms, ↑ hydration with IV dose, ↑ risk cervical cancer with genital herpes, ↑ length of treatment in immunocompromised pts

Adalimumab (Humira)
WARNING: Cases of TB have been observed, check tuberculin skin test prior to use **Uses:** Rx moderate/severe RA in patients with an inadequate response to one or more DMARDs **Action:** TNF alpha inhibitor **Dose:** 40 mg sq every other wk; increase to 40 mg every wk if not on methotrexate **Caution/Contra:** [B, ?/–], serious infections and sepsis reported **Supplied:** Prefilled 1-mL (40-mg) syringe **SE:** Injection-site reactions, serious infections, neurologic events, malignancies **Notes:** refrigerate prefilled syringe, rotate injection sites, may be used with other DMARDs **Interactions:** ↑ effects with methotrexate **Labs:** May ↑ lipids, alkaline phosphatase **NIPE:** Avoid exposure to infection; ⊘ admin live virus vaccines

Adefovir (Hepsera)
WARNING: Acute exacerbations of hepatitis may occur on discontinuation of therapy (monitor hepatic function); chronic administration may lead to nephrotoxicity, especially in patients with underlying renal dysfunction (monitor renal function); HIV resistance may emerge; lactic acidosis and severe hepatomegaly with steatosis have been reported when used alone or in combination with other antiretrovirals. **Uses:** Chronic active hepatitis B virus **Action:** Nucleotide analogue **Dose:** CrCl = 50 mL/min: 10 mg PO qd; CrCl 20–49 mL/min: 10 mg PO q48h; CrCl 10–19 mL/min: 10 mg PO q72h; Hemodialysis: 10 mg PO q7d postdialysis; adjust dose when CrCl <50 mL/min **Caution/Contra:** [C, –] **Supplied:** Tabs 10 mg **Notes/SE:** Asthenia, headache, abdominal pain, see Warning **Interactions:** See Warning **Labs:** LFTs, BUN, creatinine, creatine kinase, amylase **NIPE:** Effects on fetus & baby not known – ⊘ breast-feed; use barrier contraception

Adenosine (Adenocard)
Uses: PSVT, including associated with WPW **Action:** Class IV antiarrhythmic; slows AV node conduction **Dose:** *Adults.* 6 mg IV bolus; may repeat in 1–2 min; max 12 mg IV. *Peds.* 0.05 mg/kg IV bolus; may repeat q1–2 min to 0.25 mg/kg max **Caution/Contra:** [C, ?] 2nd- or 3rd-degree AV block or SSS (w/o pacemaker); recent MI or cerebral hemorrhage **Supplied:** Inj 6 mg/2 mL **Notes/SE:** Doses >12 mg not recommended; can cause momentary asystole when administered; caffeine and theophylline antagonize effects of adenosine; facial flushing, HA, dyspnea, chest pressure, hypotension **Interactions:** ↓ effects with theophylline, caffeine, guarana; ↑ effects with dipyridamole; ↑ risk of hypotension & chest pain with nicotine; ↑ risk of bradycardia with BBs; ↑ risk of heart block with carbamazepine; ↑ risk of ventricular fibrillation with digitalis glycosides. **Labs:** Monitor ECG during administration **NIPE:** Monitor BP & pulse during therapy, monitor respiratory status–↑ risk of bronchospasm in asthmatics, discard unused or unclear solution

Albumin (Albuminar, Buminate, Albutein)
Uses: Plasma volume expansion for shock (burns, surgery, hemorrhage, or other trauma) **Action:** Maint

of plasma colloid oncotic pressure **Dose:** *Adults.* Initially, 25 g IV; subsequent dose based on response; 250 g/48h max. *Peds.* 0.5–1.0 g/kg/dose; infuse at 0.05–0.1 g/min **Caution/Contra:** [C, ?] Severe anemia, cardiac failure; caution with cardiac, renal, or hepatic insufficiency due to added protein load and possible hypervolemia **Supplied:** Soln 5%, 25% **Notes/SE:** Contains 130–160 mEq Na$^+$/L; chills, fever, CHF, tachycardia, hypotension, hypervolemia **Interactions:** Atypical reactions with ACE Inhibitors – withhold 24 h prior to plasma administration **Labs:** ↑ alkaline phosphatase; monitor HMG, HCT, electrolytes, serum protein **NIPE:** Monitor BP & d/c if hypotensive, monitor intake & output, admin to all blood types

Albuterol (Proventil, Ventolin)
Uses: Bronchospasm in reversible obstructive airway disease; prevent exercise-induced bronchospasm **Action:** β-Adrenergic sympathomimetic bronchodilator; relaxes bronchial smooth muscle **Dose:** *Adults.* 2 inhal q4–6h PRN; 1 Rotacap inhaled q4–6h; 2–4 mg PO tid–qid; *Neb:* 1.25–5 mg (0.25–1 mL of 0.5% soln in 2–3 mL of NS tid–qid). *Peds.* 2 inhal q4–6h; 0.1–0.2 mg/kg/dose PO; max 2–4 mg PO tid; *Neb:* 0.05 mg/kg (max 2.5 mg) in 2–3 mL of NS tid–qid **Caution/Contra:** [C, +] **Supplied:** Tabs 2, 4 mg; ER tabs 4, 8 mg; syrup 2 mg/5 mL; 90-μg/dose met-dose inhaler; Rotacaps 200 μg; soln for neb 0.083, 0.5% **Notes/SE:** Palpitations, tachycardia, nervousness, GI upset **Interactions:** ↑ effects with other sympathomimetics; ↑ CV effects with MAO inhibitors, TCA, inhaled anesthetics; ↓ effects with BBs; ↓ effectiveness of insulin, oral hypoglycemics, digoxin **Labs:** Transient ↑ in serum glucose > inhalation; transient ↓ K$^+$ > inhalation **NIPE:** Monitor HR, BP, ABGs, s&s bronchospasm & CNS stimulation; instruct on use of inhaler, must use as 1st inhaler, & rinse mouth after use

Albuterol and Ipratropium (Combivent)
Uses: COPD **Action:** Combination of β-adrenergic bronchodilator and quaternary anticholinergic compound **Dose:** 2 inhal qid **Caution/Contra:** [C, +] **Supplied:** Met-dose inhaler, 18 μg ipratropium/103 μg albuterol/puff **Notes/SE:** Palpitations, tachycardia, nervousness, GI upset, dizziness, blurred vision **Interactions:** ↑ effects with anticholinergics, including ophthalmic meds; ↓ effects with herb jaborandi tree, pill-bearing spurge **NIPE:** See Albuterol; may cause transient blurred vision/irritation or urinary changes

Aldesleukin [IL-2] (Proleukin)
WARNING: Use restricted to patients with normal pulmonary and cardiac function. **Uses:** RCC, melanoma **Action:** Acts via IL-2 receptor; numerous immunomodulatory effects **Dose:** 600,000 IU/kg q8h × 14 days (FDA-approved dose/schedule for RCC). Multiple cont inf and alternate schedules (including "high dose" using 24×10^6 IU/m^2 IV q8h on days 1–5 and 12–16) **Caution/Contra:** [C, ?/–] **Supplied:** Inj 1.1 mg/mL (22×10^6 IU) **Notes/SE:** Flu-like syndrome (malaise, fever, chills), N/V/D, ↑ bilirubin; capillary leak syndrome with ↓ BP, pulmonary edema, fluid retention, and weight gain; renal toxicity and mild hematologic toxicity (anemia, thrombocytopenia, leukope-

nia) and secondary eosinophilia; cardiac toxicity (myocardial ischemia, atrial arrhythmias); neurologic toxicity (CNS depression, somnolence, rarely coma, delirium). Pruritic rashes, urticaria, and erythroderma common. Cont inf schedules less likely to cause severe hypotension and fluid retention **Interactions:** May ↑ toxicity of cardiotoxic, hepatotoxic, myelotoxic & nephrotoxic drugs; ↑ hypotension with antihypertensive drugs; ↓ effects with corticosteroids; acute reaction with iodinated contrast media up to several months > infusion; CNS effects with psychotropics **Labs:** May cause ↑ alkaline phosphatase, bilirubin, BUN, serum creatinine, LFTs. **NIPE:** Thoroughly explain serious SE of drug & that some SE are expected; ⊘ alcohol, NSAIDs, ASA

Alefacept (Amevive) WARNING: Monitor CD4 before each dose; hold if <250; d/c if <250 × 1 mon **Uses:** Moderate/severe adult chronic plaque psoriasis **Action:** fusion protein inhibitor **Dose:** *Adults.* 7.5 mg IV or 15 mg IM weekly × 12 w **Caution:** [B, ?/-] PRG registry; associated with serious infections **Contra:** Lymphopenia **Supplied:** 7.5, 15 mg vials **SE:** Chills, pharyngitis, myalgia, injection site reaction, malignancy **Notes:** Different forms for IV/IM administration; may repeat course 12 wk later if CD4 acceptable **Interactions:** No studies performed **Labs:** Monitor WBCs, CD4+T lymphocyte counts **NIPE:** ↑ risk of infection; ⊘ exposure to infections; inj site inflammation; rotate sites

Alendronate (Fosamax) **Uses:** Rx and prevention of osteoporosis, Rx of steroid-induced osteoporosis and Paget's disease **Action:** ↓Normal and abnormal bone resorption **Dose:** *Osteoporosis: Rx:* 10 mg/d PO or 70 mg/wk. *Steroid-induced osteoporosis: Rx:* 5 mg/d PO. *Prevention:* 5 mg/d PO or 35 mg/wk. *Paget's disease:* 40 mg/d PO **Caution/Contra:** [C, ?] Not recommended if CrCl <35 mL/min; abnormalities of the esophagus, inability to sit or stand upright for 30 min, hypocalcemia; caution with NSAID use **Supplied:** Tabs 5, 10, 35, 40, 70 mg **Notes/SE:** Take 1 thing in AM with water (8 oz) at least 30 min before 1st food or beverage of the day. Do not lie down for 30 min after taking. Adequate Ca and vitamin D supplement necessary; GI disturbances, HA, pain **Interactions:** ↓ absorption with antacids, calcium supplements, iron, food; ↑ risk of upper GI bleed with ASA & NSAIDs **Labs:** May cause transient ↑ serum calcium & phosphate **NIPE:** Adequate calcium & vit D suppl, ↑ wt-bearing activity, ↓ smoking, alcohol use

Alfentanil (Alfenta) [C-II] **Uses:** Adjunct in the maint of anesthesia; analgesia **Action:** Short-acting narcotic analgesic **Dose:** *Adults & Peds >12 y.* 3–75 μg/kg IV inf; total dose depends on duration of procedure **Caution/Contra:** [C, +/–] ↑ ICP, respiratory depression **Supplied:** Inj 500 μg/mL **Notes/SE:** Bradycardia, ↓ BP, cardiac arrhythmias, peripheral vasodilation, ↑ ICP, drowsiness, respiratory depression **Interactions:** ↓ effect with phenothiazines; ↑ effects with BBs, CNS depressants, erythromycin **NIPE:** Monitor HR, BP, resp rate

Alfuzosin (Uroxatral) WARNING: May prolong QTc interval **Uses:** BPH **Action:** α-blocker **Dose:** *Adults.* 10 mg PO QD immediately after the same meal **Caution:** [B, –] **Contra:** Concomitant CYP3A4 inhibitors; moderate/severe hepatic impairment **Supplied:** 10 mg tabs **SE:** Postural hypotension, dizziness, HA, fatigue **Notes:** Extended release tablet (do not cut/crush); fewest reports of ejaculatory disorders compared to other α-blockers **Interactions:** ↑ effects with atenolol, azole antifungals, cimetidine, ritonavir; ↑ effects of antihypertensives **NIPE:** Not indicated for use in women or children; take with food; ↑ risk of postural hypotension; ⊘ take other meds that prolong QT interval

Alginic Acid + Aluminum Hydroxide and Magnesium Trisilicate (Gaviscon)
Uses: Heartburn; pain from hiatal hernia **Action:** Forms protective layer blocking reflux of gastric acid **Dose:** 2–4 tabs or 15–30 mL PO qid followed by water; avoid in renal impairment or with Na-restricted diet **Caution/Contra:** [B, –] **Supplied:** Tabs, susp **Notes/SE:** Diarrhea, constipation **Interactions:** ↓ absorption of tetracyclines

Allopurinol (Zyloprim, Lopurin, Alloprim)
Uses: Gout, hyperuricemia of malignancy, and uric acid urolithiasis **Action:** Xanthine oxidase inhibitor; ↓ uric acid production **Dose:** *Adults. PO:* Initially, 100 mg/d; usual 300 mg/d; max 800 mg/d. *IV:* 200–400 mg/m²/d (max 600 mg/24 h). *Peds.* Use only for treating hyperuricemia of malignancy in <10 y: 10 mg/kg/24 h PO or 200 mg/m²/d IV ÷ q6–8h (max 600 mg/24 h); ↓ in renal impairment; take after meal with plenty of fluid **Caution/Contra:** [C, M] **Supplied:** Tabs 100, 300 mg; inj 500 mg/30 mL (Aloprim) **Notes/SE:** Aggravates acute gout; begin after acute attack resolves; administer pc; IV dose of 6 mg/mL final conc as single daily inf or ÷ 6, 8, or 12-h intervals; skin rash, N/V, renal impairment, angioedema **Interactions:** ↑ effect of theophylline, oral anticoagulants; ↑ hypersensitivity reactions with ACE inhibitors, thiazide diuretics; ↑ risk of rash with ampicillin/amoxicillin; ↑ bone marrow depression with cyclophosphamide, azathioprine, mercaptopurine; ↓ effects with alcohol **Labs:** ↑ alkaline phosphatase, bilirubin, LFTs **NIPE:** ↑ fluids to 2–3 L/day, take > meals, may ↑ drowsiness

Almotriptan (Axert)
See Table 11, page 259

Alosetron (Lotronex)
WARNING: Serious GI side effects, some fatal, including ischemic colitis, have been reported. May be prescribed only through participation in the prescribing program for Lotronex **Uses:** Treatment of severe diarrhea-predominant IBS in women who have failed conventional therapy. **Action:** Selective 5-HT₃ receptor antagonist **Dose:** *Adults.* 1 mg PO qd × 4 wk; titrate to max of 1 mg bid; DC after 4 wk at max dose if IBS symptoms not controlled **Caution/Contra:** [B, ?/–] Hx chronic or severe constipation, intestinal obstruction, strictures, toxic megacolon, GI perforation, adhesions, ischemic colitis, Crohn's disease, ulcerative colitis, diverticulitis, thrombophlebitis, or hypercoagulable state **Supplied:** 1 mg tabs **Notes/SE:** d/c immediately if constipation or symptoms of ischemic colitis develop; constipation, abdominal pain, nausea **Interactions:** ↑ risk constipation with other drugs that ↓ GI motility, inhibits N-acetyltransferase & may influence metabolism of isoniazid, procainamide, hydralazine **NIPE:** Administer w/o regard to food, eval effectiveness >4 w.

α1-Protease Inhibitor (Prolastin) **Uses:** Panacinar emphysema **Action:** Replacement of human α₁-protease inhibitor **Dose:** 60 mg/kg IV once/wk **Caution/Contra:** [C, ?] Selective IgA deficiencies with known antibodies to IgA **Supplied:** Inj 500 mg/20 mL, 1000 mg/40 mL **Notes/SE:** Fever, dizziness, flu-like symptoms, allergic reactions **NIPE:** Infuse over 30 min, do not mix with other drugs, use w/n 3 h of reconstitution

Alprazolam (Xanax) [C-IV] **Uses:** Anxiety and panic disorders + anxiety with depression **Action:** Benzodiazepine; antianxiety agent **Dose:** *Anxiety:* Initially, 0.25–0.5 mg tid; ↑ to a max of 4 mg/d in ÷ doses. *Panic:* Initially, 0.5 mg tid; may gradually ↑ to desired response; ↓ dose in elderly, debilitated, and hepatic impairment **Caution/Contra:** [D, –] **Supplied:** Tabs 0.25, 0.5, 1.0, 2.0 mg **Notes/SE:** Avoid abrupt discontinuation after prolonged use; drowsiness, fatigue, irritability, memory impairment, sexual dysfunction **Interactions:** ↑ CNS depression with alcohol, other CNS depressants, narcotics, MAO inhibitors, anesthetics, antihistamines, theophylline, & herbs: kava kava, valerian; ↑ effect with oral contraceptives, cimetidine, isoniazid, disulfiram, omeprazole, valproic acid, ciprofloxacin, erythromycin, clarithromycin, phenytoin, verapamil, grapefruit juice; ↑ risk of ketoconazole, itraconazole, & digitalis toxicity; ↓ effectiveness of levodopa; ↓ effect with carbamazepine, rifampin, rifabutin, barbiturates, cigarette smoking **Labs:** ↑ alkaline phosphatase, may cause ↓ HCT & neutropenia **NIPE:** Monitor for respiratory depression

Alprostadil [Prostaglandin E₁] (Prostin VR) **Uses:** Any state in which blood flow must be maintained through the ductus arteriosus to sustain either pulmonary or systemic circulation until surgery can be performed (eg, pulmonary atresia, pulmonary stenosis, tricuspid atresia, transposition, severe tetralogy of Fallot) **Action:** Vasodilator, platelet aggregation inhibitor; smooth muscle of the ductus arteriosus is especially sensitive **Dose:** 0.05 µg/kg/min IV; ↓ dose to lowest that maintains response **Caution/Contra:** [X, –] **Supplied:** Injectable forms **Notes/SE:** Cutaneous vasodilation, seizure-like activity, jitteriness, temperature elevation, hypocalcemia, apnea, thrombocytopenia, hypotension; may cause apnea; have an intubation kit at bedside if patient is not intubated **Interactions:** ↑ effects of anticoagulants & antihypertensives, ↓ effects of cyclosporine **Labs:** ↓ fibrinogen **NIPE:** Dilute drug before administration, refrigerate & discard >24 h, apnea & bradycardia indicates drug overdose, central line preferred, flushing indicates catheter malposition

Alprostadil, Intracavernosal (Caverject, Edex) **Uses:** Erectile dysfunction **Action:** Relaxes smooth muscles, dilates cavernosal arteries, increases lacunar spaces and entrapment of blood by compressing venules against tunica albuginea **Dose:** 2.5–60 µg intracavernosal; adjusted to individual needs **Caution/Contra:** [X, –] Conditions predisposing to priapism; anatomic deformities of the penis; penile implants; men in whom sexual activity is inadvisable **Supplied:** *Caverject:* 6–10- or 6–20-µg vials +/– diluent syringes. *Caverject Impulse:*

Self-contained syringe (29 gauge) 10 and 20 μg. *Edex:* 5-, 10-, 20-, 40-μg vials + syringes **Notes/SE:** Penile pain common; titrate dose at physician's office. Counsel patients about possible priapism, penile fibrosis, and hematoma; pain w inj **Interactions:** ↑ effects of anticoagulants & antihypertensives, ↓ effects of cyclosporine **Labs:** ↓ fibrinogen **NIPE:** Vaginal itching and burning in female partners, do not inject >3×/wk or closer than 24 h/dose

Alprostadil, Urethral Suppository (Muse)

Uses: Erectile dysfunction **Action:** Alprostadil (PGE₁) absorbed through urethral mucosa; vasodilator and smooth muscle relaxant of corpus cavernosa **Dose:** 125–1000-μg system 5–10 min prior to sexual activity **Caution/Contra:** [X, –] **Supplied:** 125, 250, 500, 1000 μg with a transurethral delivery system **Notes/SE:** Hypotension, dizziness, syncope, penile pain, testicular pain, urethral burning/bleeding, and priapism. Dose titration under physician's supervision **Interactions:** ↑ effects of anticoagulants & antihypertensives, ↓ effects of cyclosporine **Labs:** ↓ fibrinogen; **NIPE:** No more than 2 doses/pt/24 h, urinate prior to use

Alteplase, Recombinant [TPA] (Activase)

Uses: AMI, PE, and acute ischemic stroke **Action:** Thrombolytic; initiates local fibrinolysis by binding to fibrin in the thrombus **Dose:** *AMI and PE:* 100 mg IV over 3 h (10 mg over 2 min, then 50 mg over 1 h, then 40 mg over 2 h). *Stroke:* 0.9 mg/kg (max 90 mg) infused over 60 min **Caution/Contra:** [C, ?] Active internal bleeding; uncontrolled HTN (systolic BP = 185 mm Hg/diastolic = 110 mm Hg); recent (w/n 3 mon) CVA, GI bleed, trauma, surgery, prolonged external cardiac massage; intracranial neoplasm, suspected aortic dissection, AV malformation or aneurysm, bleeding diathesis, hemostatic defects, seizure at the time of stroke, suspicion of subarachnoid hemorrhage **Supplied:** Powder for inj 50, 100 mg **Notes/SE:** Bleeding, bruising (especially from venipuncture sites), hypotension; give heparin to prevent reocclusion; in AMI doses of >150 mg associated with intracranial bleeding **Interactions:** ↑ risk of bleeding with heparin, ASA, NSAIDS, abciximab, dipyridamole, eptifibtide, tirofiban; ↓ effects with nitroglycerine **Labs:** ↓ fibrinogen **NIPE:** Compress venipuncture site at least 30 min, monitor pt/PTT, bed rest during infusion

Altretamine (Hexalen)

Uses: Epithelial ovarian CA **Action:** Unknown; cytotoxic agent, possibly alkylating agent; inhibits nucleotide incorporation into DNA and RNA **Dose:** 260 mg/m²/d in 4 ÷ doses for 14–21 d of a 28-d treatment cycle; dose ↑ to 150 mg/m²/d in multiagent regimens (refer to specific protocols) **Caution/Contra:** [D, ?/–] Preexisting severe bone marrow depression or neurologic toxicity **Supplied:** Caps 50, 100 mg **Notes/SE:** N/V/D and cramps; neurologic toxicity (peripheral neuropathy, CNS depression); minimally myelosuppressive **Interactions:** ↓ effect with phenobarbital, ↓ antibody response with live virus vaccines, ↑ risk of toxicity with cimetidine & hypotension with MAO inhibitors, ↑ bone marrow depression with radiation; **Labs:** ↑ alkaline phosphatase, BUN, & serum creatinine **NIPE:** Use barrier contraception, take with food, monitor CBC

Aluminum Carbonate (Basaljel) **Uses:** Hyperacidity (peptic ulcer, GERD, etc); supplement to the Rx of hyperphosphatemia **Action:** Neutralizes gastric acid; binds phosphate **Dose:** *Adults.* 2 caps or tabs or 10 mL (in water) q2h PRN. *Peds.* 50–150 mg/kg/24 h PO ÷ q4–6h **Caution/Contra:** [C, ?] **Supplied:** Tabs, caps, susp **Notes/SE:** Constipation **Interactions:** ↓ absorption & effects of antimuscarinics, benzodiazepines, chloroquine, cimetidine, digoxin, iron salts, isoniazid, NSAIDs, phenothiazines, quinolones, tetracycline **Labs:** ↑ serum gastrin, ↓ serum phosphate **NIPE:** Separate other drug administration by 2 h, ↑ fluid intake, long-term use may cause calcium resorption & bone demineralization

Aluminum Hydroxide (Amphojel, AlternaGEL) **Uses:** Hyperacidity (peptic ulcer, hiatal hernia, etc); supplement to Rx of hyperphosphatemia **Action:** Neutralizes gastric acid; binds phosphate **Dose:** *Adults.* 10–30 mL or 2 tabs PO q4–6h. *Peds.* 5–15 mL PO q4–6h or 50–150 mg/kg/24 h PO ÷ q4–6h (hyperphosphatemia) **Caution/Contra:** [C, ?] **Supplied:** Tabs 300, 600 mg; chew tabs 500 mg; susp 320, 600 mg/5 mL **Notes/SE:** Can use in renal failure; constipation. **Interactions:** ↓ absorption & effects of allopurinol, benzodiazepines, corticosteroids, chloroquine, cimetidine, digoxin, isoniazid, phenytoin, quinolones, ranitidine, tetracycline **Labs:** ↑ serum gastrin, ↓ serum phosphate **NIPE:** Separate other drug administration by 2 h, ↑ effectiveness of liquid form

Aluminum Hydroxide + Magnesium Carbonate (Gaviscon) **Uses:** Hyperacidity (peptic ulcer, hiatal hernia, etc) **Action:** Neutralizes gastric acid **Dose:** *Adults.* 15–30 PO pc and hs. *Peds.* 5–15 mL PO qid or PRN; avoid in renal impairment; may affect absorption of some drugs **Caution/Contra:** [C, ?] **Supplied:** Liq containing aluminum hydroxide 95 mg + magnesium carbonate 358 mg/15 mL **Notes/SE:** Doses qid are best given pc and hs; may cause ↑ Mg^{2+} (with renal insufficiency), constipation, diarrhea **Interactions:** In addition to aluminum hydroxide ↓ effects of histamine blockers, hydantoins, nitrofurantoin, phenothiazines, ticlopidine, ↑ effects of quinidine, sulfonylureas **NIPE:** Avoid concurrent drug use & separate by 2 h, ↑ fiber

Aluminum Hydroxide + Magnesium Hydroxide (Maalox) **Uses:** Hyperacidity (peptic ulcer, hiatal hernia, etc) **Action:** Neutralizes gastric acid **Dose:** *Adults.* 10–60 mL or 2–4 tabs PO qid or PRN. *Peds.* 5–15 mL PO qid or PRN **Caution/Contra:** [C, ?] **Supplied:** Tabs, susp **Notes/SE:** Doses qid best given pc and hs; may cause ↑ Mg^{2+} in renal insufficiency, constipation, diarrhea **Interactions:** In addition to aluminum hydroxide, ↓ effects of digoxin, quinolones, phenytoin, iron suppl, and ketoconazole **NIPE:** Avoid concurrent drug use; separate by 2 h

Aluminum Hydroxide + Magnesium Hydroxide and Simethicone (Mylanta, Mylanta II, Maalox Plus) **Uses:** Hyperacidity with bloating **Action:** Neutralizes gastric acid **Dose:** *Adults.* 10–60 mL or 2–4 tabs PO qid or PRN. *Peds.* 5–15 mL PO qid or PRN; avoid in renal impairment; may affect absorption of some drugs **Caution/Contra:** [C, ?] **Supplied:** Tabs, susp

Notes/SE: Hypermagnesemia in renal insufficiency, diarrhea, constipation; Mylanta II contains twice the aluminum and magnesium hydroxide of Mylanta **Interactions:** in addition to aluminum hydroxide, ↓ effects of digoxin, quinolnes, phenytoin, iron suppl, and ketoconazole **NIPE:** Avoid concurrent drug use; separate by 2 h

Aluminum Hydroxide + Magnesium Trisilicate (Gaviscon, Gaviscon-2)
Uses: Hyperacidity **Action:** Neutralizes gastric acid **Dose:** Chew 2–4 tabs qid; avoid in renal impairment; concomitant administration may affect absorption of some drugs **Caution/Contra:** [C, ?] **Supplied:** *Gaviscon:* Aluminum hydroxide 80 mg and magnesium trisilicate 20 mg. *Gaviscon-2:* Aluminum hydroxide 160 mg and magnesium trisilicate 40 mg **Notes/SE:** Constipation, diarrhea **Interactions:** In addition to aluminum hydroxide, ↓ effects of digoxin, quinolines, phenytoin, iron suppl, and ketoconazole **NIPE:** Avoid concurrent drug use; separate by 2 h

Amantadine (Symmetrel)
Uses: Rx or prophylaxis for influenza A viral infections and parkinsonism **Action:** Prevents release of infectious viral nucleic acid into the host cell; releases dopamine from intact dopaminergic terminals **Dose:** *Adults.* *Influenza A:* 200 mg/d PO or 100 mg PO bid. *Parkinsonism:* 100 mg PO qd–bid. *Peds. 1–9 y:* 4.4–8.8 mg/kg/24 h to 150 mg/24 h max ÷ doses qd–bid. *10–12 y:* 100–200 mg/d in 1–2 ÷ doses; ↓ in renal impairment **Caution/Contra:** [C, M] **Supplied:** Caps 100 mg; tabs 100 mg; soln 50 mg/5 mL **Notes/SE:** Orthostatic hypotension, edema, insomnia, depression, irritability, hallucinations, dream abnormalities **Interactions:** ↑ effects with HCTZ, triamterene, amiloride, pheasant's eye herb, scopolia root, benztropine **Labs:** ↑ BUN, serum creatinine, CPK, alkaline phosphatase, bilirubin, LDH, AST, ALT **NIPE:** ⊘ discontinue abruptly, take at least 4 h before sleep if insomnia occurs, eval for mental status changes, take with meals, ⊘ alcohol

Amifostine (Ethyol)
Uses: Xerostomia prophylaxis during RT (head and neck, ovarian, or non-small-cell lung CA). Reduces renal toxicity associated with repeated administration of cisplatin **Action:** Prodrug, dephosphorylated by alkaline phosphatase to the pharmacologically active thiol metabolite **Dose:** 910 mg/m²/d as a 15-min IV inf 30 min prior to chemotherapy **Caution/Contra:** [C, +/–] **Supplied:** 500 mg vials of lyophilized drug with 500 mg of mannitol, reconstituted in sterile NS **Notes/SE:** Transient hypotension in >60%, N/V, flushing with hot or cold chills, dizziness, hypocalcemia, somnolence, and sneezing. Does not reduce the effectiveness of cyclophosphamide plus cisplatin chemotherapy **Interactions:** ↑ effects with antihypertensives **Labs:** ↓ calcium levels **NIPE:** Monitor blood pressure, ensure adequate hydration, infuse over 15 min and supine

Amikacin (Amikin)
Uses: Serious infections caused by gram– bacteria and mycobacteria **Action:** Aminoglycoside antibiotic; inhibits protein synthesis **Dose:** *Adults & Peds.* 5–7.5 mg/kg/dose ÷ q8–24h based on renal function. *Neonates <1200 g, 0–4 wk:* 7.5 mg/kg/dose q12h–18h. *Postnatal age <7 d, 1200–2000 g:* 7.5 mg/kg/dose q12h. *>2000 g:* 10 mg/kg/dose q12h. *Postnatal age*

>7 d, 1200–2000 g: 7 mg/kg/dose q8h. >2000 g: 7.5–10 mg/kg/dose q8h **Caution/Contra:** [C, +/–] **Supplied:** Inj 100, 500 mg/2 mL **Notes/SE:** May be effective against gram–bacteria resistant to gentamicin and tobramycin; monitor renal function carefully for dosage adjustments; monitor serum levels (Table 2, page 242); nephrotoxicity, ototoxicity, neurotoxicity; avoid use with potent diuretics **Interactions:** ↑ risk of ototoxicity and nephrotoxicity with acyclovir, amphotericin B, cephalosporins, cisplatin, loop diuretics, methoxyflurane, polymyxin B, vancomycine; ↑ neuromuscular blocking effect with muscle relaxants & anesthetics **Labs:** ↑ BUN, serum creatinine, AST, ALT, serum alkakine phosphatase, bilirubin, LDH **NIPE:** ↑ fluid consumption

Amiloride (Midamor)   **Uses:** HTN & CHF **Action:** K$^+$-sparing diuretic; interferes with K$^+$/Na$^+$ exchange in the distal tubules **Dose:** *Adults.* 5–10 mg/d PO. *Peds.* 0.625 mg/kg/d; ↓ in renal impairment **Caution/Contra:** [B, ?] **Supplied:** Tabs 5 mg **Notes/SE:** Hyperkalemia possible; monitor serum K$^+$ levels; HA, dizziness, dehydration, impotence **Interactions:** ↑ risk of hyperkalemia with ACEI, K$^+$-sparing diuretics, NSAIDs, & K$^+$ salt substitutes; ↑ effects of lithium, digoxin, antihypertensives, amantadine; ↑ risk of hypokalemia with licorice **NIPE:** Take with food, I&O, daily weights, avoid salt substitutes, bananas, & oranges

Aminocaproic Acid (Amicar)   **Uses:** Excessive bleeding resulting from systemic hyperfibrinolysis and urinary fibrinolysis **Action:** Inhibits fibrinolysis by inhibition of TPA substances **Dose:** *Adults.* 5 g IV or PO (1st h) followed by 1–1.25 g/h IV or PO. *Peds.* 100 mg/kg IV (1st h) (max dose/d: 30 g), then 1 g/m^2/h; max 18 g/m^2/d; ↓ in renal failure **Caution/Contra:** [C, ?] DIC, hematuria of upper urinary tract **Supplied:** Tabs 500 mg; syrup 250 mg/mL; inj 250 mg/mL **Notes/SE:** Administer for 8 h or until bleeding is controlled; not for upper urinary tract bleeding; ↓ BP, bradycardia, dizziness, HA, fatigue, rash, GI disturbance, ↓ platelet function **Interactions:** ↑ coagulation with estrogens & oral contraceptives **Labs:** ↑ K$^+$ levels, false ↑ urine amino acids **NIPE:** Creatine kinase monitoring with long-term use, eval for thrombophlebitis & difficulty uriniating

Amino-Cerv pH 5.5 Cream   **Uses:** Mild cervicitis, postpartum cervicitis/cervical tears, postcauterization, postcryosurgery, and postconization **Action:** Hydrating agent; removes excess keratin in hyperkeratotic conditions **Dose:** 1 Applicatorful intravaginally hs for 2–4 wk **Caution/Contra:** [C, ?] Use in viral skin infection **Supplied:** Vaginal cream **Notes/SE:** Also called carbamide or urea; contains 8.34% urea, 0.5% Na propionate, 0.83% methionine, 0.35% cystine, 0.83% inositol, and benzalkonium chloride; transient stinging, local irritation

Aminoglutethimide (Cytadren)   **Uses:** Adrenocortical carcinoma, Cushing's syndrome, breast and prostate CA **Action:** Inhibits adrenal steroidogenesis and adrenal conversion of androgens to estrogens **Dose:** 750–1500 mg/d in ÷ doses plus hydrocortisone 20–40 mg/d; ↓ in renal insufficiency **Caution/Contra:** [D, ?] **Supplied:** Tabs 250 mg **Notes/SE:** Adrenal insufficiency ("medical adrenalectomy"), hypothyroidism, masculinization, hypotension, vomiting, rare hepatotoxicity, rash, myalgia, fever **Interactions:** ↓ effects with dexamethasone & hydrocortisone, ↓ effects of warfarin, theophylline, medroxyprogesterone **NIPE:** Masculinization reversible due d/c drug, ⊘ PRG

Aminophylline   **Uses:** Asthma and bronchospasm **Action:** Relaxes smooth muscle of the bronchi, pulmonary blood vessels; stimulates diaphragm **Dose:** *Adults.* *Acute asthma:* Load 6 mg/kg IV, then 0.4–0.9 mg/kg/h IV cont inf. *Chronic asthma:* 24 mg/kg/24 h PO or PR ÷ q6h. *Peds.* Load 6 mg/kg IV, then 1.0 mg/kg/h IV cont inf; ↓ in hepatic insufficiency and with certain drugs (macrolide and quinolone antibiotics, cimetidine, and propranolol) **Caution/Contra:** [C, +] Uncontrolled arrhythmias, hyperthyroidism, peptic ulcers, uncontrolled seizure disorder **Supplied:** Tabs 100, 200 mg; soln 105 mg/5 mL; supp 250, 500 mg; inj 25 mg/mL **Notes/SE:** Individualize dosage; N/V, irritability, tachycardia, ventricular arrhythmias, and seizures; follow serum levels carefully (as theophylline, Table 2, page 244); aminophylline is about 85% theophylline; erratic absorption with rectal doses **Interactions:** ↓ effects of lithium, phenytoin, adenosine; ↓ effects with phenobarbital, aminoglutethamide, barbiturates, rifampin, ritonavir, thyroid meds; ↑ effects with cimetidine, ciprofloxacin, erythromycin, isoniazid, oral contraceptives, verapimil, tobacco, charcoal-broiled foods, St. John's Wort **Labs:** ↑ uric acid levels, falsely ↑ levels with furosemide, probenecid, acetaminophen, coffee, tea, cola, chocolate **NIPE:** Do not chew or crush time-released capsules & take on empty stomach, immediate release can be taken with food, ↑ fluids 2 L/, tobacco ↑ drug elimination

Amiodarone (Cordarone, Pacerone)   **Uses:** Recurrent VF or hemodynamically unstable VT, AF **Action:** Class III antiarrhythmic **Dose:** *Adults.* *Loading dose:* 800–1600 mg/d PO for 1–3 wk. *Maint:* 600–800 mg/d PO for 1 mon, then 200–400 mg/d. *IV:* 15 mg/min for 10 min, then 1 mg/min for 6 h, then maint 0.5 mg/min cont inf. *Peds.* 10–15 mg/kg/24 h ÷ q12h PO for 7–10 d, then 5 mg/kg/24 h ÷ q12h or qd (infants/neonates require a higher loading dose); ↓ in severe liver insufficiency **Caution/Contra:** [D, –] Sinus node dysfunction, 2nd- or 3rd-degree AV block, sinus bradycardia (w/o pacemaker) **Supplied:** Tabs 200 mg; inj 50 mg/mL **Notes/SE:** Half-life is 53 d; pulmonary fibrosis, exacerbation of arrhythmias, prolongs QT interval; CHF, arrhythmias, hypo-/hyperthyroidism, ↑ LFTs, liver failure, corneal microdeposits, optic neuropathy/neuritis, peripheral neuropathy, photosensitivity; IV conc of >0.2 mg/mL administered via a central catheter; alters digoxin levels, may require ↓ digoxin dose **Interactions:** ↑ serum levels of digoxin, quinidine, procainamide, flecainide, phenytoin, warfarin, theophylline, cyclosporine; ↑ levels with cimetidine, indinavir, ritonavir; ↓ levels with cholestyramine, rifampin, St. John's Wort; ↑ cardiac effects with BBs, CCB **Labs:** ↑ T4 & RT3, ANA titer, ↓ T3 **NIPE:** Monitor cardiac rhythm, BP, LFTs, thyroid function, ophthalmologic exam; ↑ photosensitivity; take with food

Amitriptyline (Elavil)   **Uses:** Depression, peripheral neuropathy, chronic pain, and tension HAs **Action:** TCA; inhibits reuptake of serotonin and norepinephrine by the presynaptic neurons **Dose:** *Adults.* Initially, 30–50 mg PO hs; may

↑ to 300 mg hs. **Peds.** Not recommended if <12 y unless for chronic pain; initially 0.1 mg/kg PO hs, advance over 2–3 wk to 0.5–2 mg/kg PO hs; caution in hepatic impairment; taper when discontinuing **Caution/Contra:** [D, +/–] With MAOIs, during acute recovery following MI, narrow-angle glaucoma **Supplied:** Tabs 10, 25, 50, 75, 100, 150 mg; inj 10 mg/mL **Notes/SE:** Strong anticholinergic side effects; overdose may be fatal, may cause urine retention and sedation, ECG changes, photosensitivity **Interactions:** ↓ effects with carbamazepine, phenobarbital, rifampin, cholestyramine, colestipol, tobacco; ↑ effects with cimetidine, quinidine, indinavir, ritonavir, CNS depressants, SSRIs, haloperidol, oral contraceptives, BBs, phenothiazines, alcohol, evening primrose oil; ↑ effects of amphetamines, anticholinergics, epinephrine, hypoglycemics, phenylephrine **Labs:** ↑ glucose, falsely ↑ carbamazepine levels **NIPE:** ↑ photosensitivity, appetite, & craving for sweets; ⊘ d/c abruptly, may turn urine blue-green

Amlodipine (Norvasc)
Uses: HTN, chronic stable angina, and vasospastic angina **Action:** Ca channel blocker; relaxation of coronary vascular smooth muscle **Dose:** 2.5–10 mg/d PO **Caution/Contra:** [C, ?] **Supplied:** Tabs 2.5, 5, 10 mg **Notes/SE:** May be taken w/o regard to meals; peripheral edema, HA, palpitations, flushing **Interactions:** ↑ hypotension with fentanyl, nitrates, alcohol, quinidine, other antihypertensives, grapefruit juice; ↑ effects with diltiazem, erythromycin, H2 blockers, proton pump inhibitors, quinidine; ↓ effects with NSAIDs, barbiturates, rifampin **NIPE:** ⊘ d/c abruptly, ↑ photosensitivity

Ammonium Aluminum Sulfate [Alum]
Uses: Hemorrhagic cystitis when bladder irrigation fails **Action:** Astringent **Dose:** 1–2% soln used with constant bladder irrigation with NS **Caution/Contra:** [+/–] **Supplied:** Powder for reconstitution **Notes/SE:** Safe to use w/o anesthesia and with vesicoureteral reflux. Encephalopathy possible; obtain aluminum levels, especially in renal insufficiency; can precipitate and occlude catheters

Amoxicillin (Amoxil, Polymox)
Uses: Infections resulting from susceptible gram+ bacteria (strept. cocci) and gram– bacteria (*H. influenzae, E. coli, P. mirabilis*) **Action:** β-Lactam antibiotic; inhibits cell wall synthesis **Dose:** **Adults.** 250–500 mg PO tid or 500–875 mg bid. **Peds.** 25–100 mg/kg/24 h PO ÷ q8h; 200–400 mg PO bid (equivalent to 125–250 mg tid); ↓ in renal impairment **Caution/Contra:** [B, +] **Supplied:** Caps 250, 500 mg; chew tabs 125, 200, 250, 400 mg; susp 50 mg/mL, 125, 250 mg/5 mL; tabs 500, 875 mg **Notes/SE:** Cross-hypersensitivity with penicillin; diarrhea; skin rash common; many hospital strains of *E. coli* are resistant **Interactions:** ↑ effects of warfarin, ↑ effects with probenecid, disulfiram, ↑ risk of rash with allopurinol, ↓ effects of oral contraceptives, ↓ effects with tetracyclines, chloramphenicol **Labs:** ↑ serum alkaline phosphatase, LDH, LFTs, false + direct Coombs test **NIPE:** Space meds over 24/h, eval for superinfection, use barrier contraception

Amoxicillin and Clavulanic Acid (Augmentin, Augmentin 600 ES, Augmentin XR)
Uses: Infections caused by β-lactamase-

producing *H. influenzae, S. aureus,* and *E. coli;* XR used for acute bacterial sinusitis and CAP **Action:** Combination of a β-lactam antibiotic and a β-lactamase inhibitor **Dose:** *Adults.* 250–500 mg PO q8h or 875 mg q12h; XR 2000 mg PO q12h. *Peds.* 20–40 mg/kg/d as amoxicillin PO ÷ q8h or 45 mg/kg/d ÷ q12h; ↓ in renal impairment; take with food **Caution/Contra:** [B, ?] **Supplied** (expressed as amoxicillin/clavulanic acid): Tabs 250/125, 500/125, 875/125 mg; chew tabs 125/31.25, 200/28.5, 250/62.5, 400/57 mg; susp 125/31.25, 250/62.5, 200/28.5, 400/57 mg/5 mL. *600-ES:* 600/42.9-mg tab. *XR:* Tab 1000/62.5 mg **Notes/SE:** Do NOT substitute two 250-mg tabs for one 500-mg tab or an overdose of clavulanic acid will occur; abdominal discomfort, N/V/D, allergic reaction, vaginitis **Interactions:** ↑ effects of warfarin, ↑ effects with probenecid, disulfiram, ↑ risk of rash with allopurinol, ↓ effects of oral contraceptives, ↓ effects with tetracyclines, chloramphenicol **Labs:** ↑ serum alkaline phosphatase, LDH, LFTs, false + direct Coombs' test **NIPE:** Space meds over 24/h, eval for superinfection, use barrier contraception

Amphotericin B (Fungizone) **Uses:** Severe, systemic fungal infections; oral and cutaneous candidiasis **Action:** Binds ergosterol in the fungal membrane, altering membrane permeability **Dose:** *Adults & Peds.* 1 mg adults or 0.1 mg/kg to 1 mg in children, then 0.25–1.5 mg/kg/24 h IV over 2–6 h (range 25–50 mg/d or qod). Total dose varies with indication. *Oral:* 1 mL qid. *Topical:* Apply bid–qid for 1–4 wk depending on infection; ↓ in renal impairment **Caution/Contra:** [B, ?] **Supplied:** Powder for inj 50 mg/vial, oral susp 100 mg/mL, cream, lotion, oint 3% **Notes/SE:** Monitor renal function/LFTs; ↓ K⁺/↓ Mg²⁺ from renal wasting; anaphylaxis reported; pretreatment with APAP and antihistamines (Benadryl) helps minimize adverse effects with IV inf (eg, fever, chills, HA, nephrotoxicity, hypotension, anemia) **Interactions:** ↑ nephrotoxic effects with antineoplastics, cyclosporine, furosemide, vancomycin, aminoglycosides, ↑ hypokalemia with corticosteroids, skeletal muscle relaxants **Labs:** ↑ serum bilirubin, serum cholesterol **NIPE:** Monitor CNS effects & ⊘ take at HS, topical cream discolors skin

Amphotericin B Cholesteryl (Amphotec) **Uses:** Refractory invasive fungal infection in persons intolerant to conventional amphotericin B **Action:** Binds to sterols in the cell membrane, altering membrane permeability **Dose:** *Adults & Peds.* Test dose 1.6–8.3 mg, over 15–20 min, followed by a dose of 3–4 mg/kg/d; 1 mg/kg/h inf; ↓ in renal insufficiency **Caution/Contra:** [B, ?] **Supplied:** Powder for inj 50 mg, 100 mg/vial (final conc 0.6 mg/mL) **Notes/SE:** Anaphylaxis reported; do not use in-line filter; monitor LFT and electrolytes; fever, chills, HA, ↓ K⁺, ↓ Mg, nephrotoxicity, ↓ BP, anemia. **See amphotericin B**

Amphotericin B Lipid Complex (Abelcet) **Uses:** Refractory invasive fungal infection in persons intolerant to conventional amphotericin B **Action:** Binds to sterols in the cell membrane, altering membrane permeability **Dose:** 5 mg/kg/d IV as a single daily dose; 2.5 mg/kg/h inf **Supplied:** Inj 5 mg/mL **Caution/Contra:** [B, ?] **Notes/SE:** Anaphylaxis reported; filter soln with a 5-mm filter needle; do not mix in electrolyte-containing solns. If inf >2 h, manually mix bag; fever, chills, HA, ↓ K+, ↓ Mg, nephrotoxicity, hypotension, anemia. **See amphotericin B**

Amphotericin B Liposomal (AmBisome)
Uses: Refractory invasive fungal infection in persons intolerant to conventional amphotericin B **Action:** Binds to sterols in the cell membrane, resulting in changes in membrane permeability **Dose:** *Adults & Peds.* 3–5 mg/kg/d, infused over 60–120 min; ↓ in renal insufficiency **Caution/Contra:** [B, ?] **Supplied:** Powder for inj 50 mg **Notes/SE:** Anaphylaxis reported; filter with no less than 1-μm filter; fever, chills, HA, ↓K+, ↓ Mg²+ nephrotoxicity, hypotension, anemia. **See amphotericin B**

Ampicillin (Amcill, Omnipen)
Uses: Susceptible gram– (*Shigella, Salmonella, E. coli, H. influenzae,* and *P. mirabilis*) and gram+ (streptococci) bacteria **Action:** β-Lactam antibiotic; inhibits cell wall synthesis **Dose:** *Adults.* 500 mg–2 g IM or IV q6h or 250–500 mg PO q6h. *Peds. Neonates <7 d:* 50–100 mg/kg/24 h IV ÷ q6–8h IV or PO. *Term infants:* 75–150 mg/kg/24 h ÷ q6–8h IV or PO. *Children >1 mo:* 100–200 mg/kg/24 h ÷ q4–6h IM or IV; 50–100 mg/kg/24 h ÷ q6h PO up to 250 mg/dose. *Meningitis:* 200–400 mg/kg/24 h ÷ q4–6h IV; ↓ in renal impairment, take on an empty stomach **Caution/Contra:** [B, M] Cross-hypersensitivity with penicillin **Supplied:** Caps 250, 500 mg; susp 100 mg/mL (reconstituted as drops), 125 mg/5 mL, 250 mg/5 mL, 500 mg/5 mL; powder for inj 125 mg, 250 mg, 500 mg, 1 g, 2 g, 10 g/vial **Notes/SE:** Diarrhea, skin rash, allergic reaction; many hospital strains of *E. coli* now resistant **Interactions:** ↓ effects of oral contraceptives & atenolol, ↓ effects with chloramphenicol, erythromycin, tetracycline, & food; ↑ effects of anticoagulants & methotrexate; ↑ risk of rash with allopurinol; ↑ effects with probenecid & disulfiram **Labs:** ↑ LFTs, serum protein, serum theophylline, serum uric acid; ↓ serum estrogen, serum cholesterol, serum folate; false + direct Coombs test, urine glucose, & urine amino acids **NIPE:** Take on empty stomach & around the clock, may cause candidal vaginitis, use barrier contraception

Ampicillin-Sulbactam (Unasyn)
Uses: Infections caused by β-lactamase-producing strains of *S. aureus, Enterococcus, H. influenzae, P. mirabilis,* and *Bacteroides* spp **Action:** Combination of a β-lactam antibiotic and a β-lactamase inhibitor **Dose:** *Adults.* 1.5–3.0 g IM or IV q6h. *Peds.* 100–200 mg ampicillin/kg/d (150–300 mg Unasyn) q6h; ↓ in renal impairment; take on an empty stomach **Caution/Contra:** [B, M] **Supplied:** Powder for inj 1.5, 3.0 g/vial **Notes/SE:** A 2:1 ratio of ampicillin: sulbactam; ↓ in renal failure; hypersensitivity reactions, rash, diarrhea, pain at inj site. **See ampicillin**

Amprenavir (Agenerase)
WARNING: Oral soln contra in children <4 y due to potential toxicity from large vol of excipient polypropylene glycol in the formulation **Uses:** HIV infection **Action:** Protease inhibitor; prevents the maturation of the virion to mature viral particle. **Dose:** *Adults.* 1200 mg bid. *Peds.* 20 mg/kg bid or 15 mg/kg tid up to 2400 mg/d **Caution/Contra:** [C, ?] CDC recommends HIV-infected mothers not breast-feed due to risk of transmission of HIV to infant; previ-

ous allergic reaction to sulfonamides **Supplied:** Caps 50, 150 mg; soln 15 mg/mL **Notes/SE:** Caps and soln contain vitamin E exceeding RDA intake amounts; avoid high-fat meals with administration; many drug interactions; life-threatening rash, hyperglycemia, hypertriglyceridemia, fat redistribution, N/V/D, depression **Interactions:** ↑ effects with abacavir, cimetidine, delavirdine, indinavir, itraconazole, ketoconazole, macrolides, ritonavir, zidovudine, grapefruit juice; ↑ effects of cisapride, clozapine, ergotamine, loratidine, nelfinavir, dapsone, pimozide, rifabutin, saquinavir, sildenafil, terfenadine, triazolam, warfarin, zidovudine, HMG-CoA reductase inhibitors; ↓ effects with antacids, barbiturates, carbamazepine, nevirapine, phenytoin, rifampin, St. John's Wort, high-fat food; ↓ effects of oral contraceptives **Labs:** ↑ serum glucose, cholesterol, & triglyceride levels **NIPE:** Use barrier contraception, may take with food other than high fat food, ⊘ take vitamin E

Amrinone [Inamrinone] (Inocor)
Uses: Short-term Rx low cardiac output states and pulmonary HTN **Action:** Positive inotropic with vasodilator activity **Dose:** *Adults & Peds.* Initial IV bolus 0.75 mg/kg over 2–3 min, then maint dose 5–10 μg/ kg/min; 10 mg/kg/d max; ↓ if CrCl <10 mL/min **Caution/Contra:** [C, ?] Hypersensitivity to sulfites **Supplied:** Inj 5 mg/mL **Notes/SE:** Incompatible with dextrose-containing solns; monitor for fluid, electrolyte, and renal changes **Interactions:** ↓ BP with disopyramide; ↓ filling pressure with diuretics **Labs:** ↑ digoxin levels, ↓ K⁺ levels **NIPE:** Monitor I&O and daily wts, IV rate and duration based on response to drug and adverse effects

Anakinra (Kineret)
WARNING: Associated with ↑ incidence of serious infections; DC with serious infection **Uses:** Reduce signs and symptoms of moderately to severely active RA, failed 1 or more disease-modifying antirheumatic drugs **Action:** Human IL-1 receptor antagonist **Dose:** 100 mg SC qd **Caution/Contra:** [B, ?]. Contra hypersensitivity to *E. coli*-derived proteins, active infection, <18 y **Supplied:** 100-mg prefilled syringes **Notes/SE:** Neutropenia especially when used with TNF-blocking agents, inj site reactions, infections **Interactions:** ↓ effects of immunizations; ↑ risk of infections if combined with tumor-necrosis-factor-blocking drugs **Labs:** ↓ WBCs, platelets, absolute neutrophil count **NIPE:** Store drug in refrig, avoid light exposure, & discard any unused portion; do not use soln if discolored or has particulate matter

Anastrozole (Arimidex)
Uses: Breast CA: postmenopausal women with metastatic breast CA, adjuvant treatment of postmenopausal women with early hormone-receptor-positive breast CA **Action:** Selective nonsteroidal aromatase inhibitor, ↓ circulating estradiol **Dose:** 1 mg/d **Caution/Contra:** [D, ?] **Supplied:** Tabs 1 mg **Notes/SE:** No detectable effect on adrenal corticosteroids or aldosterone; may ↑ cholesterol levels; diarrhea, hypertension, flushing, ↑ bone and tumor pain, HA, somnolence **Interactions:** None noted **Labs:** ↑ GTT, LFTs, alkaline phosphatase, total & LDL cholesterol **NIPE:** May ↓ fertility & cause fetal damage, eval for pain & administer adequate analgesia, may cause vaginal bleeding first few weeks

Anistreplase (Eminase) Uses: AMI Action: Thrombolytic agent; activates the conversion of plasminogen to plasmin, promoting thrombolysis Dose: 30 U IV over 2–5 min Caution/Contra: [C, ?] Active internal bleeding, Hx CVA, recent (<2 mon) intracranial or intraspinal surgery or trauma, intracranial neoplasm, AV malformation, aneurysm, bleeding diathesis, severe uncontrolled HTN; may not be effective if readministered >5 d after the previous dose of anistreplase or streptokinase, or streptococcal infection because of the production of antistreptokinase antibody. Supplied: Vials containing 30 U Notes/SE: Bleeding, hypotension, hematoma Interactions: ↑ risk of hemorrhage with warfarin, oral anticoagulants, ASA, NSAIDs, dipyridamole; ↓ effectiveness with aminocaproic acid Labs: ↓ plasminogen & fibrinogen, ↑ transaminase level, thrombin time, APTT & PT NIPE: Store powder in refrig & use w/n 30 min of reconstitution, initiate therapy ASAP >MI, monitor s/s internal bleeding

Anthralin (Anthra-Derm) Uses: Psoriasis Action: Keratolytic Dose: Apply qd Caution/Contra: [C, ?] Acutely inflamed psoriatic eruptions, use on face or genitalia Supplied: Cream, oint 0.1, 0.2, 0.25, 0.4, 0.5, 1% Notes/SE: Irritation; discoloration of hair, fingernails, skin Interactions: ↑ toxicity if used immediately >long-term topical corticosteroid therapy NIPE: May stain fabric; external use only; ⊘ sunlight-medicated areas

Antihemophilic Factor [Factor VIII] [AHF] (Monoclate) Uses: Classical hemophilia A Action: Provides factor VIII needed to convert prothrombin to thrombin Dose: *Adults & Peds.* AHF unit/kg ↑ factor VIII level ~2%. Units required = (kg) (desired factor VIII ↑ as % normal) × (0.5). Prophylax spontaneous hemorrhage = 5% normal. Hemostasis after trauma/surgery = 30% normal. Head injuries, major surgery, or bleeding = 80–100% normal. Determine patient's % of normal factor VIII before dosing Caution/Contra: [C, ?] Supplied: Check each vial for units contained Notes/SE: Not effective in controlling bleeding in von Willebrand's disease; rash, fever, HA, chills, N/V Interactions: none Labs: monitor CBC & direct Coombs test NIPE: ⊘ ASA, immunize against Hep B, d/c if tachycardiac

Apraclonidine (Iopidine) Uses: Glaucoma Action: α_2-Adrenergic agonist Dose: 1–2 gtt of 0.5% tid Caution/Contra: [C, ?] Supplied: 0.5, 1.0% soln Notes/SE: Ocular irritation, lethargy, xerostomia Interactions: ↓ intraocular pressure with pilocarpine or topical BBs NIPE: Monitor CV status of pts with CAD, potential for dizziness

Aprepitant (Emend) Uses: prevention N/V with emetogenic chemotherapy (eg cisplatin in combination with other antiemetic agents) Action: substance P/neurokinin 1(NK_1) receptor antagonist Dose: *Adults.* 125 mg PO on day 1, 1 h before chemo, then 80 mg PO qAM on d 2 & 3 Caution: [B,?/-]; substrate & moderate inhibitor of CYP3A4; inducer of CYP2C9 Contra: use with pimozide Supplied: caps 80, 125 mg SE: fatigue, asthenia, hiccups Notes: ↓ effect of oral contraceptives; decrease anticoagulant effect of warfarin Interactions: ↑ effects with clarithromycin, dilitiazem, itraconazole, ketoconazole, nefazodone, nelfinavir, ritonavir, troleandomycin; ↑ effects of alprazolam, astemizole, cisapride, dexamethasone, methylprednisolone, midazolam, pimozide, terfenadine, triazolam and chemotherapeutic agents such as docetaxel, etoposide, ifosfamide, imatinib, irinotecun, paclitaxel, vinblastine, vincristine, vinorelbine; ↓ effects with paroxetine, rifampin; ↓ effects of oral contraceptives, paroxetine, phenytoin, tolbutamide, warfarin **Labs:** ↑ ALT, AST, BUN, Alkaline phosphatase, leukocytes **NIPE:** Use barrier contraception, take w/o regard to food

Aprotinin (Trasylol) **Uses:** Reduce/prevent blood loss in patients undergoing CABG **Action:** Protease inhibitor, antifibrinolytic **Dose:** 1-mL IV test dose to assess for allergic reaction. *High dose:* 2 million KIU load, 2 million KIU to prime pump, then 500,000 KIU/h until surgery ends. *Low dose:* 1 million KIU load, 1 million KIU to prime pump, then 250,000 KIU/h until surgery ends. 7 million KIU max total **Caution/Contra:** [B, ?] Thromboembolic disease requiring anticoagulants or blood factor administration **Supplied:** Inj 1.4 mg/mL (10,000 KIU/mL) **Notes/SE:** 1000/KIU = 0.14 mg of aprotinin; AF, MI, heart failure, dyspnea, postoperative renal dysfunction **Interactions:** ↑ clotting time with heparin, ↓ effects of fibrinolytics, captopril **Labs:** Monitor aPTT, ACT, CBC, BUN, creatinine **NIPE:** Monitor cardiac and pulmonary status during infusion

Ardeparin (Normiflo) **Uses:** Prevent DVT/PE following knee replacement **Action:** LMW heparin **Dose:** 35–50 U/kg SC q12h. Begin day of surgery, continue up to 14 d; caution in ↓ renal function **Caution/Contra:** [C, ?] Active hemorrhage; hypersensitivity to pork products **Supplied:** Inj 5000, 10,000 IU/0.5 mL **Notes/SE:** Laboratory monitoring usually not necessary; bleeding, bruising, thrombocytopenia, pain at inj site, ↑ serum transaminases

Argatroban (Acova) **Uses:** Prophylaxis or Rx of thrombosis in HIT **Action:** Anticoagulant, direct thrombin inhibitor **Dose:** 2 μg/kg/min IV; adjust until aPTT 1.5–3× baseline value not to exceed 100 s; 10 μg/kg/min max; ↓ in hepatic impairment **Caution/Contra:** [B, ?] Avoid oral anticoagulants, ↑ risk of bleeding; avoid concomitant use of thrombolytics **Supplied:** Inj 100 mg/mL **Notes/SE:** AF, cardiac arrest, cerebrovascular disorder, hypotension, VT, N/V/D, sepsis, cough, renal toxicity, ↓ Hgb **Interactions:** ↑ risk of bleeding with anticoagulants, feverfew, garlic, ginger, ginkgo, ↑ risk of intracranial bleed with thrombolytics **Labs:** ↑ aPTT, PT, INR, ACT, thrombin time **NIPE:** Report ↑ bruising & bleeding, do not breast-feed

Aripiprazole (Abilify) **Uses:** Atypical antipsychotic used in the treatment of schizophrenia **Action:** Dopamine and serotonin antagonist **Dose:** *Adults.* 10–15 mg PO qd; ↓ when used in combination with potent CYP3A4 or CYP2D6 inhibitors; ↑ when used in combination with inducer of CYP3A4 **Caution/Contra:** [C, –] **Supplied:** Tabs 10, 15, 20, 30 mg **Notes/SE:** Neuroleptic malignant syndrome, tardive dyskinesia, orthostatic hypotension, cognitive and motor impairment **Interactions:** ↑ effects with ketoconazole, quinidine, fluoxetine, paroxetine,

↓ effects with carbamazepine **NIPE:** ⊘ breast-feed, consume alcohol, or use during PRG, use barrier contraception, ↑ fluid intake

Artificial Tears (Tears Naturale) **Uses:** Dry eyes **Action:** Ocular lubricant **Dose:** 1–2 gtt tid–qid **Supplied:** OTC soln

L-Asparaginase (Elspar, Oncaspar) **Uses:** ALL (in combination with other agents) **Action:** Protein synthesis inhibitor **Dose:** 500–20,000 IU/m²/d for 1–14 d (refer to specific protocols) **Caution/Contra:** [C, ?] Active or Hx pancreatitis **Supplied:** Inj 10,000 IU **Notes/SE:** Hypersensitivity reactions in 20–35% (spectrum of urticaria to anaphylaxis), test dose recommended; rare GI toxicity (mild nausea/anorexia, pancreatitis) **Interactions:** ↑ effects with prednisone, vincristine; ↓ effects of methotrexate, sulfonylureas, insulin **Labs:** ↓ thyroxine & thyroxine-binding globulin, serum albumin, total cholesterol, plasma fibrinogen; ↑ BUN, glucose, uric acid, LFTs, alkaline phosphatase **NIPE:** ↑ fluid intake, monitor for bleeding, monitor I&O and wt, ⊘ alcohol or ASA

Aspirin (Bayer, St. Joseph) **Uses:** Mild pain, HA, fever, inflammation, prevention of emboli, and prevention of MI **Action:** Prostaglandin inhibitor **Dose:** *Adults.* *Pain, fever:* 325–650 mg q4–6h PO or PR. *RA:* 3–6 g/d PO in ÷ doses. *Platelet inhibitory action:* 81–325 mg PO qd. *Prevention of MI:* 81–325 mg PO qd. *Peds.* Caution: Use linked to Reye's syndrome; avoid use with viral illness in children. *Antipyretic:* 10–15 mg/kg/dose PO or PR q4h up to 80 mg/kg/24 h. *RA:* 60–100 mg/kg/24 h PO ÷ q4–6h (monitor serum levels to maintain between 15 and 30 mg/dL); avoid use with CrCl <10 mL/min and in severe liver disease; avoid or limit alcohol intake **Caution/Contra:** [C, M] Allergy to ASA **Supplied:** Tabs 325, 500 mg; chew tabs 81 mg; EC tabs 165, 325, 500, 650, 975 mg; SR tabs 650, 800 mg; effervescent tabs 325, 500 mg; supp 120, 200, 300, 600 mg **Notes/SE:** GI upset and erosion common adverse reactions; DC use 1 wk prior to surgery to avoid postoperative bleeding complications **Interactions:** ↑ effects with anticoagulants, ammonium chloride, antibiotics, ascorbic acid, furosemide, methionine, nizatidine, NSAIDs, verapamil, alcohol, feverfew, garlic, ginkgo biloba, horse chestnut, kelpware, prickly ash, red clover; ↓ effects with antacids, activated charcoal, corticosteroids, griseofulvin, sodium bicarbonate, ginseng, food; ↑ effects of ACEI, hypoglycemics, insulin, lithium, methotrexate, phenytoin, sulfonamides, valproic acid; ↓ effects of BBs, probenecid, spironolactone, sulfinpyrazone **Labs:** False neg results of urinary glucose & urinary ketone tests, serum albumin, total serum phenytoin, T3 & T4 **NIPE:** Chronic ASA use may result in ↓ folic acid, iron-deficiency anemia, & hypernatremia; avoid foods ↑ salicylate – curry powder, paprika, licorice, prunes, raisins, tea; take ASA with food or milk, report s/s bleeding/GI pain/ringing in ears

Aspirin and Butalbital Compound (Fiorinal) [C-III] **Uses:** Tension HA, pain **Action:** Combination barbiturate and analgesic **Dose:** 1–2 PO q4h PRN, max 6 tabs/d; avoid use with CrCl <10 mL/min and in severe liver disease; or limit alcohol intake **Caution/Contra:** [C (D if used for prolonged periods

or high doses at term), ?] **Supplied:** Caps Fiorgen PF, Fiorinal. Tabs Fiorinal, Lanorinal, ASA 325 mg/butalbital 50 mg/caffeine 40 mg **Notes/SE:** Butalbital habit-forming; drowsiness, dizziness, GI upset, ulceration, bleeding; **see Aspirin. Additional Interactions:** ↑ effect of benzodiazepines, CNS depressants, chloramphenicol, methylphenidate, propoxyphene, valporic acid; ↓ effects of BBs, corticosteroids, chloramphenicol, cyclosporins, doxycycline, griseofulvin, haloperidol, oral contraceptives, phenothiazines, quinidine, TCAs, theophylline, warfarin **NIPE:** Use barrier contraception, ⊘ alcohol

Aspirin + Butalbital, Caffeine, and Codeine (Fiorinal + Codeine) [C-III]

Uses: Mild pain; HA, especially when associated with stress **Action:** Sedative analgesic, narcotic analgesic **Dose:** 1–2 tabs (caps) PO q4–6h PRN **Caution/Contra:** [D, ?] **Supplied:** Each cap or tab contains 325 mg ASA, 40 mg caffeine, 50 mg of butalbital, codeine **Notes/SE:** Drowsiness, dizziness, GI upset, ulceration, bleeding; **see Aspirin + Butalbital. Additional Interactions:** ↑ effects with narcotic analgesics, MAOI, neuromuscular blockers, ↓ effects with tobacco smoking; ↑ effects of digitoxin, phenytoin, rifampin; ↑ respiratory & CNS depression with cimetidine **Labs:** ↑ plasma amylase & lipase **NIPE:** May cause constipation, ↑ fluids & fiber, take with milk to ↓ GI upset

Aspirin + Codeine (Empirin No. 2, No. 3, No. 4) [C-III]

Uses: Mild–moderate pain **Action:** Combined effects of ASA and codeine **Dose:** *Adults.* 1–2 tabs PO q4–6h PRN. *Peds.* ASA 10 mg/kg/dose; codeine 0.5–1.0 mg/kg/dose q4h **Caution/Contra:** N/A [M] **Supplied:** Tabs 325 mg of ASA and codeine as in Notes **Notes/SE:** Codeine in No. 2 = 15 mg, No. 3 = 30 mg, No. 4 = 60 mg; drowsiness, dizziness, GI upset, ulceration, bleeding; **see Aspirin. Additional Interactions:** ↑ effects with narcotic analgesics, MAOI, neuromuscular blockers, ↓ effects with tobacco smoking; ↑ effects of digitoxin, phenytoin, rifampin; ↑ respiratory & CNS depression with cimetidine **Labs:** ↑ plasma amylase & lipase **NIPE:** May cause constipation, ↑ fluids & fiber, take with milk to ↓ GI distress

Atazanavir (Reyataz)

WARNING: Hyperbilirubinemia may require discontinuation **Uses:** HIV-1 infection **Action:** Protease inhibitor **Dose:** *Adults.* 400 mg PO QD w/food; with efavirenz 600 mg, use atazanavir 300 mg + ritonavir 100 mg QD; separate doses from buffered ddI dose; ? dose in hepatic impairment **Caution:** [B, –] **Contra:** Concomitant use of midazolam, triazolam, ergots, cisapride, pimozide **Supplied:** 100-, 150-, 200-mg caps **SE:** HA, N/V/D, rash, abdominal pain, diabetes mellitus, photosensitivity, ? PR interval **Notes:** May have less effects on cholesterol profile; ? levels of statins, sildenafil, antiarrhythmics, warfarin, cyclosporine, TCA; atazanivir ↑ by St. John's Wort **Interactions:** ↑ effects with amprenavir, clarithromycin, indinavir, lamivudine, lopinavir, ritonavir, saquinavir, stavudine, tenofovir, zalcitabine, zidovudine; ↑ effects of amiodarone, atorvastatin, CCBs, clarithromycin, cyclosporine, dilitiazem, irinotecan, lidocaine, lovastatin, oral contraceptives, rifabutin, quinidine, saquinavir, sildenafil, simvastatin, sirolimus, tacrolimus, TCAs, warfarin; ↓ effects with antacids, antimycobacterials, efavirenz, esomeprazole, H2 receptor antagonists, lansoprazole, omeprazole, rifampin, St. John's Wort **Labs:** ↑ ALT, AST, total bilirubin, amylase, lipase, serum glucose, ↓ hmg, neutrophils **NIPE:** Take with food; will not cure HIV or ↓ risk of transmission; use barrier contraception; ↑ risk of skin and/or scleral yellowing

Atenolol (Tenormin) Uses: HTN, angina, MI **Action:** Competitively blocks β-adrenergic receptors, β_1 **Dose:** *HTN and angina:* 50–100 mg/d PO. *AMI:* 5 mg IV ×2 over 10 min, then 50 mg PO bid if tolerated; adjust in renal impairment **Caution/Contra:** [D, M] Contra bradycardia, pulmonary edema; caution in DM, bronchospasm; abrupt DC can exacerbate angina and occurrence of MI **Supplied:** Tabs 25, 50, 100 mg; inj 5 mg/10 mL **Notes/SE:** Bradycardia, hypotension, 2nd- or 3rd-degree AV block, dizziness, fatigue **Interactions:** ↑ effects with other antihypertensives esp diltiazem & verapamil, nitrates, alcohol; ↑ bradycardia with adenosine, digitalis glycosides, dipyridamole, physostigmine, tacrine; ↓ effects with ampicillin, antacids, NSAIDs, salicylates; ↑ effects of lidocaine; ↓ effects of dopamine, glucagons, insulin, sulfonylureas **Labs:** ↑ ANA titers, BUN, glucose, serum lipoprotein, K^+, triglyceride, uric acid levels; ↓ HDL **NIPE:** May mask s/s hypoglycemia, may ↑ sensitivity to cold, may ↑ depression, wheezing, orthostatic hypotension

Atenolol and Chlorthalidone (Tenoretic) Uses: HTN **Action:** β-Adrenergic blockade with diuretic **Dose:** 50–100 mg/d PO; ↓ in renal impairment **Caution/Contra:** [D, M] Contra bradycardia, pulmonary edema; caution in DM, bronchospasm **Supplied:** *Tenoretic 50:* Atenolol 50 mg/chlorthalidone 25 mg; *Tenoretic 100:* Atenolol 100 mg/chlorthalidone 25 mg **Notes/SE:** Bradycardia, hypotension, 2nd- or 3rd-degree AV block, dizziness, fatigue, hypokalemia, photosensitivity; **see Atenolol. Additional Interactions:** ↑ effects with other antihypertensives; ↓ effects with cholestyramine, NSAIDs; ↑ effects of lithium, digoxin; ↓ effects of sulfonylureas **Labs:** False ↓ urine esriol; ↑ CPK, serum ammonia, amylase, calcium, chloride, cholesterol, glucose; ↓ serum chloride, magnesium, K^+, sodium **NIPE:** Take in AM to prevent nocturia, use sunblock >SPF 15, monitor s/s gout

Atomoxetine (Strattera) Uses: Treatment of ADHD **Action:** Selective norepinephrine reuptake inhibitor **Dose:** *Adults and children. >70 kg:* 40 mg × 3d, then ↑ to 80–100 mg ÷ qd–bid *Peds = 70 kg:* 0.5 mg/kg × 3d, then ↑ to max of 1.2 mg/kg given qd or bid **Caution/Contra:** [C, ? /–] Narrow-angle glaucoma, use with or w/n 2 wk of discontinuing an MAOI **Supplied:** Caps 10, 18, 25, 40, 60 mg **Notes/SE:** ↓ dose with hepatic insufficiency; ↓ dose when used in combination with inhibitors of CYP2D6; HTN, tachycardia, weight loss, sexual dysfunction

Atorvastatin (Lipitor) Uses: control ↑ cholesterol and triglycerides **Action:** HMG-CoA reductase inhibitor **Dose:** Initial dose 10 mg/d, may be ↑ to 80 mg/d **Caution/Contra:** [X, –] Active liver disease, unexplained persistent elevation of serum transaminases **Supplied:** Tabs 10, 20, 40, 80 mg **Notes/SE:** May cause myopathy, monitor LFTs regularly; HA, arthralgia, myalgia, GI upset **Interactions:** ↑ effects with azole antifungals, erythromycin, nefazodone, protease inhibitors, grapefruit juice; ↓ effects with antacids, bile acid sequestrants; ↑ effects of digoxin, levothyroxine, oral contraceptives **Labs:** ↑ LFTs, CPK, ↓ lipid levels **NIPE:** ⊘ alcohol, breast-feeding, or while pregnant

Atovaquone (Mepron) Uses: Rx and prevention mild to moderate PCP **Action:** Inhibits nucleic acid and ATP synthesis **Dose:** *Rx:* 750 mg PO bid for 21 d. *Prevention:* 1500 mg PO once/d; take with meals **Caution/Contra:** [C, ?] **Supplied:** Suspension 750 mg/5 mL **Notes/SE:** Fever, HA, anxiety, insomnia, rash, N/V **Interactions:** ↓ effects with metoclopramide, rifabutin, rifampin, tetracycline **NIPE:** ↑ absorption with meal esp ↑ fat, monitor LFTs with long-term use

Atovaquone/Proguanil (Malarone) Uses: Prevention or Rx uncomplicated *P. falciparum* malaria **Action:** Antimalarial **Dose:** *Adult. Prevention:* 1 tab PO 2 d before, during, and 7 d after leaving endemic region; *Treatment:* 4 tabs PO as single dose qd ×3 d. *Peds.* See insert **Caution/Contra:** [C, ?] **Supplied:** Tab atovaquone 250 mg/proguanil 100 mg; Ped 62.5/25 mg **Notes/SE:** HA, fever, myalgia. **See Atovaquone**

Atracurium (Tracrium) Uses: Adjunct to anesthesia to facilitate ET intubation **Action:** Nondepolarizing neuromuscular blocker **Dose:** *Adults & Peds.* 0.4–0.5 mg/kg IV bolus, then 0.08–0.1 mg/kg q20–45min PRN **Caution/Contra:** [C, ?] **Supplied:** Inj 10 mg/mL **Notes/SE:** Patient must be intubated and on controlled ventilation. Use adequate amounts of sedation and analgesia; flushing **Interactions:** ↑ effects with general anesthetics, aminoglycosides, bacitracin, BBs, β agonists, clindamycin, CCBs, diuretics, lidocaine, lithium, magnesium sulfate, narcotic analgesics, procainamide, quinidine, succinylcholine, trimethaphan, verapamil; ↓ effects with calcium, carbamazepine, phenytoin, theophylline, caffeine **Labs:** Monitor BUN, creatinine, LFTs **NIPE:** Drug does not effect consciousness or pain, inability to speak until drug wears off

Atropine Uses: Preanesthetic; symptomatic bradycardia and asystole **Action:** Antimuscarinic agent; blocks acetylcholine at parasympathetic sites **Dose:** *Adults. ECC:* 0.5–1.0 mg IV q3–5min. *Preanesthetic:* 0.3–0.6 mg IM. *Peds. ECC:* 0.01–0.03 mg/kg IV q2–5min, max 1.0 mg, min dose 0.1 mg. *Preanesthetic:* 0.01 mg/kg/dose SC/IV (max 0.4 mg) **Caution/Contra:** [C, +] **Supplied:** Tabs 0.3, 0.4, 0.6 mg; inj 0.05, 0.1, 0.3, 0.4, 0.5, 0.8, 1 mg/mL; ophth 0.5, 1, 2% **Notes/SE:** Blurred vision, urinary retention, constipation, dried mucous membranes **Interactions:** ↑ effects with amantadine, antihistamines, disopyramide, procainamide, quinidine, TCA, thiazides, betel palm, squaw vine; ↓ effects with antacids, levodopa; ↓ effects of phenothiazines **Labs:** ↓ gastric motility & emptying may effect results of upper GI series **NIPE:** Monitor I&O, ↑ fluids & oral hygiene, wear dark glasses to ↓ photophobia

Azathioprine (Imuran) Uses: Adjunct for the prevention of rejection following organ transplantation; RA; SLE **Action:** Immunosuppressive agent; antagonizes purine metabolism **Dose: *Adults & Peds.*** 1–3 mg/kg/d IV or PO; reduce in renal failure **Caution/Contra:** [D, ?] **Supplied:** Tabs 50 mg; inj 100 mg/20 mL **Notes/SE:** GI intolerance, fever, chills, leukopenia, thrombocytopenia; chronic use may ↑ neoplasia; inj should be handled with cytotoxic precautions; interaction with allopurinol **Interactions:** ↑ effects with allopurinol; ↑ effects of antineoplastic drugs, cyclosporine, myelosuppressive drugs, methotrexate; ↑ risk of severe leucopenia with ACEI; ↓ effects of nondepolarizing neuromuscular blocking drugs, warfarin **Labs:** Monitor BUN, creatinine, CBC, LFTs during therapy **NIPE:** ⊘ PRG, breast-feeding, immunizations, take with or > meals

Azithromycin (Zithromax) Uses: Community-acquired pneumonia, pharyngitis, otitis media, skin infections, nonogonococcal urethritis, and PID; Rx and prevention of MAC in HIV **Action:** Macrolide antibiotic; inhibits protein synthesis **Dose: *Adults. Oral: Respiratory tract infections:*** 500 mg day 1, then 250 mg/d PO ×4 d. *Nongonococcal urethritis:* 1 g PO single dose. *Prevention of MAC:* 1200 mg PO once/wk. *IV:* 500 mg ×2 d, then 500 mg PO ×7–10 d. ***Peds.** Otitis media:* 10 mg/kg PO day 1, then 5 mg/kg/d days 2–5. *Pharyngitis:* 12 mg/kg/d PO ×5 d **Caution/Contra:** [B, +] **Supplied:** Tabs 250, 600 mg (Z-Pack 5-day regimen); susp 1-g single-dose packet; susp 100, 200 mg/5 mL; inj 500 mg **Notes/SE:** Take susp on an empty stomach; tabs may be taken w/wo food; GI upset, photosensitivity **Interactions:** ↓ effects with aluminum & magnesium antacids, atovaquone, food (suspension); ↑ effects of alfentanil, barbiturates, bromocriptine, carbamazepine, cyclosporine, digoxin, disopyramide, ergot alkaloids, phenytoin, pimozide, terfenadine, theophylline, triazolam, warfarin; ↓ effects of penicillins **Labs:** May ↑ serum bilirubin, alkaline phosphatase, BUN, creatinine, CPK, glucose, K⁺, LFTs, LDH, PT; may ↓ WBC, platelet count, serum folate **NIPE:** Monitor s/s superinfection, use sunscreen & protective clothing

Aztreonam (Azactam) Uses: Aerobic gram− bacterial infections, including *P. aeruginosa* **Action:** Monobactam antibiotic; inhibits cell wall synthesis **Dose: *Adults.*** 1–2 g IV/IM q6–12h. ***Peds.** Premature infants:* 30 mg/kg/dose IV q12h. *Term infants, children:* 30 mg/kg/dose q6–8h; ↓ in renal impairment **Caution/Contra:** [B, +] **Supplied:** Inj 500 mg, 1 g, 2 g **Notes/SE:** No gram+ or anaerobic activity; may be given to penicillin-allergic patients; N/V/D, rash, pain at inj site **Interactions:** ↑ effects with probenecid, aminoglycosides, β-lactam antibiotics; ↓ effects with cefoxitin, chloramphenicol, imipenem **Labs:** ↑ LFTs, alkaline phosphatase, serum creatinine, PT, PTT, & + Coombs test **NIPE:** Monitor s/s superinfection, taste changes with IV administration

Bacitracin, Topical (Baciguent); Bacitracin and Polymyxin B, Topical (Polysporin); Bacitracin, Neomycin, and Polymyxin B, Topical (Neosporin Ointment); Bacitracin, Neomycin, Polymyxin B, and Hydrocortisone, Topical (Cortisporin); Bacitracin, Neomycin, Polymyxin B, and Lidocaine, Topical (Clomycin) Uses: Prevention and Rx of minor cuts, scrapes, and burns Ac-

tion:** Topical antibiotic with added effects based on components (antiinflammatory and analgesic) **Dose:** Apply sparingly bid–qid **Caution/Contra:** [C, ?] **Supplied:** Bacitracin 500 U/g oint. Bacitracin 500 U/polymyxin B sulfate 10,000 U/g oint and powder. Bacitracin 400 U/neomycin 3.5 mg/polymyxin B 5000 U/g oint (for Neosporin Cream, see Page XXX). Bacitracin 400 U/neomycin 3.5 mg/polymyxin B/10,000 U/hydrocortisone 10 mg/g oint. Bacitracin 500 U/neomycin 3.5 g/polymyxin B 5000 U/lidocaine 40 mg/g oint **Notes/SE:** Systemic and irrigation forms of bacitracin available but not generally used due to potential toxicity **Interactions:** ↑ effects with neuromuscular blocking agents, anesthetics, nephrotoxic drugs **Labs:** If systemic use - monitor BUN & creatinine **NIPE:** Monitor for superinfection & allergic contact dermatitis

Bacitracin, Ophthalmic (AK-Tracin Ophthalmic); Bacitracin and Polymyxin B, Ophthalmic (AK-Poly-Bac Ophthalmic, Polysporin Ophthalmic); Bacitracin, Neomycin, and Polymyxin B, Ophthalmic (AK Spore Ophthalmic, Neosporin Ophthalmic); Bacitracin, Neomycin, Polymyxin B, and Hydrocortisone, Ophthalmic (AK Spore HC Ophthalmic, Cortisporin Ophthalmic) **Uses:** Blepharitis, conjunctivitis, prophylactic Rx of corneal abrasions **Action:** Topical antibiotic with added effects based on components (antiinflammatory) **Dose:** Apply q3–4h into conjunctival sac **Caution/Contra:** [C, ?] **Supplied:** See Topical equivalents, Pages 249–251 **Interactions:** ↑ effects with neuromuscular blocking agents, anesthetics, nephrotoxic drugs **NIPE:** May cause blurred vision

Baclofen (Lioresal) **Uses:** Spasticity secondary to severe chronic disorders, eg, MS or spinal cord lesions, trigeminal neuralgia **Action:** Centrally acting skeletal muscle relaxant; inhibits transmission of both monosynaptic and polysynaptic reflexes at the spinal cord **Dose:** *Adults.* Initially, 5 mg PO tid; ↑ q3d to max effect; max 80 mg/d. *Peds. 2–7 y:* 10–15 mg/d ÷ q8h; titrate to effect or max of 40 mg/d. *>8 y:* Max of 60 mg/d. *IT:* Through implantable pump; ↓ in renal impairment; avoid abrupt withdrawal; take with food or milk **Caution/Contra:** [C, +] Use caution in epilepsy and neuropsychiatric disturbances; withdrawal may occur with abrupt DC **Supplied:** Tabs 10, 20 mg; IT inj 10 mg/20 mL, 10 mg/5 mL **Notes/SE:** Dizziness, drowsiness, insomnia, ataxia, weakness, hypotension **Interactions:** ↑ CNS depression with CNS depressants, MAOI, alcohol, antihistamines, opioid analgesics, sedatives, hypnotics; ↑ effects of antihypertensives, clindamycin, guanabenz; ↑ risk of respiratory paralysis & renal failure with aminoglycosides **Labs:** ↑ serum glucose, AST, ammonia, alkaline phosphatase; ↓ bilirubin **NIPE:** take oral meds with food

Balsalazide (Colazal) **Uses:** Mild–moderate ulcerative colitis **Action:** 5-Aminosalicylic acid derivative, antiinflammatory, ↓ leukotriene synthesis **Dose:** 2.25 g (3 caps) tid ×8–12 wk **Caution/Contra:** [B, ?] Contra in severe renal/hepatic failure **Supplied:** Caps 750 mg **Notes/SE:** Dizziness, HA, nausea, agranulocytosis, pancytopenia, renal impairment, allergic reactions **Interactions:** Oral antibiotics may interfere with mesalamine release in the colon **Labs:** ↑ bilirubin, CPK, LFTs, LDH, plasma fibrinogen; ↓ calcium, K^+, protein **NIPE:** ⊘ if ASA allergy, take with food & swallow capsule whole

Basiliximab (Simulect)
Uses: Prevention of acute organ transplant rejections **Action:** IL-2 receptor antagonists **Dose:** *Adults.* 20 mg IV 2 h prior to transplant, then 20 mg IV 4 d posttransplant. *Peds.* 12 mg/m² up to a max of 20 mg 2 h prior to transplant, then the same dose IV 4 d posttransplant **Caution/Contra:** [B, ?/–] Known hypersensitivity to murine proteins **Supplied:** Inj 20 mg **Notes/SE:** Murine/human monoclonal antibody; edema, HTN, HA, dizziness, fever, pain, infection, GI effects, electrolyte disturbances **Interactions:** May ↑ immunosuppression with other immunosuppressive drugs **Labs:** ↑ serum cholesterol, BUN, creatinine, uric acid; ↓ serum magnesium phosphate, platelets; ↑ or ↓ in Hgb, hct, serum glucose, K^+, calcium **NIPE:** Monitor for infection, hypersensitivity reactions, IV dose over 20–30 min

BCG [Bacillus Calmette-Guérin] (TheraCys, Tice BCG)
Uses: Bladder carcinoma, TB prophylaxis **Action:** Immunomodulator **Dose:** Bladder CA, contents of 1 vial prepared and instilled in bladder for 2 h. Repeat once weekly for 6 wk; repeat 3 weekly doses 3, 6, 12, 18, and 24 mo after initial therapy **Caution/Contra:** [C, ?] <14 d after TURBT, Hx BCG sepsis, immunosuppression, steroid use **Supplied:** Inj 27 mg (3.4 + 3 × 10⁸ CFU)/vial (TheraCys), 1–8 × 10⁸ CFU/vial (Tice BCG) **Notes/SE:** *Intravesical:* Hematuria, urinary frequency, dysuria, bacterial UTI, rare BCG sepsis; routine U.S. adult BCG immunization not recommended; occasionally used in high-risk children who are PPD– and cannot take INH **Interactions:** ↓ effects with antimicrobials, immunosuppressives, radiation **Labs:** Prior BCG may cause false + PPD **NIPE:** Monitor for s/s systemic infection, report persistant pain on urination or blood in urine

Becaplermin (Regranex Gel)
Uses: Adjunct to local wound care in diabetic foot ulcers **Action:** Recombinant PDGF, enhanced formation of granulation tissue **Dose:** Based on size of lesion; 11/3-in. ribbon from 2-g tube, 2/3-in. ribbon from 7.5- or 15-mg tube/in.² of ulcer; apply and cover with moist gauze; rinse after 12 h; do not reapply; repeat process 12 h later **Caution/Contra:** [C, ?] Neoplasm or active infection at site **Supplied:** 0.01% gel in 2-, 7.5-, 15-g tubes **Notes/SE:** Use along with good wound care; wound must be vascularized; erythema, local pain **Interactions:** None known **NIPE:** Dosage recalculated q1–2wk

Beclomethasone (Beconase, Vancenase Nasal Inhaler)
Uses: Allergic rhinitis refractory to conventional therapy with antihistamines and decongestants **Action:** Inhaled steroid **Dose:** *Adults.* 1 spray intranasally bid–qid; *aqueous inhal:* 1–2 sprays/nostril qd–bid. *Peds.* 6–12 y: 1 spray intranasally tid; **Caution/Contra:** [C, ?] **Supplied:** Nasal met-dose inhaler **Notes/SE:** Nasal spray delivers 42 μg/dose and 84 μg/dose; local irritation, burning, epistaxis; **Interac-**

tions: None noted **NIPE:** Prior use of decongestant nasal gtts if edema or secretions, may take several days for full steroid effect

Beclomethasone (Beclovent Inhaler, Vanceril Inhaler, QVAR) Uses: Chronic asthma **Action:** Inhaled corticosteroid **Dose:** *Adults.* 2–4 inhal tid–qid (max 20/d); *Vanceril double strength:* 2 inhal bid (max 10/d); *QVAR:* 1–4 inhal bid. *Peds.* 1–4 inhal tid–qid (max 10/d); *Vanceril double strength:* 2 inhal bid (max 5/d); *QVAR:* 1–4 inhal bid **Caution/Contra:** [C, ?] **Supplied:** Oral met-dose inhal 42, 84 μg/inhal; QVAR 40, 80 μg/inhal **Notes/SE:** Rinse mouth/throat after use. Not effective for acute asthmatic attacks; HA, cough, hoarseness, oral candidiasis **Interactions:** None noted **NIPE:** Use inhaled bronchodilator prior to inhaled steroid, rinse mouth after inhaled steroid

Belladonna and Opium Suppositories (B & O Supprettes) [C-II] Uses: Bladder spasms; moderate/severe pain **Action:** Antispasmodic **Dose:** Insert 1 supp PR q6h PRN. 15A = 30 mg powdered opium/16.2 mg belladonna extract. 16A = 60 mg powdered opium/16.2 mg belladonna extract **Caution/Contra:** [C, ?] **Supplied:** Supp 15A, 16A **Notes/SE:** Anticholinergic side effects (sedation, urinary retention, and constipation) **Interactions:** ↑ effects with CNS depressants, TCAs; ↓ effects with phenothiazines **Labs:** ↑ LFTs **NIPE:** Do not refrigerate, moisten finger & supp < insertion, may cause blurred vision

Benazepril (Lotensin) Uses: HTN, DN, CHF **Action:** ACE inhibitor **Dose:** 10–40 mg/d PO **Caution/Contra:** [C (1st trimester), D (2nd and 3rd trimesters), +] **Supplied:** Tabs 5, 10, 20, 40 mg **Notes/SE:** Symptomatic hypotension with diuretics; dizziness, HA, hyperkalemia, nonproductive cough **Interactions:** ↑ effects with α-blockers, diuretics, capsaicin; ↓ effects with NSAIDs, ASA; ↑ effects of insulin, lithium; ↑ risk of hyperkalemia with trimethoprim & K⁺-sparing diuretics **Labs:** ↑ BUN, serum creatinine, K⁺; ↓ hemoglobin; ECG changes **NIPE:** Persistant cough and/or taste changes may develop, ⊘ PRG, d/c if angioedema

Benzocaine and Antipyrine (Auralgan) Uses: Analgesia in severe otitis media **Action:** Anesthetic and local decongestant **Dose:** Fill the ear and insert a moist cotton plug; repeat 1–2 h PRN **Caution/Contra:** [C, ?] **Supplied:** Soln **Notes/SE:** Do not use with perforated eardrum; local irritation **Interactions:** May ↓ effects of sulfonamides

Benzonatate (Tessalon Perles) Uses: Symptomatic relief of cough **Action:** Anesthetizes the stretch receptors in the respiratory passages **Dose:** *Adults & Peds >10 y.* 100 mg PO tid **Caution/Contra:** [C, ?] **Supplied:** Caps 100 mg **Notes/SE:** Do not chew or puncture the caps; sedation, dizziness, GI upset **Interactions:** ↑ CNS depression with antihistamines, alcohol, hypnotics, opioids, sedatives **NIPE:** ↑ fluid intake to liquefy secretions

Benztropine (Cogentin) Uses: Parkinsonism and drug-induced extrapyramidal disorders **Action:** Partially blocks striatal cholinergic receptors **Dose:** *Adults.* 0.5–6 mg PO, IM, or IV in ÷ doses/d. *Peds >3 y.* 0.02–0.05 mg/kg/dose

1–2/d **Caution/Contra:** [C, ?] **Supplied:** Tabs 0.5, 1.0, 2.0 mg; inj 1 mg/mL
Notes/SE: Anticholinergic side effects; physostigmine 1–2 mg SC/IV can reverse
severe symptoms **Interactions:** ↑ sedation and depressant effects with alcohol &
CNS depressants; ↑ anticholinergic effects with antihistamines, phenothiazines,
quinidine, disopyramide, TCAs, MAOIs; ↑ effect of digoxin; ↓ effect of levodopa;
↓ effects with antacids and antidiarrheal drugs **NIPE:** May ↑ susceptibility to heat
stroke, take with meals to < GI upset

Bepridil (Vascor)   **Uses:** Chronic stable angina **Action:** CCB agent **Dose:**
200–400 mg/d PO **Caution/Contra:** [C, ?] QT interval prolongation, Hx ventricular arrhythmias, sick sinus syndrome, hypotension (DBP <90 mm Hg) **Supplied:**
Tabs 200, 300, 400 mg **Notes/SE:** Dizziness, nausea, agranulocytosis, bradycardia,
and serious ventricular arrhythmias, including torsades de pointes **Interactions:** ↑
effects with amprenavir, ritonavir, moxifloxacin, gatifloxacin, sparfloxacin; ↑ effects of digitalis glycoside, cyclosporine, BBs; ↑ QT prolongation with procainamide, quinidine, TCAs **Labs:** ↑ LFTs, CPK, LDH **NIPE:** Take with food if
GI upset, monitor K^+ & ECG

Beractant (Survanta)   **Uses:** Prevention and Rx of RDS in premature infants **Action:** Replacement of pulmonary surfactant **Dose:** 100 mg/kg administered
via ET tube. May be repeated 3 more × q6h for a max of 4 doses/48 h
Caution/Contra: [N/A, N/A] **Supplied:** Suspension 25 mg of phospholipid/mL
Notes/SE: Administer via 4-quadrant method; transient bradycardia, oxygen desat-
uration, apnea **Interactions:** None noted **NIPE:** ↑ risk of nosocomial sepsis after
treatment with this drug

Betaxolol (Kerlone)   **Uses:** HTN **Action:** Competitively blocks β-adrenergic receptors, β_1 **Caution/Contra:** [C (1st trimester), D (2nd or 3rd trimester),
+/–] Sinus bradycardia, AV conduction abnormalities, cardiac failure **Dose:** 10–20
mg/d **Supplied:** Tabs 10, 20 mg **Notes/SE:** Dizziness, HA, bradycardia, edema,
CHF **Interactions:** ↑ effects with anticholinergics, verapamil, general anesthetics;
↓ effects with thyroid drugs, amphetamine, cocaine, ephedrine, epinephrine, norepinephrine, phenylephrine, pseudoephedrine, NSAIDs; ↑ effects of insulin, digitalis glycosides; ↓ effects of theophylline, dopamine, glucagon **Labs:** ↑ BUN,
serum lipoprotein, glucose, K^+, triglyceride, uric acid, ANA titers **NIPE:** May ↑
sensitivity to cold, ⊘ d/c abruptly

Betaxolol, Ophthalmic (Betoptic)   **Uses:** Glaucoma **Action:** Competitively blocks β-adrenergic receptors, β_1 **Dose:** 1 gt bid **Caution/Contra:**
[C (1st trimester), D (2nd or 3rd trimester), ?/–] **Supplied:** Soln 0.5%; susp 0.25%
Notes/SE: Local irritation, photophobia; see Betaxolol **NIPE:** Use sunglasses to
avoid exposure, may cause photophobia, review installation procedures

Bethanechol (Urecholine, Duvoid, others)   **Uses:** Neurogenic
bladder atony with retention, acute postoperative and postpartum functional
(nonobstructive) urinary retention **Action:** Stimulates cholinergic smooth-muscle
receptors in bladder and GI tract **Dose:** *Adults.* 10–50 mg PO tid–qid or 2.5–5 mg

SC tid–qid and PRN. **Peds.** 0.6 mg/kg/24 h PO ÷ tid–qid or 0.15–2 mg/kg/d SC ÷ 3–4×; on empty stomach **Caution/Contra:** [C, ?/–] Bladder outlet obstruction, PUD, epilepsy, hyperthyroidism, bradycardia, COPD, AV conduction defects, parkinsonism, hypotension, vasomotor instability **Supplied:** Tabs 5, 10, 25, 50 mg; inj 5 mg/mL **Notes/SE:** Do not administer IM or IV; abdominal cramps, diarrhea, salivation, hypotension **Interactions:** ↑ effects with BBs, tacrine, cholinesterase inhibitors; ↓ effects with atropine, anticholinergic drugs, procainamide, quinidine, epinephrine **Labs:** ↑ in serum AST, ALT, amylase, lipase, bilirubin **NIPE:** May cause blurred vision, reduced I&O, take on an empty stomach

Bicalutamide (Casodex)
Uses: Advanced prostate CA (in combination with GnRH agonists such as leuprolide or goserelin) **Action:** Nonsteroidal antiandrogen **Dose:** 50 mg/d **Caution/Contra:** [X, ?/–] **Supplied:** Caps 50 mg **Notes/SE:** Hot flashes, loss of libido, impotence, diarrhea, N/V, gynecomastia, and ↑ LFT **Interactions:** ↑ effects of anticoagulants, TCAs, phenothiazides; ↓ effects of antipsychotic drugs **Labs:** ↑ LFTs, alkaline phosphatase, bilirubin, BUN, creatinine; ↓ Hgb, WBCs **NIPE:** Monitor PSA, may experience hair loss

Bicarbonate (See Sodium Bicarbonate, page 206)

Bisacodyl (Dulcolax)
Uses: Constipation; preoperative bowel preparation **Action:** Stimulates peristalsis **Dose:** **Adults.** 5–15 mg PO or 10 mg PR PRN. **Peds.** <2 y: 5 mg PR PRN. >2 y: 5 mg PO or 10 mg PR PRN; do not chew tabs; do not give w/n 1 h of antacids or milk **Caution/Contra:** [B, ?] Acute abdomen or bowel obstruction **Supplied:** EC tabs 5 mg; supp 10 mg **Notes/SE:** Abdominal cramps, proctitis, and inflammation with suppositories **Interactions:** antacids & milk ↑ dissolution of enteric coating causing abdominal irritation **Labs:** False ↓ urine glucose **NIPE:** ↑ fluid intake & high fiber foods, ⊘ take with milk or antacids

Bismuth Subsalicylate (Pepto-Bismol)
Uses: N/V/D; combination for treatment of *H. pylori* infection **Action:** Antisecretory and antiinflammatory effects **Dose:** **Adults.** 2 tabs or 30 mL PO PRN (max 8 doses/24 h). **Peds.** *3–6 y:* 1/3 tab or 5 mL PO PRN (max 8 doses/24 h). *6–9 y:* 2/3 tab or 10 mL PO PRN (max 8 doses/24 h). *9–12 y:* 1 tab or 15 mL PO PRN (max 8 doses/24 h); avoid in patients with renal failure **Caution/Contra:** [C, D (3rd trimester), –] Contra with influenza or chickenpox (↑ risk of Reye's syndrome) **Supplied:** Chew tabs 262 mg; liq 262, 524 mg/15 mL **Notes/SE:** May turn tongue and stools black **Interactions:** ↑ effects of ASA, methotrexate, valproic acid; ↓ effects of tetracyclines, quinolones, probenecid; ↓ effects with corticosteroids **Labs:** Falsely ↑ uric acid, AST; may interfere with GI tract xrays; ↓ K+, T3, & T4 **NIPE:** May darken tongue & stool, chew tab, do not swallow whole

Bisoprolol (Zebeta)
Uses: HTN **Action:** Competitively blocks β_1-adrenergic receptors **Dose:** 5–10 mg/d (max dose 20 mg/d); ↓ in renal impairment **Caution/Contra:** [C (D 2nd and 3rd trimesters), +/–] Sinus bradycardia, AV conduction abnormalities, cardiac failure **Supplied:** Tabs 5, 10 mg **Notes/SE:** Fa-

tigue, lethargy, HA, bradycardia, edema, CHF; not dialyzed **Interactions:** ↑ bradycardia with adenosine, amiodarone, digoxin, dipyridamole, neostigmine, physostigmine, tacrine; ↑ effects with cimetidine, fluoxetine, prazosin; ↓ effects with NSAIDs, rifampin; ↓ effects of theophylline, glucagon **Labs:** ↑ thyroxine, cholesterol, glucose, triglycerides, uric acid; ↓ HDL **NIPE:** ⊘ d/c abruptly, may mask s/s hypoglycemia, take w/o regard to food

Bitolterol (Tornalate) **Uses:** Prophylaxis and Rx of asthma and reversible bronchospasm **Action:** Sympathomimetic bronchodilator; stimulates β₂-adrenergic receptors in the lungs **Dose:** *Adults & Peds >12 y.* 2 inhal q8h **Caution/Contra:** [C, ?] **Supplied:** Aerosol 0.8% **Notes/SE:** Dizziness, nervousness, trembling, HTN, palpitations **Interactions:** ↑ cardiac effects of theophylline; ↑ hypokalemia with furosemide; ↑ effects with other β-adrenergic bronchodilators, MAOI, TCA, inhaled anesthetics; ↓ effects with β-adrenergic blockers; **Labs:** ↑ AST, ↓ platelets, WBCs, proteinuria **NIPE:** Wait 15 min after use of this drug before using an adrenocorticoid inhaler. Shake inhaler well before use

Bivalirudin (Angiomax) **Uses:** Anticoagulant used with ASA in unstable angina undergoing PTCA **Action:** Anticoagulant, direct thrombin inhibitor **Dose:** 1 mg/kg IV bolus, then 2.5 mg/kg/h over 4 h; if needed, use 0.2 mg/kg/h for up to 20 h; give with aspirin 300–325 mg/day; start pre-PTCA **Caution/Contra:** [B, ?] Contra in major bleeding **Supplied:** Powder for inj **Notes/SE:** Bleeding, back pain, nausea, HA **Interactions:** ↑ risk of bleeding with thrombolytics, heparin, warfarin; d/c heparin 8+ h < giving this drug **Labs:** ↑ PT, APTT, ACT, thrombin time **NIPE:** Drug given with ASA—avoid other ASA-containing drugs or NSAIDs.

Bleomycin Sulfate (Blenoxane) **Uses:** Testicular carcinomas; Hodgkin's and NHLs; cutaneous lymphomas; and squamous cell carcinomas of the head and neck, larynx, cervix, skin, penis; sclerosing agent for malignant pleural effusion **Action:** Induces breakage (scission) of single- and double-stranded DNA **Dose:** 10–20 mg (U)/m² 1–2/wk (refer to specific protocols); ↓ in renal impairment **Supplied:** Inj 15 mg (15 U) **Caution/Contra:** [D, ?] Contra severe pulmonary disease **Notes/SE:** Hyperpigmentation (skin staining) and hypersensitivity (rash to anaphylaxis); test dose of 1 mg (U) recommended, especially in lymphoma patients; fever in 50%; lung toxicity (idiosyncratic and dose-related); pneumonitis may progress to fibrosis; lung toxicity likely when the total dose >400 mg (U); Raynaud's phenomenon, N/V **Interactions:** ↑ effects with cisplatin & other antineoplastic drugs; ↓ effects of digoxin & phenytoin **Labs:** Monitor CBC, LFTs, BUN, creatinine; pulmonary function tests **NIPE:** ⊘ immunizations, breast-feeding; use contraception method

Bortezomib (Velcade) **WARNING:** May worsen preexisting neuropathy **Uses:** Progression of multiple myeloma despite two previous treatments **Action:** Proteasome inhibitor **Dose:** *Adults.* 1.3 mg/m² bolus IV twice weekly for 2 wk, w/10-day rest (= 1 cycle); ↓ dose for hematologic toxicity, neuropathy. *Peds.* Safety and effectiveness have not yet been established **Caution:** [D, ?/–] Contra:

Pts with hypersensitivity to bortezomib, boron or mannitol **Supplied:** 3.5-mg vial **SE:** Asthenia, GI upset, anorexia, dyspnea, HA, orthostatic hypotension, edema, insomnia, dizziness, rash, pyrexia, arthralgia, neuropathy **Notes:** May interact with drugs metabolized via CYP450 system **Interactions:** ↑ risk of peripheral neuropathy and/or hypotension with amiodarone, antivirals, isoniazid, nitrofurantoin, statins **Labs:** Monitor for ↑ uric acid, ↓ K+, calcium, neutrophils, platelets **NIPE:** ⊘ PRG or breast feeding; use contraception; caution with driving due to fatigue/dizziness; ↑ fluids if c/o N/V

Brimonidine (Alphagan) **Uses:** Open-angle glaucoma **Action:** α₂-Adrenergic agonist **Dose:** 1 gt in eye(s) tid; wait 15 min to insert contacts **Caution/Contra:** [B, ?] MAOI therapy **Supplied:** 0.2% soln **Notes/SE:** Local irritation, HA, fatigue **Interactions:** ↑ effects of antihypertensives, BBs, cardiac glycosides, CNS depressants; ↓ effects with TCA **NIPE:** ⊘ alcohol, insert soft contact lenses 15+ min after drug use

Brinzolamide (Azopt) **Uses:** Open-angle glaucoma **Action:** Carbonic anhydrase inhibitor **Dose:** 1 gt in eye(s) tid **Caution/Contra:** [C, ?] **Supplied:** 1.0% susp **Notes/SE:** Blurred vision, dry eye, blepharitis, taste disturbance **Interactions:** ↑ effects with oral carbonic anhydrase inhibitors **Labs:** Check LFTs, BUN, creatinine **NIPE:** ⊘ use drug if impaired renal & hepatic studies or allergies to sulfonamides; shake well before use; insert soft contact lenses 15+ min after drug use; wait 10 min <use of other topical ophthalmic drugs

Bromocriptine (Parlodel) **Uses:** Parkinson's syndrome, hyperprolactinemia, acromegaly **Action:** Direct-acting on the striatal dopamine receptors; ↓ prolactin secretion **Dose:** Initially, 1.25 mg PO bid; titrate to effect **Caution/Contra:** [C, ?] Severe ischemic heart disease or peripheral vascular disease **Supplied:** Tabs 2.5 mg; caps 5 mg **Notes/SE:** Hypotension, Raynaud's phenomenon, dizziness, nausea, hallucinations **Interactions:** ↑ effects with erythromycin, fluvoxamine, nefazodone, sympathomimetics; ↓ effects with phenothiazines, antipsychotics; **Labs:** ↑ BUN, AST, ALT, CPK, alkaline phosphatase, uric acid **NIPE:** ⊘ breastfeeding, PRG, oral contraceptives; drug may cause intolerance to alcohol, return of menses & suppression of galactorrhea may take 6–8 wk

Budesonide (Rhinocort, Pulmicort) **Uses:** Allergic and nonallergic rhinitis, asthma **Action:** Steroid **Dose:** *Adults.* *Intranasal:* 2 sprays/nostril bid or 4 sprays/nostril/d. *Aqueous:* 1 spray/nostril/d. *Oral inhaled:* 1–4 inhal bid. *Peds.* 1–2 inhal bid; rinse mouth after oral use **Caution/Contra:** [C, ?/–] **Supplied:** Met-dose Turbuhaler, nasal inhaler, and aqueous spray **Notes/SE:** HA, cough, hoarseness, *Candida* infection, epistaxis **Interactions:** ↑ effects with ketoconazole, itraconazole, ritonavir, indinavir, saquinavir, erythromycine, and grapefruit juice **NIPE:** Shake inhaler well < use, rinse mouth & wash inhaler > use, swallow capsules whole, ⊘ exposure chickenpox or measles.

Bumetanide (Bumex) **Uses:** Edema from CHF, hepatic cirrhosis, and renal disease **Action:** Loop diuretic; inhibits reabsorption of Na and chloride in the ascending loop of Henle and the distal renal tubule **Dose:** *Adults.* 0.5–2 mg/d PO; 0.5–1 mg IV q8–24h (max 10 mg/d). *Peds.* 0.015–0.1 mg/kg/d PO, IV, or IM ÷ q6–24h **Caution/Contra:** [D, ?] Anuria or increasing azotemia **Supplied:** Tabs 0.5, 1, 2 mg; inj 0.25 mg/mL **Notes/SE:** Monitor fluid and electrolyte status during treatment; hypokalemia, hyperuricemia, hypochloremia, hyponatremia, dizziness, ↑ serum creatinine, ototoxicity **Interactions:** ↑ effects with antihypertensives, thiazides, nitrates, alcohol, clofibrate; ↑ effects of lithium, warfarin, thrombolytic drugs, anticoagulants; ↑ K⁺ loss with carbenoxolone, corticosteroids, terbutaline; ↑ ototoxicity with aminoglycosides, cisplatin; ↓ effects with cholestyramine, colestipol, NSAIDs, probenecid, barbiturates, phenytoin **Labs:** ↑ thyroxine, T3, BUN, serum glucose, creatinine uric acid; ↓ serum K⁺, calcium, magnesium **NIPE:** Take drug with food, take early to prevent nocturia, daily wts

Bupivacaine (Marcaine) Uses: Peripheral nerve block **Action:** Local anesthetic **Dose:** *Adults & Peds.* Dose-dependent on procedure (ie, tissue vascularity, depth of anesthesia, etc) (Table 3, page 247) **Caution/Contra:** [C, ?] **Supplied:** Inj 0.25, 0.5, 0.75% **Notes/SE:** Hypotension, bradycardia, dizziness, anxiety **Interactions:** ↑ effects with BBs, hyaluronidase, ergot-type oxytocics, MAOI, TCAs, phenothiazines, vasopressors, CNS depressants; ↓ effects with chloroprocaine **NIPE:** Anesthetized area has temporary loss of sensation & function

Buprenorphine (Buprenex) [C-V] Uses: Moderate/severe pain **Action:** Opiate agonist–antagonist **Dose:** 0.3–0.6 mg IM or slow IV push q6h PRN **Caution/Contra:** [C, ?/–] **Supplied:** Inj 0.324 mg/mL (= 0.3 mg of buprenorphine) **Notes/SE:** May induce withdrawal syndrome in opioid-dependent patients; sedation, hypotension, respiratory depression **Interactions:** ↑ effects of respiratory & CNS depression with alcohol, opiates, benzodiazepines, TCAs, MAOIs, other CNS depressants **Labs:** ↑ serum amylase and lipase **NIPE:** ⊘ alcohol & other CNS depressants

Bupropion (Wellbutrin, Wellbutrin SR, Zyban) Uses: Depression, adjunct to smoking cessation **Action:** Weak inhibitor of neuronal uptake of serotonin and norepinephrine; inhibits the neuronal reuptake of dopamine **Dose:** *Depression:* 100–450 mg/d ÷ bid–tid. *Smoking cessation:* 150 mg/d ×3 d, then 150-mg bid ×8–12 wk; ↓ in renal/hepatic impairment **Caution/Contra:** [B, ?/–] Seizure disorder, prior diagnosis of anorexia nervosa or bulimia **Supplied:** Tabs 75, 100 mg; SR tabs 100, 150 mg **Notes/SE:** Associated with seizures; avoid use of alcohol and other CNS depressants; agitation, insomnia, HA, tachycardia **Interactions:** ↑ effects with cimetidine, levodopa, MAOIs; ↑ risk of seizures with alcohol, phenothiazines, antidepressants, theophylline, TCAs, abrupt withdrawal of corticosteroids, benzodiazepines **Labs:** ↓ prolactin level **NIPE:** Drug may cause seizures, take 3–4 w for full effect, ⊘ alcohol or abrupt d/c.

Buspirone (BuSpar) Uses: Short-term relief of anxiety **Action:** Antianxiety agent; selectively antagonizes CNS serotonin receptors **Dose:** 5–10 mg PO tid; ↑ to desired response; usual dose 20–30 mg/d; max 60 mg/d; ↓ in severe hepatic/renal insufficiency **Caution/Contra:** [B, ?/–] **Supplied:** Tabs 5, 10, 15 mg **Notes/SE:** No abuse potential or physical or psychologic dependence; drowsiness, dizziness; HA, nausea **Interactions:** ↑ effects with erythromycin, clarithromycin, itraconazole, ketoconazole, diltiazem, verapamil, grapefruit juice; ↓ effects with carbamazepine, rifampin, phenytoin, dexamethasone, phenobarbital, fluoxetine **Labs:** ↑ AST, ALT, growth hormone, prolactin **NIPE:** ↑ sedation with alcohol, therapeutic effects may take up to 4 wk

Busulfan (Myleran, Busulfex) **Uses:** CML, preparative regimens for allogeneic and ABMT in high doses **Action:** Alkylating agent **Dose:** 4–12 mg/d for several wk; 16 mg/kg once or 4 mg/kg/d for 4 d in conjunction with another agent in transplant regimens. Refer to specific protocol **Caution/Contra:** [D, ?] **Supplied:** Tabs 2 mg; inj 60 mg/10 mL **Notes/SE:** Myelosuppression, pulmonary fibrosis, nausea (high-dose therapy), gynecomastia, adrenal insufficiency, and skin hyperpigmentation **Interactions:** ↑ effects with acetaminophen; ↑ bone-marrow suppression with antineoplastic drugs & radiation therapy; ↑ uric acid levels with probenecid & sulfinpyrazone; ↓ effects with itraconazole, phenytoin **Labs:** ↑ uric acid; monitor CBC, LFTs **NIPE:** ⊘ immunizations, PRG, breast-feeding; ↑ fluids; use barrier contraception; ↑ risk of hair loss, rash, darkened skin pigment; ↑ susceptability to infection

Butorphanol (Stadol) [C-IV] **Uses:** Moderate–severe pain and HAs **Action:** Opiate agonist–antagonist with central analgesic actions **Dose:** 1–4 mg IM or IV q3–4h PRN. *HAs:* 1 spray in 1 nostril, may repeat ×1 if pain not relieved in 60–90 min; ↓ in renal impairment **Caution/Contra:** [C (D if used in high doses or for prolonged periods at term), +] **Supplied:** Inj 1, 2 mg/mL; nasal spray 10 mg/mL **Notes/SE:** Drowsiness, dizziness, nasal congestion; may induce withdrawal in opioid-dependent patients **Interactions:** ↑ effects with alcohol, antihistamines, cimetidine, CNS depressants, phenothiazines, barbiturates, skeletal-muscle relaxants, MAOIs; ↓ effects of opioids **Labs:** ↑ serum amylase & lipase **NIPE:** ⊘ alcohol or other CNS depressants

Calcipotriene (Dovonex) **Uses:** Plaque psoriasis **Action:** Keratolytic **Dose:** Apply bid **Caution/Contra:** [C, ?] **Supplied:** Cream; oint; soln 0.005% **Notes/SE:** Skin irritation, dermatitis **Interactions:** None noted **Labs:** Monitor serum calcium **NIPE:** Wash hands >application or wear gloves to apply, d/c drug if ↑ calcium

Calcitonin (Cibacalcin, Miacalcin) **Uses:** Paget's disease of bone; hypercalcemia; osteogenesis imperfecta, postmenopausal osteoporosis **Action:** Polypeptide hormone **Dose:** *Paget's salmon form:* 100 U/d IM/SC initially, 50 U/d or 50–100 U q1–3d maint. *Paget's human form:* 0.5 mg/d initially; maint 0.5 mg 2–3×/wk or 0.25 mg/d, max 0.5 mg bid. *Hypercalcemia salmon calcitonin:* 4 U/kg IM/SC q12h; ↑ to 8 U/kg q12h, max q6h. *Osteoporosis salmon calcitonin:* 100 U/d IM/SC; intranasal 200 U = 1 nasal spray/d **Caution/Contra:** [C, ?] **Supplied:** Spray, nasal 200 U/activation; inj, human (Cibacalcin) 0.5 mg/vial, salmon

200 U/mL (2 mL) **Notes/SE:** Human (Cibacalcin) and salmon forms; human only approved for Paget's bone disease; facial flushing, nausea, edema at inj site. nasal irritation, polyuria **Interactions:** None noted **Labs:** ↑ serum lithium **NIPE:** Allergy skin test prior to use

Calcitriol (Rocaltrol) **Uses:** ↓ Elevated PTH levels, hypocalcemia associated with dialysis **Action:** 1,25-Dihydroxycholecalciferol, a vitamin D analogue **Dose:** *Adults. Renal failure:* 0.25 μg/d PO, ↑ 0.25 μg/d q4–6wk PRN; 0.5 μg 3×/wk IV, ↑ PRN. *Hyperparathyroidism:* 0.5–2 μg/d. *Peds. Renal failure:* 15 ng/kg/d, ↑ PRN; typical maint 30–60 ng/kg/d. *Hyperparathyroidism:* <5 y, 0.25–0.75 μg/d; >6 y, 0.5–2 μg/d **Caution/Contra:** [C, ?] **Supplied:** Inj 1, 2 μg/mL (in 1-mL vol); caps 0.25, 0.5 μg **Notes/SE:** Monitor dosing to keep Ca⁺ wnl; hypercalcemia possible **Interactions:** ↑ effect with thiazide diuretics; ↓ effect with cholestyramine, colestipol **Labs:** ↑ calcium, cholesterol, magnesium, BUN, AST, ALT; ↓ alkaline phosphatase; **NIPE:** ⊘ magnesium-containing antacids or supplements

Calcium Acetate (Calphron, Phos-Ex, PhosLo) **Uses:** ESRD-associated hyperphosphatemia **Action:** Ca supplement to treat ESRD hyperphosphatemia w/o aluminum **Dose:** 2–4 tabs PO with meals **Caution/Contra:** [C, ?] **Supplied:** Caps Phos-Ex 500 mg (125 mg Ca); tabs Calphron and PhosLo 667 mg (169 mg Ca) **Notes/SE:** Can cause ↑ Ca²⁺, monitor Ca²⁺ levels; hypophosphatemia, constipation **Interactions:** ↑ effects of quinidine; ↓ effects with large intake of dietary fiber, spinach, rhubarb; ↓ effects of atenolol, CCB, etidronate, tetracyclines, fluoroquinolones, phenytoin, iron salts **Labs:** ↑ calcium; ↓ magnesium **NIPE:** ⊘ alcohol, caffeine, tobacco; separate calcium supplements and other meds by 1–2 h

Calcium Carbonate (Tums, Alka-Mints) **Uses:** Hyperacidity associated with peptic ulcer disease, hiatal hernia, GERD **Action:** Neutralizes gastric acid **Dose:** 500 mg–2 g PO PRN; ↓ in renal impairment **Caution/Contra:** [C, ?] **Supplied:** Chew tabs 350, 420, 500, 550, 750, 850 mg; susp **Notes/SE:** Hypercalcemia, hypophosphatemia, constipation **Interactions:** ↓ effect of tetracyclines, fluoroquinolones, iron salts, and ASA; ↓ calcium absorption with high intake of dietary fiber **Labs:** ↑ calcium; ↓ magnesium **NIPE:** ↑ fluids, may cause constipation, ⊘ alcohol, caffeine, tobacco; separate calcium supplements and other meds by 1–2 h, chew tablet well

Calcium Glubionate (Neo-Calglucon) [OTC] **Uses:** Rx and prevention of Ca deficiency **Action:** Oral Ca supplementation **Dose:** *Adults.* 6–18 g/d ÷ doses. *Peds.* 600–2000 mg/kg/d ÷ qid (9 g/d max); ↓ in renal impairment **Caution/Contra:** [C, ?] **Supplied:** OTC syrup 1.8 g/5 mL = Ca 115 mg/5 mL **Notes/SE:** Hypercalcemia, hypophosphatemia, constipation **Interactions:** ↑ effects of quinidine; ↓ effect of tetracyclines; ↓ calcium absorption with high intake of dietary fiber; **Labs:** ↑ calcium, ↓ magnesium **NIPE:** ⊘ alcohol, caffeine, tobacco, separate calcium supplements and other meds by 1–2 h, chew tab well

Calcium Salts (Chloride, Gluconate, Gluceptate) **Uses:** Ca replacement, VF, Ca blocker toxicity, Mg²⁺ intoxication, tetany, hyperphosphatemia in

ESRD Action: Ca supplementation/replacement **Dose:** *Adults.* *Replacement:* 1–2 g/d PO. *Cardiac emergencies:* CaCl 0.5–1.0 g IV q10 min or Ca gluconate 1–2 g IV q10 min. *Tetany:* 1 g CaCl over 10–30 min; repeat in 6 h PRN. *Peds. Replacement:* 200–500 mg/kg/24 h PO or IV ÷ qid. *Cardiac emergency:* 100 mg/kg/dose IV of gluconate salt q10 min. *Tetany:* 10 mg/kg CaCl over 5–10 min; repeat in 6 h or use inf (200 mg/kg max). *Adult & Peds. Hypocalcemia due to citrated blood inf:* 0.45 mEq Ca/100 mL citrated blood infused; ↓ in renal impairment **Caution/Contra:** [C, ?] **Supplied:** CaCl inj 10% = 100 mg/mL = Ca 27.2 mg/mL = 10-mL amp. Ca gluconate inj 10% = 100 mg/mL = Ca 9 mg/mL; tabs 500 mg = 45 mg Ca, 650 mg = 58.5 mg Ca, 975 mg = 87.75 mg Ca, 1 g = 90 mg Ca. Ca gluceptate inj 220 mg/mL = 18 mg/mL Ca **Notes/SE:** CaCl contains 270 mg (13.6 mEq) elemental Ca/g, and Ca gluconate contains 90 mg (4.5 mEq) Ca/g. *RDA for Ca: Adults.* 800 mg/d. *Peds. <6 mon:* 360 mg/d. *6 mon–1 y:* 540 mg/d. *1–10 y:* 800 mg/d. *10–18 y:* 1200 mg/d; bradycardia, cardiac arrhythmias, hypercalcemia **Interactions:** ↑ effects of quinidine and digitalis; ↓ effects of tetracyclines, quinolones, verapamil, CCBs, iron salts, ASA, atenolol; ↓ calcium absorption with high intake of dietary fiber **Labs:** ↑ calcium, ↓ magnesium **NIPE:** ⊘ alcohol, caffeine, tobacco; separate calcium supplements and other meds by 1–2 h, chew tablet well

Calfactant (Infasurf) **Uses:** Prevention and Rx of RDS in infants **Action:** Exogenous pulmonary surfactant **Dose:** 3 mL/kg instilled into lungs. Can retreat for a total of 3 doses given 12 h apart **Caution/Contra:** [?, ?] **Supplied:** Intratracheal susp 35 mg/mL **Notes/SE:** Monitor for cyanosis, airway obstruction, bradycardia during administration **Interactions:** None noted **NIPE:** ⊘ Reconstitute, dilute, or shake vial; refrigerate & keep away from light; no need to warm solution prior to use

Candesartan (Atacand) **Uses:** HTN, DN, CHF **Action:** Angiotensin II receptor antagonist **Dose:** 2–32 mg/d (usual 16 mg/d) **Caution/Contra:** [X, –] Primary hyperaldosteronism; bilateral renal artery stenosis **Supplied:** Tabs 4, 8, 16, 32 mg **Notes/SE:** Dizziness, HA, flushing, angioedema **Interactions:** ↑ effects with cimetidine; ↑ risk of hyperkalemia with amiloride, spironolactone, triamterene, K⁺ supplements, trimethoprim; ↑ effects of lithium; ↓ effects with phenobarbital, rifampin **Labs:** ↑ creatine phosphatase; monitor for albuminuria, hyperglycemia, triglyceridemia, uricemia. **NIPE:** ⊘ breast-feeding or PRG, use barrier contraception, may take 4–6 wk for full effect, adequate fluid intake, take w/o regard to food

Capsaicin (Capsin, Zostrix, others) [OTC] **Uses:** Pain due to postherpetic neuralgia, chronic neuralgia, arthritis, diabetic neuropathy, postoperative pain, psoriasis, intractable pruritus **Action:** Topical analgesic **Dose:** Apply tid–qid **Caution/Contra:** [?, ?] **Supplied:** OTC creams; gel; lotions; roll-ons **Notes/SE:** Local irritation, neurotoxicity, cough **Interactions:** May ↑ cough with ACEI **NIPE:** External use only, ⊘ contact with eyes or broken/irritated skin, apply with gloves, transient stinging/burning

Captopril (Capoten, others) Uses: HTN, CHF, LVD, DN Action: ACE inhibitor Dose: *Adults. HTN:* Initially, 25 mg PO bid–tid; ↑ to maint q1–2 wk by 25-mg increments/dose (max 450 mg/d) to effect. *CHF:* Initially, 6.25–12.5 mg PO tid; titrate PRN. *LVD:* 50 mg PO tid. *DN:* 25 mg PO tid. **Peds.** *Infants <2 mon:* 0.05–0.5 mg/kg/dose PO q8–24h. *Children:* Initially, 0.3–0.5 mg/kg/dose PO; ↑ to 6 mg/kg/d max; take 1 h before meals **Caution/Contra:** [C (1st trimester; D 2nd and 3rd trimesters), +] **Supplied:** Tabs 12.5, 25, 50, 100 mg; ? in renal impairment **Notes/SE:** Rash, proteinuria, cough, ↑ K⁺ **Interactions:** ↑ effects with antihypertensives, diuretics, nitrates, probenecid, black catechu; ↓ effects with antacids, ASA, NSAIDs, food; ↑ effects of digoxin, insulin, oral hypoglycemics, lithium **Labs:** False + urine acetone; may ↑ urine protein, serum BUN, creatinine, K⁺, prolactin, LFTs; may ↓ FBS **NIPE:** ⊘ PRG, breast-feeding, K⁺-sparing diuretics; take w/o food, may take 2 wk for full therapeutic effect

Carbamazepine (Tegretol) WARNING: Aplastic anemia and agranulocytosis have been reported with carbamazepine Uses: Epilepsy, trigeminal neuralgia, alcohol withdrawal Action: Anticonvulsant Dose: *Adults.* Initially, 200 mg PO bid; ↑ by 200 mg/d; usual 800–1200 mg/d in ÷ doses. *Peds.* **<6 y:** 5 mg/kg/d, ↑ to 10–20 mg/kg/d ÷ in 2–4 doses. **6–12 y:** Initially, 100 mg PO bid or 10 mg/kg/24 h PO ÷ qd–bid; ↑ to a maint of 20–30 mg/kg/24 h ÷ tid–qid; ↓ in renal impairment; take with food **Caution/Contra:** [D, +] **Supplied:** Tabs 200 mg; chew tabs 100 mg; XR tabs 100, 200, 400 mg; susp 100 mg/5 mL **Notes/SE:** Monitor CBC and serum levels (Table 2, page 243; generic products not interchangeable; drowsiness, dizziness, blurred vision, N/V, rash, ↓ Na⁺, leukopenia, agranulocytosis **Interactions:** ↑ effects with cimetidine, clarithromycine, danazol, diltiazem, felbamate, fluconazole, fluoxetine, fluvoxamine, isoniazid, itraconazole, ketoconazole, macrolides, metronidazole, propoxyphene, protease inhibitors, valporic acid, verapamil, grapefruit juice; ↑ effects of lithium, MAOIs; ↓ effects with phenobarbital, phenytoin, primidone, plantain; ↓ effects of benzodiazepines, corticosteroids, cyclosporine, doxycycline, felbamate, haloperidol, oral contraceptives, phenytoin, theophylline, thyroid hormones, TCAs, warfarin **Labs:** ↑ BUN, LFTs, bilirubin, alkaline phosphatase; ↓ calcium, T3, T4, sodium; false neg PRG test & uric acid **NIPE:** Take with food, may cause photosensitivity, use barrier contraception, abrupt withdrawal may cause seizures, ⊘ breast-feeding or PRG

Carbidopa/Levodopa (Sinemet) Uses: Parkinson's disease Action: ↑ CNS levels of dopamine Dose: 25/100 mg bid–qid; ↑ as needed (max 200/2000 mg/d) Caution/Contra: [C, ?] Narrow-angle glaucoma, suspicious skin lesion (may activate melanoma) **Supplied:** Tabs (mg carbidopa/mg levodopa) 10/100, 25/100, 25/250; tabs SR (mg carbidopa/mg levodopa) 25/100, 50/200 **Notes/SE:** Psychiatric disturbances, orthostatic hypotension, dyskinesias, cardiac arrhythmias **Interactions:** ↑ effects with antacids; ↓ effects with anticonvulsants, benzodiazepines, haloperidol, iron, methionine, papaverine, phenothiazines, phenytoin, pyridoxine, spiramycin, tacrine, thioxanthenes, high protein food **Labs:** ↑ urine amino acids, serum acid phosphatase, aspartate aminotransferase; ↓ serum bilirubin, BUN, creatinine, glucose, uric acid **NIPE:** Darkened urine & sweat may result, do not crush or chew sustained release tabs, take w/o food

Carboplatin (Paraplatin)

Uses: Ovarian, lung, head and neck, testicular, and brain CAs and allogeneic and ABMT in high doses **Action:** DNA cross-linker; forms DNA-platinum adducts **Dose:** 360 mg/m² (ovarian carcinoma); AUC dosing 4–7 mg/mL (using Culvert's formula: mg = AUC × [25 + calculated GFR]); adjusted based on pretreatment platelet count, CrCl, and BSA (Egorin's formula); up to 1500 mg/m² used in ABMT setting (refer to specific protocols) **Caution/Contra:** [D, ?] Severe bone marrow suppression, excessive bleeding **Supplied:** Inj 50, 150, 450 mg **Notes/SE:** Physiologic dosing based on either Culvert's or Egorin's formula allows ↑ doses with ↓ toxicity; myelosuppression, N/V/D, nephrotoxicity, hematuria, neurotoxicity, ↑ LFTs **Interactions:** ↑ myelosuppression with myelosuppressive drugs; ↑ hematologic effects with bone-marrow suppressants; ↑ bleeding with ASA; ↑ nephrotoxicity with nephrotoxic drugs; ↓ effects of phenytoin; ↓ effects with food and with aluminum **Labs:** ↓ magnesium, K⁺, sodium, calcium; ↑ LFTs **NIPE:** ⊘ use with aluminum needles or IV administration sets, PRG, breast-feeding; antiemetics prior to admin may prevent N/V, maintain adequate food & fluid intake

Carisoprodol (Soma)

Uses: Adjunct to sleep and physical therapy for the relief of painful musculoskeletal conditions **Action:** Centrally acting muscle relaxant **Dose:** 350 mg PO tid–qid **Caution/Contra:** [C, M] Caution in renal/hepatic impairment **Supplied:** Tabs 350 mg **Notes/SE:** Avoid alcohol and other CNS depressants; available in combination with ASA or codeine; drowsiness, dizziness **Interactions:** ↑ effects with CNS depressants, phenothiazines, alcohol **NIPE:** ⊘ breast-feeding, take with food if GI upset

Carmustine [BCNU] (BiCNU)

Uses: Primary brain tumors, melanoma, Hodgkin's and NHLs, multiple myeloma, and induction for allogeneic and ABMT in high doses **Action:** Alkylating agent; nitrosourea forms DNA cross-links; inhibitor of DNA synthesis **Dose:** 75–100 mg/m²/d for 2 d; 200 mg/m² in a single dose; 450–900 mg/m² in BMT setting (refer to specific protocols); ↓ in hepatic impairment **Caution/Contra:** [D, ?] Contra in myelosuppression **Supplied:** Inj 100 mg; wafer 7.7 mg **Notes/SE:** Myelosuppression (especially leukocytes and platelets), phlebitis, facial flushing, hepatic and renal dysfunction, pulmonary fibrosis, optic neuroretinitis. Hematologic toxicity may persist up to 4–6 wk after dose **Interactions:** ↑ bleeding with ASA, anticoagulants; ↑ hepatic dysfunction with etoposide; ↑ myelosuppression with cimetidine; ↑ suppression of bone marrow with radiation or additional antineoplastics; ↓ effects of phenytoin, digoxin; ↓ pulmonary function **Labs:** ↑ AST, alkaline phosphatase, bilirubin; monitor CBC, platelets, LFTs, PFTs **NIPE:** ⊘ PRG, breast-feeding, exposure to infections, ASA products

Carteolol (Cartrol, Ocupress Ophthalmic)

Uses: HTN, ↑ intraocular pressure **Action:** Competitively blocks β-adrenergic receptors, β₁, β₂, ISA

Dose: PO 2.5–5 mg/d; ophth 1 gt in eye(s) bid **Caution/Contra:** [C (1st trimester; D 2nd and 3rd trimesters), ?/–] Bradycardia, AV conduction abnormalities, cardiac failure, asthma **Supplied:** Tabs 2.5, 5 mg; ophth soln 1% **Notes/SE:** Drowsiness, sexual dysfunction, bradycardia, edema, CHF; *ocular:* conjunctival hyperemia, anisocoria, keratitis, eye pain **Interactions:** ↑ effects with amiodarone, adenosine, barbiturates, CCBs, digoxin, dipyridamole, fluoxetine, rifampin, tacrine, nitrates, alcohol; ↑ α-adrenergic effects with amphetamines, cocaine, ephedrine, epinephrine, phenylephrine; ↑ effects of theophylline; ↓ effects with antacids, NSAIDs, thyroid drugs, clonidine; ↓ effects of hypoglycemics, theophylline, dopamine **Labs:** ↑ BUN, uric acid, K⁺, serum lipoprotein, triglycerides, glucose, ANA titers **NIPE:** Ophthalmic drug may cause photophobia & risk of burning; may ↑ cold sensitivity, mental confusion

Carvedilol (Coreg)

Uses: HTN and CHF **Action:** Competitively blocks adrenergic receptors, β_1, β_2, α **Dose:** *HTN:* 6.25–12.5 mg bid. *CHF:* 3.125–25 mg bid; take with food to minimize hypotension **Caution/Contra:** [C (1st trimester; D 2nd and 3rd trimesters), ?/–] Bradycardia, AV conduction abnormalities, uncompensated CHF, severe hepatic impairment, asthma **Supplied:** Tabs 3.125, 6.25, 12.5, 25 mg **Notes/SE:** Chest pain, dizziness, fatigue, hyperglycemia, bradycardia, edema, hypercholesterolemia; do not DC abruptly; increases digoxin levels **Interactions:** ↑ effects with cimetidine, clonidine, MAOIs, reserpine, verapamil, fluoxetine, paroxetine; ↑ effects of digoxin, hypoglycemics, cyclosporine, CCBs; ↓ effects with rifampine, NSAIDs; **Labs:** ↑ LFTs, K⁺, triglycerides, uric acid, BUN, creatinine, alkaline phosphatase; ↓ HDL **NIPE:** Food slows absorption, may cause dry eyes with contact lenses

Caspofungin (Cancidas)

Uses: Invasive aspergillosis refractory/intolerant to standard therapy **Action:** An echinocandin; inhibits fungal cell wall synthesis **Dose:** 70 mg IV load day 1, 50 mg/d IV; slow inf **Caution/Contra:** [C, ?/–] Do not use with cyclosporine. **Supplied:** IV inf **Notes/SE:** Fever, N/V, thrombophlebitis at inj site, altered LFTs **Interactions:** ↑ effects with cyclosporine; ↓ effects with carbamazepine, dexamethasone, efavirenz, nelfinavir, nevirapine, phenytoin, rifampin; ↓ effect of tacrolimus **Labs:** ↑ LFTs, serum alkaline phosphatase, eosinophils, PT, urine protein & RBCs; ↓ K⁺, albumin, WBCs, Hgb, Hct, platelets, neutrophils; **NIPE:** Infuse slowly over 1 h & do not mix with other drugs

Cefaclor (Ceclor)

Uses: Infections caused by susceptible bacteria involving the upper and lower respiratory tract, skin, bone, urinary tract, abdomen, and gynecologic system **Action:** 2nd-gen. cephalosporin; inhibits cell wall synthesis **Dose:** *Adults.* 250–500 mg PO tid. *Peds.* 20–40 mg/kg/d PO ÷ tid; adjust in renal impairment **Caution/Contra:** [B, +] **Supplied:** Caps 250, 500 mg; ER tabs 375, 500 mg; susp 125, 187, 250, 375 mg/5 mL **Notes/SE:** More gram-activity than 1st-gen. cephalosporins; diarrhea, rash, eosinophilia, ↑ transaminases **Interactions:** ↑ bleeding with anticoagulants; ↑ nephrotoxicity with aminoglycosides, loop diuretics; ↑ effects with probenecid; ↓ effects with antacids, chloramphenicol **Labs:** Positive direct Coombs test; ↑ LFTs, alkaline phosphatase, bilirubin, LDH, BUN, creatinine; false positive of serum or urine creatinine, false positive urine glucose **NIPE:** Food with extended release tabs ↑ absorption, monitor for superinfection, ⊘ breast-feeding

Cefadroxil (Duricef, Ultracef)   **Uses:** Infections caused by *Streptococcus, Staphylococcus, E. coli, Proteus,* and *Klebsiella* involving skin, bone, upper and lower respiratory tract, and urinary tract **Action:** 1st-gen. cephalosporin; inhibits cell wall synthesis **Dose:** *Adults.* 500–1000 mg PO bid–qd. *Peds.* 30 mg/kg/d ÷ bid; ↓ in renal impairment **Caution/Contra:** [B, +] **Supplied:** Caps 500 mg; tabs 1 g; susp 125, 250, 500 mg/5 mL **Notes/SE:** Diarrhea, rash, eosinophilia, ↑ transaminases; **see Cefaclor Additonal NIPE:** Give w/o regard to food

Cefazolin (Ancef, Kefzol)   **Uses:** Infections caused by *Streptococcus, Staphylococcus, E. coli, Proteus,* and *Klebsiella* involving the skin, bone, upper and lower respiratory tract, and urinary tract **Action:** 1st-gen. cephalosporin; inhibits cell wall synthesis **Dose:** *Adults.* 1–2 g IV q8h. *Peds.* 50–100 mg/kg/d IV ÷ q8h; ↓ in renal impairment **Caution/Contra:** [B, +] **Supplied:** Inj **Notes/SE:** Widely used for surgical prophylaxis; diarrhea, rash, eosinophilia, ↑ transaminases, pain at inj site; **see Cefaclor NIPE:** Monitor renal function, I&O

Cefdinir (Omnicef)   **Uses:** Infections involving the respiratory tract, skin, bone, and urinary tract **Action:** 3rd-gen. cephalosporin; inhibits cell wall synthesis **Dose:** *Adults.* 300 mg PO bid or 600 mg PO qd. *Peds.* 7 mg/kg PO bid or 14 mg/kg/d PO; ↓ in renal impairment **Caution/Contra:** [B, +] **Supplied:** Caps 300 mg; susp 125 mg/5 mL **Notes/SE:** Cross-reactions with penicillin, anaphylaxis, diarrhea, rare pseudomembranous colitis; **see Cefaclor Additional Interactions:** ↓ effects with iron supplements **NIPE:** Stools may initially turn red in color, sucrose in suspension

Cefditoren (Spectracef)   **Uses:** Acute exacerbations of chronic bronchitis, pharyngitis, tonsillitis; skin infections **Action:** 3rd-gen. cephalosporin **Dose:** *Adults & Peds >12 y. Skin:* 200 mg PO bid × 10 days. *Chronic bronchitis, pharyngitis, tonsillitis:* 400 mg PO bid × 10 days; avoid antacids w/n 2 h; ↓ dose in renal impairment **Caution/Contra:** [B, ?] Contra cephalosporin/penicillin allergy, carnitine deficiency, milk sensitivities, or renal failure. **Supplied:** 200-mg tabs **Notes/SE:** HA, N/V/D, colitis, nephrotoxicity, hepatic dysfunction, Stevens-Johnson syndrome, toxic epidermal necrolysis, hypersensitivity reactions; **see Cefaclor. Additional NIPE:** ⊘ take if sensitive to milk protein, monitor for seizure activity

Cefepime (Maxipime)   **Uses:** UTI and pneumonia due to *S. pneumoniae, S. aureus, K. pneumoniae, E. coli, P. aeruginosa,* and *Enterobacter* spp **Action:** 4th-gen. cephalosporin; inhibits cell wall synthesis **Dose:** 1–2 g IV q12h; ↓ in renal impairment **Caution/Contra:** [B, +] **Supplied:** Inj 500 mg, 1, 2 g **Notes/SE:** Rash, pruritus, N/V/D, fever, HA, positive Coombs' test w/o hemolysis; **see Cefaclor. Additional Interactions:** ↓ effects of oral contraceptives **NIPE:** ⊘ use alcohol with drug or w/n 3 d of taking drug

Cefixime (Suprax) **Uses:** Infections caused by susceptible bacteria involving the respiratory tract, skin, bone, and urinary tract **Action:** 3rd-gen. cephalosporin; inhibits cell wall synthesis **Dose:** *Adults.* 200–400 mg PO qd-bid. *Peds.* 8 mg/kg/d PO ÷ qd-bid; ↓ in renal impairment **Caution/Contra:** [B, +] **Supplied:** Tabs 200, 400 mg; susp 100 mg/5 mL **Notes/SE:** Use susp for otitis media; N/V/D, flatulence, abdominal pain; **see Cefaclor. Additional Interactions:** ↓ effects of oral contraceptives

Cefmetazole (Zefazone) **Uses:** Infections involving the upper and lower respiratory tract, skin, bone, urinary tract, abdomen, and gynecologic system **Action:** 2nd-gen. cephalosporin; inhibits cell wall synthesis **Dose:** *Adults.* 1–2 mg IV q8h; ↓ in renal impairment **Caution/Contra:** [B, +] **Supplied:** Inj 1, 2 g **Notes/SE:** Has more gram– activity than 1st-gen. cephalosporins; has anaerobic activity; ↑ risk of bleeding; rash, diarrhea; **see Cefaclor. Additional NIPE:** ⊘ use alcohol with drug or w/n 3 d of taking drug

Cefonicid (Monocid) **Uses:** Susceptible bacterial infections (respiratory tract, skin, bone and joint, urinary tract, gynecologic, sepsis) **Action:** 2nd-gen. cephalosporin **Dose:** *Adults.* 1 g/24 h IM/IV; ↓ in renal impairment **Caution/Contra:** [B, +] **Supplied:** Powder for inj 500 mg, 1 g **Notes/SE:** Diarrhea, rash, eosinophilia, ↑ transaminases; **see Cefaclor**

Cefoperazone (Cefobid) **Uses:** Susceptible bacterial infections (respiratory, skin, urinary tract, sepsis); as a 3rd-gen. cephalosporin, cefoperazone has activity against gram– organisms (eg, *E. coli, Klebsiella*) and variable activity against *Streptococcus* and *Staphylococcus* spp; active against *P. aeruginosa* but less than ceftazidime **Action:** 3rd-gen. cephalosporin **Dose:** *Adults.* 2–4 g/d IM/IV ÷ q12h (12 g/d max). *Peds.* 100–150 mg/kg/d IM/IV ÷ bid-tid; ↓ in renal impairment **Caution/Contra:** [B, +] **Supplied:** Powder for inj 1, 2 g **Notes/SE:** Diarrhea, rash, eosinophilia, ↑ LFTs, hypoprothrombinemia, and bleeding (due to MTT side chain); **see Cefaclor. Additional NIPE:** ⊘ use alcohol with drug or w/n 3 d of taking drug

Cefotaxime (Claforan) **Uses:** Infections involving the respiratory tract, skin, bone, urinary tract, meningitis, sepsis **Action:** 3rd-gen. cephalosporin; inhibits cell wall synthesis **Dose:** *Adults.* 1–2 g IV q4–12h. *Peds.* 100–200 mg/kg/d IV ÷ q6–8h; ↓ in renal impairment **Caution/Contra:** [B, +] **Supplied:** Powder for inj 500 mg, 1, 2 g **Notes/SE:** Diarrhea, rash, eosinophilia, ↑ transaminases; **see Cefaclor. Additional NIPE:** ⊘ use alcohol with drug or w/n 3 d of taking drug

Cefotetan (Cefotan) **Uses:** Infections involving the upper and lower respiratory tract, skin, bone, urinary tract, abdomen, and gynecologic system **Action:** 2nd-gen. cephalosporin; inhibits cell wall synthesis **Dose:** *Adults.* 1–2 g IV q12h. *Peds.* 40–80 mg/kg/d IV ÷ q12h; ↓ in renal impairment **Caution/Contra:** [B, +] **Supplied:** Powder for inj 1, 2 g **Notes/SE:** More gram– activity than 1st-gen. cephalosporins; has anaerobic activity; diarrhea, rash, eosinophilia, ↑ transaminases, hypoprothrombinemia, bleeding (due to MTT side chain); **see Cefaclor. Additional NIPE:** ⊘ use alcohol with drug or w/n 3 d of taking drug

Cefoxitin (Mefoxin) **Uses:** Infections involving the upper and lower respiratory tract, skin, bone, urinary tract, abdomen, and gynecologic system **Action:** 2nd-gen. cephalosporin; inhibits cell wall synthesis **Dose:** *Adults.* 1–2 mg IV q6h. *Peds.* 80–160 mg/kg/d ÷ q4–6h; ↓ in renal impairment **Caution/Contra:** [B, +] **Supplied:** Powder for inj 1, 2 g **Notes/SE:** More gram– activity than 1st-gen. cephalosporins; has anaerobic activity; diarrhea, rash, eosinophilia, ↑ transaminases; **see Cefaclor**

Cefpodoxime (Vantin) **Uses:** Infections involving the respiratory tract, skin, and urinary tract **Action:** 3rd-gen. cephalosporin; inhibits cell wall synthesis **Dose:** *Adults.* 200–400 mg PO q12h. *Peds.* 10 mg/kg/d PO ÷ bid; ? in renal impairment; take with food **Caution/Contra:** [B, +] **Supplied:** Tabs 100, 200 mg; susp 50, 100 mg/5 mL **Notes/SE:** Drug interactions with agents that increase gastric pH; diarrhea, rash, eosinophilia, ↑ transaminases; **see Cefaclor. Additional Interactions:** ↑ effects if taken with food

Cefprozil (Cefzil) **Uses:** Infections involving the upper and lower respiratory tract, skin, and urinary tract **Action:** 2nd-gen. cephalosporin; inhibits cell wall synthesis **Dose:** *Adults.* 250–500 mg PO qd–bid. *Peds.* 7.5–15 mg/kg/d PO ÷ bid; ↓ in renal impairment **Caution/Contra:** [B, +] **Supplied:** Tabs 250, 500 mg; susp 125, 250 mg/5 mL **Notes/SE:** More gram– activity than 1st-gen. cephalosporins; use higher doses for otitis and pneumonia; diarrhea, rash, eosinophilia, ↑ transaminases; **see Cefaclor**

Ceftazidime (Fortaz, Ceptaz, Tazidime, Tazicef) **Uses:** Infections involving the respiratory tract, skin, bone, urinary tract, meningitis, and septicemia **Action:** 3rd-gen. cephalosporin; inhibits cell wall synthesis **Dose:** *Adults.* 1–2 g IV q8h. *Peds.* 30–50 mg/kg/d IV ÷ q8h; ↓ in renal impairment **Caution/Contra:** [B, +] **Supplied:** Powder for inj 1, 2 g **Notes/SE:** Diarrhea, rash, eosinophilia, ↑ transaminases; **see Cefaclor. Additional NIPE:** ⊘ use alcohol with drug w/n 3 d of taking drug

Ceftibuten (Cedax) **Uses:** Infections involving the respiratory tract, skin, and urinary tract **Action:** 3rd-gen. cephalosporin; inhibits cell wall synthesis **Dose:** *Adults.* 400 mg/d PO. *Peds.* 9 mg/kg/d PO; ↓ in renal impairment; take on an empty stomach **Caution/Contra:** [B, +] **Supplied:** Caps 400 mg; susp 90, 180 mg/5 mL **Notes/SE:** Little activity against *Streptococcus;* diarrhea, rash, eosinophilia, ↑ transaminases; **see Cefaclor. Additional NIPE:** ⊘ use alcohol with drug w/n 3 d of taking drug

Ceftizoxime (Cefizox) **Uses:** Infections involving the respiratory tract, skin, bone, urinary tract, meningitis, and septicemia **Action:** 3rd-gen cephalosporin; inhibits cell wall synthesis **Dose:** *Adults.* 1–2 g IV q8–12h. *Peds.* 150–200 mg/kg/d IV ÷ q6–8h; ÷ in renal impairment **Caution/Contra:** [B, +] **Supplied:** Inj 500 mg, 1, 2 g **Notes/SE:** Diarrhea, rash, eosinophilia, ↑ transaminases; see Cefaclor

Ceftriaxone (Rocephin) **Uses:** Respiratory tract, skin, bone, urinary tract infections, meningitis, and septicemia; pneumonia and GC **Action:** 3rd-gen.

cephalosporin; inhibits cell wall synthesis **Dose:** *Adults.* 1–2 g IV q12–24h. *Peds.* 50–100 mg/kg/d IV ÷ q12–24h; ↓ in renal impairment **Caution/Contra:** [B, +] **Supplied:** Powder for inj 250 mg, 1, 2 g **Notes/SE:** Diarrhea, rash, eosinophilia, ↑ transaminases; see Cefaclor. **Additional NIPE:** ⊘ use alcohol with drug or w/n 3 d of taking drug, ⊘ mix with other antimicrobials

Cefuroxime (Ceftin [oral], Zinacef [parenteral]) Uses: Upper and lower respiratory tract, skin, bone, urinary tract, abdomen, and gynecologic infections **Action:** 2nd-gen. cephalosporin; inhibits cell wall synthesis **Dose:** *Adults.* 750 mg–1.5 g IV q8h or 250–500 mg PO bid. *Peds.* 100–150 mg/kg/d IV ÷ q8h or 20–30 mg/kg/d PO ÷ bid; adjust in renal impairment; take with food **Caution/Contra:** [B, +] **Supplied:** Tabs 125, 250, 500 mg; susp 125, 250 mg/5 mL; powder for inj 750 mg, 1.5, 7.5 g **Notes/SE:** ↑ Gram– activity over 1st-gen. cephalosporins; IV crosses blood–brain barrier; diarrhea, rash, eosinophilia, ↑ LFTs; see Cefaclor **Additional NIPE:** ⊘ use alcohol with drug or w/n 3 d of taking drug, food will ↓ GI distress & ↑ absorption, swallow tabs whole

Celecoxib (Celebrex) Uses: Osteoarthritis and RA; acute pain, primary dysmenorrhea; preventive in familial adenomatous polyposis **Action:** NSAID; inhibits the COX-2 pathway **Dose:** 100–200 mg/d or bid; caution in renal impairment; ↓ with hepatic impairment **Caution/Contra:** [C, ?] Allergy to sulfonamides **Supplied:** Caps 100, 200 mg **Notes/SE:** GI upset, HTN, edema, renal failure, HA, no effect on platelets/bleeding time; can affect drugs metabolized by P-450 pathway **Interactions:** ↑ effects with fluconazole; ↑ effects of lithium; ↑ risks of GI upset &/or bleeding with ASA, NSAIDs, warfarin, alcohol; ↓ effects with aluminum- & magnesium-containing antacids; ↓ effects of thiazide diuretics, loop diuretics, ACEIs **Labs:** ↑ LFTs, BUN, creatinine, CPK, alkaline phosphatase; monitor for hypercholesterolemia, hyperglycemia, hypokalemia, hypophosphatemia, albuminuria, hematuria **NIPE:** Take with food if GI distress

Cephalexin (Keflex, Keftab) Uses: Infections due to *Streptococcus, Staphylococcus, E. coli, Proteus,* and *Klebsiella* involving skin, bone, upper and lower respiratory tract, and urinary tract **Action:** 1st-gen. cephalosporin; inhibits cell wall synthesis **Dose:** *Adults.* 250–500 mg PO qid. *Peds.* 25–100 mg/kg/d PO ÷ qid; ↓ in renal impairment; take on an empty stomach **Caution/Contra:** [B, +] **Supplied:** Caps 250, 500 mg; tabs 250, 500, 1000 mg; susp 125, 250 mg/5 mL **Notes/SE:** Diarrhea, rash, eosinophilia, ↑ LFTs

CefaclorCephradine (Velosef) Uses: Various bacterial infections (includes group A β-hemolytic strep) **Action:** 1st-gen. cephalosporin; inhibits cell wall synthesis **Dose:** *Adults.* 2–4 g/d PO/IV ÷ qid (8 g/d max). *Peds >9 mon.* 25–100 mg/kg/d ÷ bid–qid (4 g/d max); ↓ in renal impairment **Caution/Contra:** [B, +] **Supplied:** Caps 250, 500 mg; powder for susp 125, 250 mg/5 mL, injectable **Notes/SE:** Diarrhea, rash, eosinophilia, ↑ LFTs; see Cefaclor. **Additional NIPE:** ⊘ use alcohol with drug or w/n 3 d of taking drug, ⊘ take with any other antibiotic, take with food

Cetirizine (Zyrtec) **Uses:** Allergic rhinitis and chronic urticaria **Action:** Nonsedating antihistamine **Dose:** *Adults & Children >6 y:* 5–10 mg/d. *Peds: 6–11 mon:* 2.5 mg/d. *12–23 mon:* 2.5 mg qd–bid; ↓ in renal/hepatic impairment **Caution/Contra:** [B, ?/–] **Supplied:** Tabs 5, 10 mg; syrup 5 mg/5 mL **Notes/SE:** HA, drowsiness, xerostomia **Interactions:** ↑ effects with anticholinergics, CNS depressants, theophylline, alcohol **Labs:** May cause false negatives with allergy skin tests **NIPE:** ⊘ take with alcohol or CNS depressants

Charcoal, Activated (Superchar, Actidose, Liqui-Char) **Uses:** Emergency treatment in poisoning by most drugs and chemicals **Action:** Adsorbent detoxicant **Dose:** Also give 70% sorbitol solution (2 mL/kg body weight) *Adults. Acute intoxication:* 30–100 g/dose. *GI dialysis:* 25–50 g q4–6h. *Peds. Acute intoxication:* 1–2 g/kg/dose. *GI dialysis:* 5–10 g/dose q4–8h **Caution/Contra:** [C, ?] Iron, lithium, lead, alkali, acid poisonings **Supplied:** Powder, liq **Notes/SE:** Some liq dosage forms in sorbitol base (a cathartic). If sorbitol used, monitor for hypokalemia and hypomagnesemia. Protect the airway in lethargic or comatose patients; vomiting, diarrhea, black stools **Interactions:** ↓ effects if taken with ice cream, milk, or sherbert; ↓ effects of digoxin & absorption of other oral meds, ↓ effects of syrup of ipecac **NIPE:** Most effective if given w/n 30 min of acute poisoning, only give to conscious patients

Chloral Hydrate [C-IV] **Uses:** Nocturnal and preoperative sedation **Action:** Sedative hypnotic **Dose:** *Adults. Hypnotic:* 500 mg–1 g PO or PR 30 min hs or before procedure. *Sedative:* 250 mg PO or PR tid. *Peds. Hypnotic:* 20–40 mg/kg/24 h PO or PR 30 min hs or before procedure. *Sedative:* 25–50 mg/kg/d q6–8h; avoid use in CrCl <50 mL/min or severe hepatic impairment **Caution/Contra:** [C, +] **Supplied:** Caps 500 mg; syrup 250, 500 mg/5 mL; supp 324, 500, 648 mg **Notes/SE:** Mix syrup in water or fruit juice; drowsiness, ataxia, dizziness, nightmares, rash **Interactions:** ↑ effects with antihistamines, barbiturates, paraldehyde, CNS depressants, opioid analgesics, alcohol; ↑ effects of anticoagulants **Labs:** false positive of urine glucose, may interfer with tests for catecholamines and urinary 17-hydroxycorticosteroids **NIPE:** ⊘ take with alcohol, CNS depressants; ⊘ chew or crush capsules

Chlorambucil (Leukeran) **Uses:** CLL, Hodgkin's disease, Waldenström's macroglobulinemia **Action:** Alkylating agent **Dose:** 0.1–0.2 mg/kg/d for 3–6 wk or 0.4 mg/kg q2wk (refer to specific protocol) **Caution/Contra:** [D, ?] **Supplied:** Tabs 2 mg **Notes/SE:** Myelosuppression, CNS stimulation, N/V, drug fever, skin rash, chromosomal damage that can result in secondary leukemias, alveolar dysplasia, pulmonary fibrosis, hepatotoxicity **Interactions:** ↑ bone marrow suppression with antineoplastic drugs and immunosuppressants; ↑ risk of bleeding with ASA, anticoagulants **Labs:** ↑ urine and serum uric acid, ALT, alkaline phosphatase **NIPE:** ⊘ PRG, breast-feeding; infection; ↑ fluids to 2–3 L/day; monitor lab work periodically & CBC with differential weekly during drug use, may cause hair loss

Chlordiazepoxide (Librium) [C-IV]   Uses: Anxiety, tension, alcohol withdrawal, and preoperative apprehension Action: Benzodiazepine; antianxiety agent Dose: *Adults. Mild anxiety:* 5–10 mg PO tid–qid or PRN. *Severe anxiety:* 25–50 mg IM, IV, or PO q6–8h or PRN. *Alcohol withdrawal:* 50–100 mg IM or IV; repeat in 2–4 h if needed, up to 300 mg in 24 h; gradually taper the daily dosage. *Peds >6 y:* 0.5 mg/kg/24 h PO or IM ÷ q6–8h; ↓ in renal impairment, elderly; avoid in hepatic impairment Caution/Contra: [D, ?] Supplied: Caps 5, 10, 25 mg; tabs 10, 25 mg; inj 100 mg Notes/SE: Erratic IM absorption; drowsiness, fatigue, memory impairment, xerostomia, weight gain Interactions: ↑ effects with antidepressants, antihistamines, anticonvulsants, barbiturates, general anesthetics, MAOIs, narcotics, phenothiazines cimetidine, disulfiram, fluconazole, itraconazole, ketoconazole, oral contraceptives, isoniazid, metoprolol, propoxyphene, propranolol, valproic acid, alcohol, grapefruit juice, kava kava, valerian; ↑ effects of digoxin, phenytoin; ↓ effects with aminophylline, antacids, carbamazepine, dyphylline, oxitriphylline, theophylline, rifampin, rifabutin, tobacco; ↓ effects of levodopa Labs: ↑ LFTs, alkaline phosphatase, bilirubin, triglycerides; false ↑ urine 5-HIAA, urine 17-ketosteroids; false + urine PRG test; false ↓ urine 17 ketogenic steroids; ↓ HDL NIPE: ⊘ alcohol, PRG, breast-feeding; risk of photosensitivity, orthostatic hypotension, tachycardia

Chlorothiazide (Diuril)   Uses: HTN, edema Action: Thiazide diuretic Dose: *Adults.* 500 mg–1 g PO or IV qd–bid. *Peds.* 20–30 mg/kg/24 h PO ÷ bid Caution/Contra: [D, +] Contra in cross-sensitivity to thiazides/sulfonamides, anuria Supplied: Tabs 250, 500 mg; susp 250 mg/5 mL; inj 500 mg/vial Notes/SE: Hypokalemia, hyponatremia, dizziness, hyperglycemia, hyperuricemia, hyperlipidemia, photosensitivity Interactions: ↑ effects with ACEI, amphotericin B, corticosteroids; ↑ effects of diazoxide, lithium, methotrexate; ↓ effects with colestipol, cholestyramine, NSAIDs; ↓ effects of hypoglycemics Labs: ↑ CPK, ammonia, amylase, calcium, chloride, cholesterol, glucose, chloride, magnesium, K⁺, sodium, uric acid NIPE: Monitor for gout, hyperglycemia, photosensitivity, I&O, wt

Chlorpheniramine (Chlor-Trimeton, others)   Uses: Allergic reactions Action: Antihistamine Dose: *Adults.* 4 mg PO q4–6h or 8–12 mg PO bid of SR. *Peds.* 0.35 mg/kg/24 h PO ÷ q4–6h or 0.2 mg/kg/24 h SR Caution/Contra: [C, ?/–] Supplied: Tabs 4 mg; chew tabs 2 mg; SR tabs 8, 12 mg; syrup 2 mg/5 mL; inj 10, 100 mg/mL Notes/SE: Anticholinergic SE and sedation common, orthostatic hypotension, QT changes, extrapyramidal reactions, photosensitivity Interactions: ↑ effects with other CNS depressants, alcohol, opioids, sedatives, MAOIs, atropine, haloperidol, phenothiazines, quinidine, disopyramide; ↑ effects of epinephrine; ↓ effects of heparin, sulfonylureas Labs: False negatives with allergy testing NIPE: Stop drug 4 d prior to allergy testing, take with food if GI distress

Chlorpromazine (Thorazine)   Uses: Psychotic disorders, apprehension, intractable hiccups, N/V Action: Phenothiazine antipsychotic; antiemetic Dose: *Adults. Psychosis:* 10–25 mg PO or PR bid–tid (usual 30–800 mg/d in ÷ doses).

Children. *Psychosis & N/V:* 0.5–1 mg/kg/dose PO q4–6h or IM/IV q6–8h. *Severe symptoms:* 25 mg IM; can repeat in 1 h; then 25–50 mg PO or PR tid. *Hiccups:* 25–50 mg PO bid–tid; avoid in severe hepatic impairment **Caution/Contra:** [C, ?/–] **Supplied:** Tabs 10, 25, 50, 100, 200 mg; SR caps 30, 75, 150 mg; syrup 10 mg/5 mL; conc 30, 100 mg/mL; supp 25, 100 mg; inj 25 mg/mL **Notes/SE:** Extrapyramidal SE and sedation; α-adrenergic blocking properties; prolongs QT interval **Interactions:** ↑ effects with amodiaquine, chloroquine, sulfadoxine-pyrimethamine, antidepressants, narcotic analgesics, propranolol, quinidine, BBs, MAOIs, TCAs, alcohol, kava kava; ↑ effects of anticholinergics, centrally acting antihypertensives, propranolol, valproic acid; ↓ effects with antacids, antidiarrheals, barbiturates, lithium, tobacco; ↓ effects of anticonvulsants, guanethidine, levodopa, lithium, warfarin **Labs:** False + for amylase, phenylketonuria, urine bilirubin, urine protein, uroporphyrins, urobilinogen, PRG test; ↑ plasma cholesterol **NIPE:** Risk of photosensitivity & tardive dyskinesia, take with food if GI upset, may darken urine

Chlorpropamide (Diabinese)
Uses: Type 2 DM **Action:** Sulfonylurea; ↑ release of insulin from pancreas; ↑ insulin sensitivity at peripheral sites; ↓ hepatic glucose output **Dose:** 100–500 mg/d; avoid use in CrCl <50 mL/min; ↓ in hepatic impairment; take with food, avoid alcohol (disulfiram-like reaction) **Caution/Contra:** [C, ?/–] **Supplied:** Tabs 100, 250 mg **Notes/SE:** HA, dizziness, rash, photosensitivity, hypoglycemia, SIADH **Interactions:** ↑ effects with ASA, NSAIDs, anticoagulants, BBs, chloramphenicol, guanethidine, insulin, MAOIs, phenytoin, probenecid, rifampin, sulfonamides, alcohol, juniper berries, ginseng, garlic, fenugreek, coriander, dandelion root, celery, bitter melon, ginkgo biloba; ↑ effects of anticoagulants, phenytoin, ASA, NSAIDs; ↓ effects with diazoxide, thiazide diuretics **Labs:** False ↑ serum calcium

Chlorthalidone (Hygroton)
Uses: HTN **Action:** Thiazide diuretic **Dose:** *Adults.* 50–100 mg/d PO qd. *Peds.* 2 mg/kg/dose PO 3×/wk or 1–2 mg/kg/d PO; ↓ in renal impairment **Caution/Contra:** [D, +] Anuria **Supplied:** Tabs 15, 25, 50, 100 mg **Notes/SE:** Hypokalemia, dizziness, photosensitivity, hyperglycemia, hyperuricemia, sexual dysfunction **Interactions:** ↑ effects with ACEIs, diazoxide; ↑ effects of digoxin, lithium, methotrexate; ↓ effects with cholestyramine, colestipol, NSAIDs; ↓ effects of hypoglycemics; ↓ K⁺ with amphotericin B, carbenoxolone, corticosteroids **Labs:** ↑ CPK, amylase, calcium, chloride, cholesterol, glucose, uric acid; ↓ chloride, magnesium, K⁺, sodium **NIPE:** May take with food, take early in day, use sunscreen

Chlorzoxazone (Paraflex, Parafon Forte DSC)
Uses: Adjunct to rest and physical therapy for the relief of discomfort associated with acute, painful musculoskeletal conditions **Action:** Centrally acting skeletal muscle relaxant **Dose:** *Adults.* 250–500 mg PO tid–qid. *Peds.* 20 mg/kg/d in 3–4 ÷ doses **Caution/Contra:** [C, ?] Contra in severe liver disease **Supplied:** Tabs 250, 500 mg; caps 250, 500 mg **Notes/SE:** Drowsiness, tachycardia, dizziness, hepatotoxicity, angioedema **Interactions:** ↑ effects with antihistamines, CNS depressants,

MAOIs, TCAs, opioids, alcohol, watercress **Labs:** Monitor LFTs **NIPE:** Urine may turn reddish purple or orange

Cholecalciferol [Vitamin D₃] (Delta D)   **Uses:** Dietary supplement for treatment of vitamin D deficiency **Action:** Enhances intestinal Ca absorption **Dose:** 400–1000 IU/d PO **Caution/Contra:** [A (D, doses above the RDA), +] Hypercalcemia **Supplied:** Tabs 400, 1000 IU **Notes/SE:** 1 mg of cholecalciferol = 40,000 IU of vitamin D activity; vitamin D toxicity (renal failure, HTN, psychosis)

Cholestyramine (Questran)   **Uses:** Hypercholesterolemia; Rx pruritus associated with partial biliary obstruction **Action:** Binds intestinal bile acids to form insoluble complexes **Dose:** *Adults.* Individualize: 4 g/d–bid (↑ to max 24 g/d and 6 doses/d). *Peds.* 240 mg/kg/d in 3 ÷ doses **Caution/Contra:** [C, ?] **Supplied:** 4 g of cholestyramine resin/9 g of powder; *with aspartame:* 4 g resin/5 g of powder **Notes/SE:** Mix 4 g of cholestyramine in 2–6 oz of noncarbonated beverage; take other meds 1–2 h before or 6 h after cholestyramine; constipation, abdominal pain, bloating, HA **Interactions:** ↓ effects of acetaminophen, amiodarone, anticoagulants, ASA, cardiac glycosides, clindamycin, corticosteroids, diclofenac, fat-soluble vitamins, gemfibrozil, glipizide, iron salts, methotrexate, methyldopa, nicotinic acid, penicillins, phenobarbital, phenytoin, propranolol, thiazide diuretics, tetracyclines, thyroid drugs, troglitazone, ursodial, valproic acid, warfarin **Labs:** ↑ LFTs, PT, phosphorus, chloride, alkaline phosphatase, ↓ serum calcium, sodium, K⁺, cholesterol **NIPE:** ↑ fluids, take other drugs 1 h < or 4–6 h >

Ciclopirox (Loprox)   **Uses:** Tinea pedis, tinea cruris, tinea corporis, cutaneous candidiasis, tinea versicolor **Action:** Antifungal antibiotic **Dose:** *Adults & Peds >10 y.* Massage into affected area bid **Caution/Contra:** [B, ?] **Supplied:** Cream; gel; lotion 1% **Notes/SE:** Pruritus, local irritation **Interactions:** None noted **NIPE:** Nail lacquer may take 6 mo to see improvement, cream/gel/lotion see improvement by 4 wk

Cidofovir (Vistide)   **WARNING:** Renal impairment is the major toxicity. Follow administration instructions **Uses:** CMV retinitis **Action:** Selective inhibition of viral DNA synthesis **Dose:** *Rx:* 5 mg/kg IV once/wk for 2 wk; administered with probenecid. *Maint:* 5 mg/kg IV once/2 wk; administered with probenecid. *Probenecid:* 2 g PO 3 h prior to cidofovir, and then 1 g PO at 2 h and 8 h after cidofovir; ↓ in renal impairment **Caution/Contra:** [C –] SCr >1.5 mg/dL or CrCl <55 mL/min or urine protein >100 mg/dL; other nephrotoxic drugs, hypersensitivity to probenecid or sulfa **Supplied:** Inj 75 mg/mL **Notes/SE:** Hydrate with NS prior to each inf; renal toxicity, renal function; chills, fever, HA, N/V/D, thrombocytopenia, neutropenia **Interactions:** ↑ nephrotoxicity with aminoglycosides, amphotericin B, foscarnet, IV pentamidine, NSAIDs, vancomycine; ↑ effects with zidovudine **Labs:** ↑ serum creatinine, BUN, alkaline phosphatase, LFTs, urine protein, WBCs; monitor for hematuria, glycosuria, hypocalcemia, hyperglycemia, hypokalemia, hyperlipidemia **NIPE:** Coadminister oral probenecid with each dose, possible hair loss

Cimetidine (Tagamet)   **Uses:** Duodenal ulcer; ulcer prophylaxis in hypersecretory states, eg, trauma, burns, surgery; GERD **Action:** H₂ receptor antagonist **Dose:** *Adults. Active ulcer:* 2400 mg/d IV cont inf or 300 mg IV q6h; 400 mg PO bid or 800 mg hs. *Maint:* 400 mg PO hs. *GERD:* 800 mg PO bid; maint 800 mg PO hs. *Peds. Infants:* 10–20 mg/kg/24 h PO or IV ÷ q6–12h. *Children:* 20–40 mg/kg/24 h PO or IV ÷ q6h; ↑ dosing interval with renal insufficiency; ↓ dose in the elderly **Caution/Contra:** [B, +] Many drug interactions **Supplied:** Tabs 200, 300, 400, 800 mg; liq 300 mg/5 mL; inj 300 mg/2 mL **Notes/SE:** Dizziness, agitation, thrombocytopenia, gynecomastia **Interactions:** ↑ effects of benzodiazepines, disulfram, flecainide, isoniazid, lidocaine, oral contraceptives, sulfonylureas, warfarin, theophylline, phenytoin, metronidazole, triamterene, procainamide, quinidine, propranolol, diazepam, nifedipine, TCA, procainamide, tacrine, carbamazepine, valproic acid, xanthines; ↓ effects with antacids, tobacco; ↓ effects of digoxin, ketoconazole, cefpodoxime, indomethacin, tetracyclines **Labs:** ↑ creatinine, LFTs, false + hemoccult **NIPE:** Take with meals, monitor for gynecomastia, breast pain, impotence

Ciprofloxacin (Cipro)   **Uses:** Broad-spectrum activity against a variety of gram+ and gram– aerobic bacteria **Action:** Quinolone antibiotic; inhibits DNA gyrase **Dose:** *Adults.* 250–750 mg PO q12h or 200–400 mg IV q12h; ↓ in renal impairment; avoid antacids; reduce/restrict caffeine intake **Caution/Contra:** [C, ?/–] Children <18 y **Supplied:** Tabs 100, 250, 500, 750 mg; susp 5, 10 g/100 mL; inj 200, 400 mg **Notes/SE:** Little activity against streptococci; interactions with theophylline, caffeine, sucralfate, warfarin, antacids; restlessness, N/V/D, rash, ruptured tendons, ↑ LFTs **Interactions:** ↑ effects with probenecid; ↑ effects of diazepam, theophylline, caffeine, metoprolol, propranolol, phenytoin, warfarin; ↓ effects with antacids, didanosine, iron salts, magnesium, sucralfate, sodium bicarbonate, zinc **Labs:** ↑ LFTs, alkaline phosphatase, serum bilirubin, LDH, BUN, serum creatinine, amylase, uric acid, K⁺, PT, triglycerides, cholesterol; ↓ HMG, HCT; **NIPE:** ⊘ give to children <18 y, ↑ fluids to 2–3 L/d, may cause photosensitivity

Ciprofloxacin, Ophthalmic (Ciloxan)   **Uses:** Rx and prevention of ocular infections, eg, conjunctivitis, blepharitis, cornea; abrasions **Action:** Quinolone antibiotic; inhibits DNA gyrase **Dose:** 1–2 gtt in eye(s) q2h while awake for 2 d, then 1–2 gtt q4h while awake for 5 d **Caution/Contra:** [C, ?/–] **Supplied:** Soln 3.5 mg/mL **Notes/SE:** Local irritation **Interactions:** None reported **NIPE:** Limited systemic absorption

Ciprofloxacin, Otic (Cipro HC Otic)   **Uses:** Otitis externa **Action:** Quinolone antibiotic; inhibits DNA gyrase **Dose:** *Adults & Peds >1 mon.* 1–2 gtt in ear(s) bid for 7 d **Caution/Contra:** [C, ?/–] Perforated tympanic membrane, viral infections of the external canal **Supplied:** Susp ciprofloxacin 0.2% and hydrocortisone 1% **Notes/SE:** HA, pruritus **NIPE:** With diabetics, first choice therapy for otitis externa

Cisplatin (Platinol AQ) **Uses:** Testicular, small-cell and non-small-cell lung, bladder, ovarian, breast, head and neck, and penile CAs; osteosarcoma; pediatric brain tumors **Action:** DNA-binding; intrastrand cross-linking; formation of DNA adducts **Dose:** 20 mg/m²/d for 5 d q3wk; 120 mg/m² q3–4wk; 100 mg/m² on days 1 and 8 q20d (refer to specific protocols); ↓ in renal impairment **Caution/Contra:** [D, –] Preexisting renal insufficiency, myelosuppression, hearing impairment **Supplied:** Inj 1 mg/mL **Notes/SE:** Allergic reactions, N/V, nephrotoxicity (exacerbated by concurrent administration of other nephrotoxic drugs and minimized by NS inf and mannitol diuresis), high-frequency hearing loss in 30%, peripheral "stocking glove"-type neuropathy, cardiotoxicity (ST-,T-wave changes), hypomagnesemia, mild myelosuppression, hepatotoxicity; renal impairment is dose-related and cumulative **Interactions:** ↑ effects of antineoplastic drugs and radiation therapy; ↑ ototoxicity with loop diuretics; ↑ nephrotoxicity with aminoglycosides, amphotericin B, vancomycin; ↓ effects with sodium thiosulfate; ↓ effects of phenytoin **Labs:** ↑ BUN, creatinine, serum bilirubin, AST; ↓ calcium, magnesium, phosphate, sodium, K⁺ **NIPE:** Drug ineffective with aluminum needles or equipment, may cause infertility, ⊘ immunizations

Citalopram (Celexa) **Uses:** Depression **Action:** SSRI **Dose:** Initial 20 mg/d, may be ↑ to 40 mg/d **Caution/Contra:** [C, +/–] Contra if used with MAOI or w/n 14 d of MAOI administration **Supplied:** Tabs 20, 40 mg **Notes/SE:** Somnolence, insomnia, anxiety, xerostomia, sexual dysfunction **Interactions:** ↑ effects with azole antifungals, cimetidine, lithium, macroloids, alcohol; ↑ effects of BBs, carbamazepine, warfarin; ↓ effects with carbamazepine; ↓ effects of phenytoin; may cause fatal reaction with MAOIs **Labs:** ↑ LFTs, alkaline phosphatase **NIPE:** ⊘ PRG, breast-feeding, use barrier contraception

Cladribine (Leustatin) **Uses:** HCL **Action:** Induces DNA strand breakage; interferes with DNA repair/synthesis **Dose:** 0.09 mg/kg/d cont IV inf for 7 d (refer to specific protocols) **Caution/Contra:** [D, ?/–] **Supplied:** Inj 1 mg/mL **Notes/SE:** Myelosuppression; T-lymphocyte suppression may be prolonged (26–34 wk); fever in 46% (possibly tumor lysis); infections (especially lung and IV sites); rash (50%) **Interactions:** ↑ risk of bleeding with anticoagulants, NSAIDs, salicylates, ↑ risk of nephrotoxicity with amphotericin B; **Labs:** Monitor CBC, LFTs, serum creatinine; **NIPE:** ⊘ PRG, breast-feeding

Clarithromycin (Biaxin) **Uses:** Upper and lower respiratory tract infections, skin and skin structure infections, *H. pylori* infections, and infections caused by nontuberculosis (atypical) *Mycobacterium*; prevention of MAC infections in HIV-infected individuals. **Action:** Macrolide antibiotic; inhibits protein synthesis **Dose:** *Adults.* 250–500 mg PO bid or 1000 mg (2 × 500 mg ER tab)/d. *Mycobacterium:* 500–1000 mg PO bid. *Peds.* 7.5 mg/kg/dose PO bid; ↓ in renal/hepatic impairment **Caution/Contra:** [C, ?] **Supplied:** Tabs 250, 500 mg; susp 125, 250 mg/ 5 mL; 500 mg ER tab **Notes/SE:** Increases theophylline and carbamazepine levels; prolongs QT interval; multiple drug interactions; causes metallic taste, diarrhea, nausea, abdominal pain, HA **Interactions:** ↑ effects with amprenavir, indinavir, nelfinavir, ritonavir; ↑ effects of atorvastatin, buspirone, clozapine, colchicine, diazepam, felodipine, itraconazole, lovastatin, simvastatin, methylprednisolone, theophylline, phenytoin, quinidine, digoxin, carbamazepine, triazolam, warfarin, ergotamine, alprazolam, valproic acid; ↓ effects with alcohol; ↓ effects of penicillin, zafirlukast **Labs:** ↑ serum AST, ALT, GTT, alkaline phosphatase, LDH, total bilirubin, BUN, creatinine, PT; ↓ WBC **NIPE:** May take with food

Clemastine Fumarate (Tavist)   **Uses:** Allergic rhinitis **Action:** Antihistamine **Dose:** *Adults & Peds >12 y.* 1.34 mg bid–2.68 mg tid; max 8.04 mg/d. *<12 y:* 0.4 mg PO bid **Caution/Contra:** [C, M] Narrow-angle glaucoma **Supplied:** Tabs 1.34, 2.68 mg; syrup 0.67 mg/5 mL **Notes/SE:** Drowsiness **Interactions:** ↑ effects with CNS depressants, MAOIs, alcohol; ↓ effects of heparin, sulfonylureas

Clindamycin (Cleocin, Cleocin-T)   **Uses:** Susceptible strains of streptococci, pneumococci, staphylococci, and gram+ and gram– anaerobes; no activity against gram– aerobes; bacterial vaginosis; topical for severe acne and vaginal infections **Action:** Bacteriostatic; interferes with protein synthesis **Dose:** *Adults.* 150–450 mg PO qid; 300–600 mg IV q6h or 900 mg IV q8h. *Vaginal:* 1 applicatorful hs for 7 d. *Topical:* Apply 1% gel, lotion, or soln bid. *Peds. Neonates:* 10–15 mg/kg/24 h ÷ q8–12h. *Children >1 mon:* 10–30 mg/kg/24 h ÷ q6–8h, to a max of 1.8 g/d oral or 4.8 g/d IV. *Topical:* Apply 1%, gel, lotion, or soln bid; adjust in severe hepatic impairment **Caution/Contra:** [B, +] **Supplied:** Caps 75, 150, 300 mg; susp 75 mg/5 mL; inj 300 mg/2 mL; vaginal cream 2% **Notes/SE:** Diarrhea may be pseudomembranous colitis caused by *C. difficile;* rash, ↑ LFTs **Interactions:** ↑ effects of neuromuscular blockage with tubocurarine, pancuronium; ↓ effects with erythromycin, kaolin, foods with sodium cyclamate **Labs:** Monitor CBC, LFTs, BUN, creatinine; false ↑ serum theophylline **NIPE:** ⊘ intercourse, tampons, douches while using vaginal cream; take oral meds with 8 oz water

Clofazimine (Lamprene)   **Uses:** Leprosy and combination therapy for MAC in AIDS **Action:** Bactericidal; inhibits DNA synthesis **Dose:** *Adults.* 100–300 mg PO qd. *Peds.* 1 mg/kg/d; take with meals **Caution/Contra:** [C, +/–] **Supplied:** Caps 50 mg **Notes/SE:** Pink to brownish-black discoloration of the skin and conjunctiva, dry skin, GI intolerance **Interactions:** ↑ effects with isoniazid, food, ↓ effect with dapsone **Labs:** ↑ effects of AST, serum bilirubin, albumin, glucose, ESR **NIPE:** Take with food

Clonazepam (Klonopin) [C-IV]   **Uses:** Lennox-Gastaut syndrome, akinetic and myoclonic seizures, absence seizures, panic attacks **Action:** Benzodiazepine; anticonvulsant **Dose:** *Adults.* 1.5 mg/d PO in 3 ÷ doses; ↑ by 0.5–1.0 mg/d q3d PRN up to 20 mg/d. *Peds.* 0.01–0.03 mg/kg/24 h PO ÷ tid; ↑ to 0.1–0.2 mg/kg/24 h tid; avoid abrupt withdrawal **Caution/Contra:** [D, M] Severe hepatic impairment, narrow-angle glaucoma **Supplied:** Tabs 0.5, 1.0, 2.0 mg **Notes/ SE:** CNS side effects, including drowsiness, dizziness, ataxia, memory impairment

Interactions: ↑ effects with anticonvulsants, antihistamines, cimetidine, ciprofloxacin, clarithromycin, clozapine, CNS depressants, diltiazem, disulfiram, digoxin, erythromycin, fluconazole, fluoxetine, isoniazid, itraconazole, ketoconazole, labetalol, levodopa, metoprolol, opioids, ritonavir, valproic acid, verapmil, alcohol, kava kava, valerian; ↑ effects of phenytoin; ↓ effects with barbiturates, carbamazepine, phenytoin, rifampin, rifabutin; ↓ effects of levodopa **NIPE:** ⊘ d/c abruptly

Clonidine, Oral (Catapres)
Uses: HTN; opioid, alcohol, and tobacco withdrawal **Action:** Centrally acting α-adrenergic stimulant **Dose:** *Adults.* 0.10 mg PO adjust daily by 0.1- to 0.2-mg increments (max 2.4 mg/d). *Peds.* 5–10 μg/kg/d ÷ q8–12h (max 0.9 mg/d) **Caution/Contra:** [C, +/–] Avoid with β-blocker **Supplied:** Tabs 0.1, 0.2, 0.3 mg **Notes/SE:** More effective for HTN if combined with diuretics; rebound HTN with abrupt cessation of doses >0.2 mg bid; drowsiness, orthostatic hypotension, xerostomia, constipation; bradycardia **Interactions:** ↑ effects with BBs, neuroleptics, nitroprusside, alcohol; ↓ effects of barbiturates; ↓ effects with MAOIs, TCAs, tolazoline, antidepressants, prazosin, capsicum; ↓ effects of levodopa **Labs:** ↑ glucose, phosphatase, CPK **NIPE:** Tolerance develops with long-term use

Clonidine, Transdermal (Catapres TTS)
Uses: HTN **Action:** Centrally acting α-adrenergic stimulant **Dose:** Apply 1 patch q7–10d to hairless area (upper arm/torso); titrate to effect; ↓ in severe renal impairment, do not DC abruptly (rebound HTN) **Caution/Contra:** [C, +/–] Avoid with BBs **Supplied:** TTS-1, TTS-2, TTS-3 (delivers 0.1, 0.2, 0.3 mg, respectively, of clonidine/d for 1 wk) **Notes/SE:** Doses >2 TTS-3 usually not associated with ↑ efficacy; steady state in 3 d; drowsiness, orthostatic hypotension, xerostomia, constipation, bradycardia; **see Clonidine. NIPE:** Rotate transdermal site weekly

Clopidogrel (Plavix)
Uses: Reduction of atherosclerotic events **Action:** Inhibits platelet aggregation **Dose:** 75 mg/d **Caution/Contra:** [B, ?] Active bleeding **Supplied:** Tabs 75 mg **Notes/SE:** Prolongs bleeding time, use with caution in persons at risk of bleeding from trauma and other causes; GI intolerance, HA, dizziness, rash, thrombocytopenia, leukopenia; platelet aggregation returns to baseline ~5 d after DC; platelet transfusion reverses effects acutely **Interactions:** ↑ risk of GI bleed with ASA, NSAIDs, heparin, warfarin, feverfew, garlic, ginger, ginkgo biloba; ↑ effects of phenytoin, tamoxifen, tolbutamide **Labs:** ↑ LFTs; ↓ platelets, neutrophils **NIPE:** d/c drug 1 wk prior to surgery

Clorazepate (Tranxene) [C-IV]
Uses: Acute anxiety disorders, acute alcohol withdrawal symptoms, adjunctive therapy in partial seizures **Action:** Benzodiazepine; antianxiety agent **Dose:** *Adults.* 15–60 mg/d PO single or ÷ doses. *Elderly and debilitated patients:* Start at 7.5–15 mg/d in ÷ doses. *Alcohol withdrawal:* Day 1: Initially, 30 mg; then 30–60 mg in ÷ doses. *Day 2:* 45–90 mg in ÷ doses. *Day 3:* 22.5–45 mg in ÷ doses. *Day 4:* 15–30 mg in ÷ doses. *Peds.* 3.75–7.5 mg/dose bid to 60 mg/d max ÷ bid–tid; monitor patients with renal/he-

patic impairment; avoid abrupt withdrawal **Caution/Contra:** [D, ?/–] **Supplied:** Tabs 3.75, 7.5, 11.25, 15, 22.5 mg **Notes/SE:** Monitor patients with renal/hepatic impairment (drug may accumulate); CNS depressant effects (drowsiness, dizziness, ataxia, memory impairment), hypotension **Interactions:** ↑ effects with antidepressants, antihistamines, barbiturates, MAOIs, narcotics, phenothiazines; cimetidine, disulfiram, alcohol; ↓ effects of levodopa; ↓ effects with ginkgo, tobacco **Labs:** ↓ HCT, abnormal LFTs, BUN, creatinine **NIPE:** ⊘ d/c abruptly

Clotrimazole (Lotrimin, Mycelex) **Uses:** Candidiasis and tinea infections **Action:** Antifungal agent; alters cell wall permeability **Dose:** *Oral:* One troche dissolved in mouth 5 ×/d for 14 d. *Vaginal:* Cream 1 applicatorful hs for 7–14 d. Tabs 100 mg vaginally hs for 7 d or 200 mg (2 tabs) vaginally hs for 3 d or 500-mg tabs vaginally hs once. *Topical:* Apply bid for 10–14 d **Caution/Contra:** [B, (C if oral)/?] **Supplied:** 1% cream; soln; lotion; troche 10 mg; vaginal tabs 100, 500 mg; vaginal cream 1% **Notes/SE:** Oral prophylaxis common in immunosuppressed patients; *topical SE:* Local irritation; *oral:* N/V, ↑ LFTs **Interactions:** ↑ effects of cyclosporine, tacrolimus; ↓ effects of spermicides

Clotrimazole and Betamethasone (Lotrisone) **Uses:** Fungal skin infections **Action:** Imidazole antifungal and antiinflammatory **Dose:** Apply and massage into area bid for 2–4 wk **Caution/Contra:** [C, ?] Children, varicella infection **Supplied:** Cream 15, 45 g **Notes/SE:** Local irritation, rash

Clozapine (Clozaril) **WARNING:** Myocarditis, agranulocytosis, seizures, and orthostatic hypotension have been associated with clozapine. **Uses:** Refractory severe schizophrenia **Action:** Tricyclic "atypical" antipsychotic **Dose:** Initially, 25 mg qd–bid; ↑ to 300–450 mg/d over 2 wk. Maintain at the lowest dose possible; do not DC abruptly **Caution/Contra:** [B, +/–] WBC count = 3500 cells/mm³ before Rx or <3000 cells/mm³ during Rx **Supplied:** Tabs 25, 100 mg **Notes/SE:** CBC weekly for the 1st 6 mo, then every other wk; tachycardia, drowsiness, weight gain, constipation, urinary incontinence, rash, seizures **Interactions:** ↑ effects with clarithromycin, cimetidine, erythromycin, fluoxetine, paroxetine, quinidine, sertraline; ↑ depressant effects with CNS depressants, alcohol; ↑ effects of digoxin, warfarin; ↓ effects with carbamazepine, phenytoin, primidone, phenobarbital, valproic acid, St. John's Wort, nutmeg, caffeine; ↓ effects of phenytoin **Labs:** Monitor WBCs **NIPE:** ↑ risk of developing agranulocytosis

Cocaine [C-II] **Uses:** Topical anesthetic for mucous membranes **Action:** Narcotic analgesic, local vasoconstrictor **Dose:** Apply lowest amount of topical soln that provides relief; 1 mg/kg max **Caution/Contra:** [C, ?] **Supplied:** Topical soln and viscous preparations 4, 10%; powder, soluble tabs (135 mg) for soln **Notes/SE:** CNS stimulation, nervousness, loss of taste/smell, chronic rhinitis **Interactions:** ↑ effects with MAOIs, ↑ risk of HTN & arrhythmias with epinephrine

Codeine [C-II] **Uses:** Mild–moderate pain; symptomatic relief of cough **Action:** Narcotic analgesic; depresses cough reflex **Dose:** *Adults. Analgesic:* 15–60 mg PO or IM qid PRN. *Antitussive:* 10–20 mg PO q4h PRN; max 120 mg/d. *Peds.*

Analgesic: 0.5–1 mg/kg/dose PO or IM q4–6h PRN. *Antitussive:* 1–1.5 mg/kg/24 h PO ÷ q4h; max 30 mg/24 h; ↓ in renal/hepatic impairment **Caution/Contra:** [C, (D if prolonged use or high doses at term), +] **Supplied:** Tabs 15, 30, 60 mg; soln 15 mg/5 mL; inj 30, 60 mg/mL **Notes/SE:** Usually combined with APAP for pain or with agents (eg, terpin hydrate as an antitussive); 120 mg IM = 10 mg IM morphine; drowsiness, constipation **Interactions:** ↑ CNS depression with CNS depressants, antidepressants, MAOIs, TCAs, barbiturates, benzodiazepines, muscle relaxants, phenothiazines, cimetidine, antihistamines, sedatives, alcohol; ↑ effects of digitoxin, phenytoin, rifampin; ↓ effects with nalbuphine, pentazocine, tobacco **Labs:** False ↑ amylase, lipase, ↑ urine morphine

Colchicine **Uses:** Acute gout **Action:** Inhibits migration of leukocytes; reduces production of lactic acid by leukocytes **Dose:** *Initially:* 0.5–1.2 mg PO, then 0.5–0.6 mg q1–2h until relief or GI side effects develop (max 8 mg/d); do not repeat for 3 d. *IV:* 1–3 mg, then 0.5 mg q6h until relief (max 4 mg/d); do not repeat for 7 d. *Prophylaxis:* PO 0.5–0.6 mg/d or 3–4 d/wk; ↓ renal impairment; caution in elderly **Caution/Contra:** [D, +] Serious renal, hepatic, cardiac, or GI disorder **Supplied:** Tabs 0.5, 0.6 mg; inj 1 mg/2 mL **Notes/SE:** Colchicine 1–2 mg IV w/in 24–48 h of an acute attack diagnostic/therapeutic in monoarticular arthritis; N/V/D, abdominal pain, bone marrow suppression, hepatotoxicity **Interactions:** ↑ GI effects with NSAIDs; ↑ effects of sympathomimetics, CNS depressants, bone marrow depressants, radiation therapy; ↓ effects of vitamin B_{12} **Labs:** Monitor CBC, BUN, creatinine; false + urine Hgb & RBCs **NIPE:** ⊘ alcohol

Colesevelam (Welchol) **Uses:** Reduction of LDL and total cholesterol **Action:** Bile acid sequestrant **Dose:** 3 tabs PO bid with meals **Caution/Contra:** [B, ?] Bowel obstruction **Supplied:** Tabs 625 mg **Notes/SE:** Constipation, dyspepsia, myalgia **Interactions:** ↓ effects of verapamil **Labs:** Monitor lipids **NIPE:** Take with food and liquid

Colestipol (Colestid) **Uses:** Adjunct to ↓ serum cholesterol in primary hypercholesterolemia **Action:** Binds intestinal bile acids to form an insoluble complex **Dose:** *Granules:* 5–30 g/d ÷ into 2–4 doses; *tabs:* 2–16 g/d qd–bid **Caution/Contra:** [C, ?] Avoid in patients with high triglycerides **Supplied:** Tabs 1 g; granules **Notes/SE:** Do NOT use dry powder; mix with beverages, soups, cereals, etc; constipation, abdominal pain, bloating, HA **Interactions:** ↓ absorption of numerous drugs esp anticoagulants, cardiac glycosides, digitoxin, digoxin, phenobarbital, penicillin G, tetracycline, thiazide diuretics, thyroid drugs **Labs:** ↓ serum cholesterol, ↑ PT **NIPE:** Take other meds 1 h < or 4 h > colestipol

Colfosceril Palmitate (Exosurf Neonatal) **Uses:** Prophylaxis and Rx for RDS in infants **Action:** Synthetic lung surfactant **Dose:** 5 mL/kg/dose through ET tube as soon after birth as possible and again at 12 and 24 h **Caution/Contra:** [?, ?] **Supplied:** Suspension 108 mg **Notes/SE:** Monitor pulmonary compliance and oxygenation carefully; pulmonary hemorrhage possible in infants weighing <700 g at birth; mucous plugging **Interactions:** None noted

Cortisone   See **Steroids**, Tables 4 and 5 (pages 248 and 249)

Cromolyn Sodium (Intal, Nasalcrom, Opticrom)   **Uses:** Adjunct to the Rx of asthma; prevent exercise-induced asthma; allergic rhinitis; ophth allergic manifestations **Action:** Antiasthmatic; mast cell stabilizer **Dose:** *Adults & Children >12 y.* Inhal: 20 mg (as powder in caps) inhaled qid or met-dose inhal 2 puffs qid. *Oral:* 200 mg qid 15–20 min ac, up to 400 mg qid. *Nasal instillation:* Spray once in each nostril 2–6×/d. *Ophth:* 1–2 gtt in each eye 4–6×/d. *Peds.* Inhal: 2 puffs qid of met-dose inhal. *Oral: Infants <2 y:* 20 mg/kg/d in 4 ÷ doses. *2–12 y:* 100 mg qid ac **Caution/Contra:** [B, ?] **Supplied:** Oral conc 100 mg/5 mL; soln for neb 20 mg/2 mL; met-dose inhal; nasal soln 40 mg/mL; ophth soln 4% **Notes/SE:** No benefit in acute Rx; 2–4 wk for maximal effect in perennial allergic disorders; unpleasant taste, hoarseness, coughing **Interactions:** None noted **Labs:** Monitor pulmonary function tests

Cyanocobalamin [Vitamin B₁₂]   **Uses:** Pernicious anemia and other vitamin B_{12} deficiency states **Action:** Dietary supplement of vitamin B_{12} **Dose:** *Adults.* 100 µg IM or SC qd for 5–10 d, then 100 µg IM 2×/wk for 1 mon, then 100 µg IM monthly. *Peds.* 100 µg/d IM or SC for 5–10 d, then 30–50 µg IM q4wk **Caution/Contra:** [A (C if dose exceeds RDA), +] **Supplied:** Tabs 25, 50, 100, 250, 500, 1000 µg; inj 30, 100, 1000 µg/mL **Notes/SE:** Oral absorption erratic, altered by many drugs, and not recommended; for use with hyperalimentation; itching, diarrhea **Interactions:** ↓ effects with aminosalicylic acid, chloramphenicol, cholestyramine, cimetidine, colchicines, neomycin, amino salicylate, alcohol **Labs:** Antibiotics, methotrexate, pyrimethamine invalidate blood assays of vitamin B_{12} and folic acid

Cyclobenzaprine (Flexeril)   **Uses:** Relief of muscle spasm **Action:** Centrally acting skeletal muscle relaxant; reduces tonic somatic motor activity **Dose:** 10 mg PO 2–4×/d (2–3 wk max) **Caution/Contra:** [B, ?] **Supplied:** Tabs 10 mg **Notes/SE:** Sedative and anticholinergic **Interactions:** ↑ effects of CNS depression with CNS depressants, TCAs, barbiturates, alcohol; ↑ risk of HTN & convulsions with MAOIs **NIPE:** ↑ fluids & fiber for constipation

Cyclopentolate (Cyclogyl)   **Uses:** Diagnostic procedures requiring cycloplegia and mydriasis **Action:** Cycloplegic and mydriatic agent (can last up to 24 h) **Dose:** 1 gtt then another in 5 min **Caution/Contra:** [C, ?] Narrow-angle glaucoma **Supplied:** Soln, 0.5, 1, 2% **Notes/SE:** Blurred vision, ↑ sensitivity to light, tachycardia, restlessness **Interactions:** ↓ effects of carbachol, cholinesterase inhibitors, pilocarpine **NIPE:** Burning when instilled

Cyclophosphamide (Cytoxan, Neosar)   **Uses:** Hodgkin's and NHLs, multiple myeloma, small-cell lung, breast, and ovarian CAs, mycosis fungoides, neuroblastoma, retinoblastoma, acute leukemias, CA, and allogeneic and ABMT in high doses; severe rheumatologic disorders **Action:** Converted to acrolein and phosphoramide mustard, the active alkylating moieties **Dose:**

500–1500 mg/m^2 as a single dose at 2–4-wk intervals; 1.8 g/m^2 to 160 mg/kg (or $\cong$12 g/m^2 in a 75-kg individual) in the BMT setting (refer to specific protocols); ↓ in renal/hepatic impairment **Caution/Contra:** [D, ?] **Supplied:** Tabs 25, 50 mg; inj 100 mg **Notes/SE:** Myelosuppression (leukopenia and thrombocytopenia); hemorrhagic cystitis, SIADH, alopecia, anorexia; N/V; hepatotoxicity and rarely interstitial pneumonitis; irreversible testicular atrophy possible; cardiotoxicity rare; 2nd malignancies (bladder CA and acute leukemias); cumulative risk 3.5% at 8 y, 10.7% at 12 y. Hemorrhagic cystitis prophylaxis: continuous bladder irrigation and mesna uroprotection **Interactions:** ↑ effects with allopurinol, cimetidine, phenobarbital, rifampin; ↑ effects of succinylcholine,warfarin; ↓ effects of digoxin **Labs:** May inhibit + reactions to skin tests for PPD, risk of false + Pap smear results **NIPE:** May cause sterility, hair loss, ⊘ PRG, breast-feeding, immunizations

Cyclosporine (Sandimmune, Neoral)
Uses: Organ rejection in kidney, liver, heart, and BMT with steroids; RA; psoriasis **Action:** Immunosuppressant; reversible inhibition of immunocompetent lymphocytes **Dose:** *Adults & Peds.* *Oral:* 15 mg/kg/d 12 h pretransplant; after 2 wk, taper by 5 mg/wk to 5–10 mg/kg/d. *IV:* If NPO, give 1/3 oral dose IV; ↓ in renal/hepatic impairment **Caution/Contra:** [C, ?] **Supplied:** Caps 25, 50, 100 mg; oral soln 100 mg/mL; inj 50 mg/mL **Notes/SE:** May ↑ BUN and creatinine and mimic transplant rejection; administer in glass containers; many drug interactions; Neoral and Sandimmune not interchangeable; HTN; interaction with St. John's Wort. See Table 2, page 246 **Interactions:** ↑ effects with azole antifungals, allopurinol, amiodarone, anabolic steroids, CCBs, cimetidine, chloroquine, clarithromycin, clonidine, diltiazem, macrolides, metoclopramide, nicardipine, NSAIDs, oral contraceptives, ticlopidine, grapefruit juice; ↑ nephrotoxicity with aminoglycosides, amphotericin B, acyclovir, colchine, enalapril, ranitidine, sulfonamides; ↑ risk digoxin toxicity; ↑ risk of hyperkalemia with diuretics, ACEIs; ↓ effects with barbiturates, carbamazepine, isoniazid, nafcillin, pyrazinamide, phenytoin, rifampin, sulfonamides, St. John's Wort, alfalfa sprouts, astragalus, echinacea, licorice; ↓ effects immunizations **Labs:** ↑ serum creatinine, BUN, total bilirubin, K$^+$, alkaline phosphatase, lipids **NIPE:** Monitor for hyperglycemia, hyperkalemia, hyperuricemia, risk of photosensitivity

Cyproheptadine (Periactin)
Uses: Allergic reactions; itching **Action:** Phenothiazine antihistamine **Dose:** *Adults.* 4–20 mg PO + q8h; max 0.5 mg/kg/d. *Peds.* *2–6 y:* 2 mg bid–tid (max 12 mg/24 h). *7–14 y:* 4 mg bid–tid; ↓ in hepatic impairment **Caution/Contra:** [B, ?] **Supplied:** Tabs 4 mg; syrup 2 mg/5 mL **Notes/SE:** Anticholinergic, drowsiness, may stimulate appetite **Interactions:** ↑ effects with CNS depressants, MAOIs, alcohol; ↓ effects of epinephrine, fluoxetine **Labs:** False neg skin testing; false + urine TCA assay; ↑ serum amylase, prolactin; ↓ FBS **NIPE:** ↑ risk photosensitivity, take with food if GI distress

Cytarabine [ARA-C] (Cytosar-U)
Uses: Acute leukemias, CML, NHL; IT administration for leukemic meningitis or prophylaxis **Action:** Antimetabolite; interferes with DNA synthesis **Dose:** 100–150 mg/m^2/d for 5–10 d

(low dose); 3 g/m^2 q12h for 8–12 doses (high dose); 1 mg/kg 1–2×/wk (SC maint regimens); 5–70 mg/m2 up to 3×/wk IT (refer to specific protocols); ↓ in renal/hepatic impairment **Caution/Contra:** [D, ?] **Supplied:** Inj 100, 500 mg, 1, 2 g **Notes/SE:** Myelosuppression, N/V/D, stomatitis, flu-like syndrome, rash on palms/soles, hepatic dysfunction; toxicity of high-dose regimens (conjunctivitis) ameliorated by corticosteroid ophth soln; cerebellar dysfunction, noncardiogenic pulmonary edema; neuropathy **Interactions:** ↑ effects with alkylating drugs and radiation therapy; ↓ effects of digoxin, gentamicin, methotrexate, flucytosine **Labs:** ↑ uric acid, monitor CBC, BUN, creatinine, LFTs **NIPE:** ⊘ alcohol, NSAIDs, ASA, PRG, breast-feeding, immunizations

Cytarabine Liposomal (DepoCyt)
Uses: Lymphomatous meningitis **Action:** Antimetabolite; interferes with DNA synthesis **Dose:** 50 mg IT q14d for 5 doses, then 50 mg IT q28d for 4 doses; use dexamethasone prophylaxis **Caution/Contra:** [D, ?] **Supplied:** IT inj 50 mg/5 mL **Notes/SE:** Neck pain/rigidity, HA, confusion, somnolence, fever, back pain, N/V, edema, neutropenia, thrombocytopenia, anemia **Interactions:** None noted, perhaps because of limited systemic exposure **Labs:** May interfere with CSF interpretation **NIPE:** ⊘ PRG, use contraception

Cytomegalovirus Immune Globulin [CMV-IG IV] (CytoGam)
Uses: Attenuation of primary CMV disease associated with transplantation **Action:** Exogenous IgG antibodies to CMV **Dose:** Administer for 16 wk posttransplant; see product information for dosing schedule **Caution/Contra:** [C, ?] **Supplied:** Inj 50–10 mg/mL **Notes/SE:** Flushing, N/V, muscle cramps, wheezing, HA, fever **Interactions:** ↓ effects of live virus vaccines **NIPE:** Admin immunizations at least 3 mo after CMV-IG

Dacarbazine (DTIC)
Uses: Melanoma, Hodgkin's disease, sarcoma **Action:** Alkylating agent; antimetabolite activity as a purine precursor; inhibits synthesis of protein, RNA, and especially DNA **Dose:** 2–4.5 mg/kg/d for 10 consecutive d or 250 mg/m^2/d for 5 d (refer to specific protocols); ↓ in renal impairment **Caution/Contra:** [C, ?] **Supplied:** Inj 100, 200, 500 mg **Notes/SE:** Myelosuppression, severe N/V, hepatotoxicity, flu-like syndrome, hypotension, photosensitivity, alopecia, facial flushing, facial paresthesias, urticaria, phlebitis at inj site **Interactions:** ↑ effects with amphotericin B, anticoagulants, ASA, bonemarrow suppressants; ↑ effects of phenobarbital, phenytoin **Labs:** ↑ AST, ALT **NIPE:** Risk of photosensitivity, hair loss, infection

Daclizumab (Zenapax)
Uses: Prevents acute organ rejection **Action:** IL-2 receptor antagonist **Dose:** 1 mg/kg IV/dose; 1st dose pretransplant, then 4 doses 14 d apart posttransplant **Caution/Contra:** [C, ?] **Supplied:** Inj 5 mg/mL **Notes/SE:** Hyperglycemia, edema, HTN, hypotension, constipation, HA, dizziness, anxiety, nephrotoxicity, pulmonary edema, pain **Interactions:** ⊘ give echinacea **NIPE:** ⊘ immunizations, infections, ↑ fluid intake

Dactinomycin (Cosmegen) **Uses:** Choriocarcinoma, Wilms' tumor, Kaposi's sarcoma, Ewing's sarcoma, rhabdomyosarcoma, testicular CA **Action:** DNA intercalating agent **Dose:** 0.5 mg/d for 5 d; 2 mg/wk for 3 consecutive wk; 15 μg/kg or 0.45 mg/m²/d (max 0.5 mg) for 5 d q3–8wk in pediatric sarcoma (refer to specific protocols); ↓ in renal impairment **Caution/Contra:** [C, ?] **Supplied:** Inj 0.5 mg **Notes/SE:** Myelosuppression, immunosuppression, severe N/V, alopecia, acne, hyperpigmentation, radiation recall phenomenon, tissue damage with extravasation, hepatotoxicity **Interactions:** ↑ effects bone marrow suppressants, radiation therapy; ↓ effects of vitamin K **Labs:** ↑ uric acid; monitor CBC with differential & platelets, LFTs, BUN, creatinine **NIPE:** ⊘ PRG, breast-feeding; risk of irreversible infertility, reversible hair loss, ↑ fluids to 2–3 L/d

Dalteparin (Fragmin) **Uses:** Unstable angina, non-Q-wave MI, prevention of ischemic complications due to clot formation in patients on concurrent ASA, prevention and Rx of DVT following surgery **Action:** LMW heparin **Dose:** *Angina/MI:* 120 IU/kg (max 10,000 IU) SC q12h with ASA. *DVT prophylaxis:* 2500–5000 IU SC 1–2 h preop, then qd for 5–10 d. *Systemic anticoagulation:* 200 IU/kg/d SC or 100 IU/kg bid SC **Caution/Contra:** [B, ?] Active hemorrhage, cerebrovascular disease, cerebral aneurysm, severe uncontrolled HTN **Supplied:** Inj 2500 IU (16 mg/0.2 mL), 5000 IU (32 mg/0.2 mL), 10,000 IU (64 mg/mL) **Notes/SE:** Predictable antithrombotic effects eliminate need for laboratory monitoring; bleeding, pain at inj site, thrombocytopenia **Interactions:** ↑ bleeding with oral anticoagulants, platelet inhibitors, penicillins, cephalosporins, garlic, ginger, ginkgo biloba, ginseng, chamomile, vitamin E **Labs:** ↑ AST, ALT, monitor CBC and platelets **NIPE:** ⊘ give orally or IM; give deep SC

Dantrolene (Dantrium) **Uses:** Clinical spasticity due to upper motor neuron disorders, eg, spinal cord injuries, strokes, CP, MS; Rx of malignant hyperthermia **Action:** Skeletal muscle relaxant **Dose:** *Adults. Spasticity:* Initially, 25 mg PO qd; ↑ to effect by 25 mg to a max dose of 100 mg PO qid PRN. *Peds.* Initially, 0.5 mg/kg/dose bid; ↑ by 0.5 mg/kg to effect to a max dose of 3 mg/kg/dose qid PRN. *Adults & Peds. Malignant hyperthermia: Treatment:* Continuous rapid IV push beginning at 1 mg/kg until symptoms subside or 10 mg/kg is reached. *Post-crisis follow-up:* 4–8 mg/kg/d in 3–4 ÷ doses for 1–3 d to prevent recurrence **Caution/Contra:** [C, ?] Active hepatic disease **Supplied:** Caps 25, 50, 100 mg; powder for inj 20 mg/vial **Notes/SE:** Monitor transaminases; drowsiness, dizziness, rash, muscle weakness, pleural effusion with pericarditis, diarrhea, blurred vision, hepatitis **Interactions:** ↑ effects with CNS depressants, antihistamines, opioids, alcohol; ↑ risk of hepatotoxicity with estrogens; ↑ risk of CV collapse & ventricular fib with CCBs; ↓ plasma protein binding with clofibrate, warfarin **Labs:** ↑ AST, ALT, alkaline phosphatase, LDH, BUN, total serum bilirubin **NIPE:** ↑ risk of photosensitivity

Dapsone (Avlosulfon) **Uses:** Rx and prevent PCP; toxoplasmosis prophylaxis; leprosy **Action:** Unknown; bactericidal **Dose:** *Adults. Prophylaxis of*

PCP: 50–100 mg/d PO; *Rx of PCP:* 100 mg/d PO with TMP 5 mg/kg for 21 d. **Peds.** *Prophylaxis of PCP:* 1–2 mg/kg/24 h PO qd; max 100 mg/d **Caution/Contra:** [C, +] Caution in G6PD deficiency **Supplied:** Tabs 25, 100 mg **Notes/SE:** Absorption ↑ by an acidic environment; with leprosy, combine with rifampin and other agents; hemolysis, methemoglobinemia, agranulocytosis, rash, cholestatic jaundice **Interactions:** ↑ effects with probenecid, trimethoprim; ↓ effects with activated charcoal, rifampin **Labs:** monitor CBC, LFTs **NIPE:** ↑ risk of photosensitivity

Darbepoetin Alfa (Aranesp)
Uses: Anemia associated with CRF **Action:** Stimulates erythropoiesis, recombinant variant of erythropoietin **Dose:** 0.45 μg/kg single IV or SC qwk; titrate dose, do not exceed target Hgb of 12 g/dL; see insert for converting from Epogen **Caution/Contra:** [C, ?] Contra uncontrolled hypertension, allergy to components **Supplied:** 25, 40, 60, 100 μg/mL, in polysorbate or albumin excipient **Notes/SE:** Longer 1/2-life than Epogen; follow weekly CBC until stable; may ↑ risk of cardiac events, chest pain, hypo-/hypertension, N/V/D, myalgia, arthralgia, dizziness, edema, fatigue, fever; ↑ risk of infection **Interactions:** None noted **Labs:** Monitor CBC with differential & platelets, BUN, creatinine, serum phosphorus, K+, iron stores **NIPE:** Monitor BP & for seizure activity, shaking vial inactivates drug

Daunorubicin (Daunomycin, Cerubidine)
WARNING: Cardiac function should be monitored due to potential risk for cardiac toxicity and CHF **Uses:** Acute leukemias **Action:** DNA intercalating agent; inhibits topoisomerase II; generates oxygen free radicals **Dose:** 45–60 mg/m²/d for 3 consecutive d; 25 mg/m²/wk (refer to specific protocols); ↓ in renal/hepatic impairment **Caution/Contra:** [D, ?] **Supplied:** Inj 20 mg **Notes/SE:** Myelosuppression, mucositis, N/V, alopecia, radiation recall phenomenon, hepatotoxicity (hyperbilirubinemia), tissue necrosis on extravascular extravasation, and cardiotoxicity (1–2% CHF risk with 550 mg/m² cumulative dose); prevent cardiotoxicity with dexrazoxane **Interactions:** ↑ risk of cardiotoxicity with cyclophosphamide; ↑ myelosuppression with antineoplastic agents; ↓ response to live virus vaccines **Labs:** ↑ serum alkaline phosphatase, bilirubin, AST, monitor uric acid, CBC, LFTs **NIPE:** ⊘ ASA, NSAIDs, alcohol, PRG, breastfeeding, immunizations; risk of hair loss

Delavirdine (Rescriptor)
Uses: HIV infection **Action:** Nonnucleoside reverse transcriptase inhibitor **Dose:** 400 mg PO tid; avoid antacids **Caution/Contra:** [C, ?] CDC recommends HIV-infected mothers not breast-feed due to risk of HIV transmission to infant **Supplied:** Tabs 100 mg **Notes/SE:** Inhibits cytochrome P-450 enzymes. Numerous drug interactions; HA, fatigue, rash, ↑ serum transaminases, N/V/D **Interactions:** ↑ effects with fluoxetine; ↑ effects of astemizole, benzodiazepines, cisapride, clarithromycin, dapsone, ergotamines, indinavir, lovastatin, midazolam, nifedipine, quinidine, ritonavir, simvastatin, terfenadine, triazolam, warfarin; ↓ effects with antacids, barbiturates, carbamazepine, cimetidine, famotidine, lansoprazole, nizatidine, phenobarbital, phenytoin, ranitidine, rifabutin, ri-

fampin; ↓ effects of didanosine **Labs:** ↑ AST, ALT, ↓ neutrophil counts **NIPE:** Take w/o regard to food

Demeclocycline (Declomycin) **Uses:** SIADH **Action:** Antibiotic; antagonizes action of ADH on renal tubules **Dose:** 300–600 mg PO q12h on an empty stomach; ↓ in renal failure; avoid antacids **Caution/Contra:** [D, +] Avoid use in hepatic/renal dysfunction **Supplied:** Caps 150 mg; tabs 150, 300 mg **Notes/SE:** Diarrhea, abdominal cramps, photosensitivity, DI **Interactions:** effects of digoxin, anticoagulants; ↓ effects with antacids, bismuth salts, iron, sodium bicarbonate, barbiturates, carbamazepine, hydantoins, food; ↓ effects of oral contraceptives, penicillin **Labs:** false neg urine glucose; monitor CBC, LFTs, BUN, creatinine **NIPE:** risk of photosensitivity

Desipramine (Norpramin) **Uses:** Endogenous depression, chronic pain, and peripheral neuropathy **Action:** TCA; increases synaptic conc of serotonin or norepinephrine in CNS **Dose:** 25–200 mg/d single or ÷ doses; usually a single hs dose (max 300 mg/d) **Caution/Contra:** [C, ?/–] Caution in cardiovascular disease, seizure disorder, hypothyroidism **Supplied:** Tabs 10, 25, 50, 75, 100, 150 mg; caps 25, 50 mg **Notes/SE:** Anticholinergic (blurred vision, urinary retention, xerostomia); prolongs QT interval; numerous drug interactions **Interactions:** ↑ effects with cimetidine, diltiazem, fluoxetine, indinavir, MAOIs, paroxetine, propoxyphene, quinidine, ritonavir ranitidine, alcohol, grapefruit juice; ↑ effects of lithium, sulfonylureas; ↓ effects with barbiturates, carbamazepine rifampine, tobacco **NIPE:** Full effect of drug may take 4 wk, risk of photosensitivity

Desloratadine (Clarinex) **Uses:** Symptoms of seasonal and perennial allergic rhinitis; chronic idiopathic urticaria **Action:** The active metabolite of Claritin, H_1-antihistamine, blocks inflammatory mediators **Dose:** *Adults & Peds >12 y.* 5 mg PO qid; hepatic/renal impairment, 5 mg PO qod **Caution/Contra:** [C, ?/–] **Supplied:** Tabs 5 mg **Notes/SE:** Hypersensitivity reactions, anaphylaxis somnolence, HA, dizziness, fatigue, pharyngitis, xerostomia, nausea, dyspepsia, myalgia **Labs:** ↑ LFTs, bilirubin **NIPE:** Take w/o regard to food

Desmopressin (DDAVP, Stimate) **Uses:** DI (intranasal and parenteral); bleeding due to uremia, hemophilia A, and type I von Willebrand's disease (parenteral) **Action:** Synthetic analogue of vasopressin, a naturally occurring human ADH; ↑ factor VIII **Dose:** *DI: Intranasal: Adults.* 0.1–0.4 mL (10–40 µg)/d in 1–4 ÷ doses. *Peds 3 mon–12 y.* 0.05–0.3 mL/d in 1 or 2 doses. *Parenteral: Adults.* 0.5–1 mL (2–4 µg)/d in 2 ÷ doses. If converting from nasal to parenteral, use 1/2 nasal dose. *Oral: Adults.* 0.05 mg bid; ↑ to max of 1.2 mg. *Hemophilia A and von Willebrand's disease (type I): Adults & Peds >10 kg.* 0.3 µg/kg in 50 mL NS, infuse over 15–30 min. *Peds <10 kg.* As above with dilution to 10 mL with NS. *Nocturnal enuresis: Peds >6 y.* 20 µg intranasally hs. **Caution/Contra:** [B, M] **Supplied:** Tabs 0.1, 0.2 mg; inj 4 µg/mL; nasal soln 0.1, 1.5 mg/mL **Notes/SE:** In very young and old patients, ↓ fluid intake to avoid water intoxication and hyponatremia; facial flushing, HA, dizziness, vulval pain, nasal congestion, pain at inj site, hyponatremia, water intoxication **Interactions:** ↑ antidiuretic effects with carbamazepine, chlorpropamide, clofibrate; ↑ effects of vasopressors; ↓ antidiuretic effects with demeclocycline, lithium, norepinephrine **NIPE:** Monitor I&O, ⊘ ETOH, overhydration

Dexamethasone, Nasal (Dexacort Phosphate Turbinaire)
Uses: Chronic nasal inflammation or allergic rhinitis **Action:** Antiinflammatory corticosteroid **Dose:** *Adult and Peds >12 y.* 2 sprays/nostril bid–tid, max 12 sprays/d. *Peds 6–12 y.* 1–2 sprays/nostril, bid, max 8 sprays/d **Caution/Contra:** [C, ?] **Supplied:** Aerosol, 84 µg/activation **Notes/SE:** Local irritation **NIPE:** Use decongestant nose gtt 1st if nasal congestion

Dexamethasone, Ophthalmic (AK-Dex Ophthalmic, Decadron Ophthalmic)
Uses: Inflammatory or allergic conjunctivitis **Action:** Antiinflammatory corticosteroid **Dose:** Instill 1–2 gtt tid–qid **Caution/Contra:** [C, ?/–] Contra in active untreated bacterial, viral, and fungal eye infections **Supplied:** Susp and soln 0.1%; oint 0.05% **Notes/SE:** Long-term use associated with cataract formation **NIPE:** Eval intraocular pressure and lens if prolonged use

Dexamethasone, Systemic, Topical (Decadron) See Steroids, Systemic, Page 248, and Table 4, Page 209, and Steroids, Topical, Page 249, and Table 5, Page 210
Interactions: ↑ effects with cyclosporine, estrogens, oral contraceptives, macrolides; ↑ effects of cyclosporine; ↓ effects with aminoglutethimide, antacids, barbiturates, carbamazepine, cholestyramine, colestipol, phenytoin, phenobarbital, rifampin; ↓ effects of anticoagulants, hypoglycemics, isoniazid, toxoids, salicylates, vaccines **Labs:** false neg allergy skin tests **NIPE:** ⊘ vaccines, breast-feeding, use on broken skin

Dexpanthenol (Ilopan-Choline Oral, Ilopan)
Uses: Minimizes paralytic ileus, Rx postop distention **Action:** Cholinergic agent **Dose:** *Adults. Relief of gas:* 2–3 tabs PO tid. *Prevent postop ileus:* 250–500 mg IM stat, repeat in 2 h, then q6h PRN. *Ileus:* 500 mg IM stat, repeat in 2 h, followed by doses q6h, if needed **Caution/Contra:** [C, ?] Hemophilia, mechanical obstruction **Supplied:** Inj; tabs 50 mg; cream **Notes/SE:** GI cramps

Dexrazoxane (Zinecard)
Uses: Prevents anthracycline-induced cardiomyopathy **Action:** Chelates heavy metals; binds intracellular iron and prevents anthracycline-induced free radicals **Dose:** 10:1 ratio dexrazoxane:doxorubicin 30 min prior to each dose **Caution/Contra:** [C, ?] **Supplied:** Inj 10 mg/mL **Notes/SE:** Myelosuppression (especially leukopenia), fever, infection, stomatitis, alopecia, N/V/D; mild ↑ transaminase, pain at inj site **Interactions:** ↑ length of muscle relaxation with succinylcholine

Dextran 40 (Rheomacrodex)
Uses: Shock, prophylaxis of DVT and thromboembolism, adjunct in peripheral vascular surgery **Action:** Expands plasma volume; ↓ blood viscosity **Dose:** *Shock:* 10 mL/kg infused rapidly; 20 mL/kg max

in the 1st 24 h; beyond 24 h 10 mL/kg max; DC after 5 d. *Prophylaxis of DVT and thromboembolism:* 10 mL/kg IV day of surgery, then 500 mL/d IV for 2–3 d, then 500 mL IV q2–3d based on risk for up to 2 wk **Caution/Contra:** [C, ?] **Supplied:** 10% dextran 40 in 0.9% NaCl or 5% dextrose **Notes/SE:** Hypersensitivity/anaphylactoid reaction (observe patient closely during 1st min of inf), arthralgia, cutaneous reactions, fever; monitor renal function and electrolytes **Interactions:** ↑ bleeding times with antiplatelet agents or anticoagulants **Labs:** False ↑ serum glucose, urinary protein, bilirubin assays, & total protein assays **NIPE:** Draw blood before administration of drug, pt should be well hydrated prior to infusion

Dextromethorphan (Mediquell, Benylin DM, PediaCare 1, others)
Uses: Controlling nonproductive cough **Action:** Depresses the cough center in the medulla **Dose:** *Adults.* 10–30 mg PO q4h PRN. *Peds. 7 mon–1 y:* 2.5–7.5 mg q6–8h; *2–6 y:* 2.5–7.5 mg q4–8h (max 30 mg/24 h). *7–12 y:* 5–10 mg q4–8h (max 60 mg/24h) **Caution/Contra:** [C,?/–] **Supplied:** Caps 30 mg; lozenges 2.5, 5, 7.5, 15 mg; syrup 15 mg/15 mL, 10 mg/5 mL; liq 10 mg/15 mL, 3.5, 7.5, 15 mg/5 mL; sustained-action liq 30 mg/5 mL **Notes/SE:** May be found in combination products with guaifenesin; GI disturbances **Interactions:** ↑ effects with amiodarone, fluoxetin, quinidine, terbinafine; ↑ risk of serotonin syndrome with sibutramine, MAOIs; ↑ CNS depression with antihistamines, antidepressants, sedative, opioids, alcohol **NIPE:** ↑ fluids, humidity to environment, stop MAOIs for 2 wk before administering drug

Dezocine (Dalgan)
Uses: Moderate–severe pain **Action:** Narcotic agonist–antagonist **Dose:** 5–20 mg IM or 2.5–10 mg IV q2–4h PRN; ↓ in renal impairment **Caution/Contra:** [C, ?] Not recommended for patients <18 y **Supplied:** Inj 5, 10, 15 mg/mL **Notes/SE:** Withdrawal possible in patients dependent on narcotics **Interactions:** ↑ effects with CNS depressants, ⊘ MAOIs **NIPE:** ↑ resp depression greatest 1st h >admin

Diazepam (Valium) [C-IV]
Uses: Anxiety, alcohol withdrawal, muscle spasm, status epilepticus, panic disorders, amnesia, preoperative sedation **Action:** Benzodiazepine **Dose:** *Adults. Status epilepticus:* 5–10 mg q10–20 min to 30 mg max in 8-h period. *Anxiety, muscle spasm:* 2–10 mg PO bid–qid or IM/IV q3–4h PRN. *Preop:* 5–10 mg PO or IM 20–30 min or IV just prior to procedure. *Alcohol withdrawal:* Initial 2–5 mg IV, then 5–10 mg q5–10min, 100 mg in 1 h max. May require up to 1000 mg in 24-h period for severe withdrawal. Titrate to agitation; avoid excessive sedation; may lead to aspiration or respiratory arrest. *Peds. Status epilepticus:* <5 y: 0.05–0.3 mg/kg/dose IV q15–30 min up to a max of 5 mg. >5 y: Give up to max of 10 mg. *Sedation, muscle relaxation:* 0.04–0.3 mg/kg/dose q2–4h IM or IV to max of 0.6 mg/kg in 8 h, or 0.12–0.8 mg/kg/24 h PO ÷ tid–qid; ↓ in hepatic impairment; avoid abrupt withdrawal **Caution/Contra:** [D, ?/–] **Supplied:** Tabs 2, 5, 10 mg; soln 1, 5 mg/mL; inj 5 mg/mL; rectal gel 5 mg/mL **Notes/SE:** Do not exceed 5 mg/min IV in adults or 1–2 mg/min in peds because respiratory arrest possible; IM absorption erratic; sedation, amnesia, bradycardia, hypotension, rash,

decreased respiratory rate **Interactions:** ↑ effects with antihistamines, azole anti-fungals, BBs, CNS depressants, cimetidine, ciprofloxin, disulfiram, isoniazid, oral contraceptives, omeprazole, phenytoin, valproic acid, verapimil, alcohol, kava kava, valerian; ↑ effects of digoxin, diuretics; ↓ effects with barbiturates, car-bamzepine, theophylline, ranitidine, tobacco; ↓ effects of haloperidol, levodopa **Labs:** False neg urine glucose; monitor LFTs, BUN, creatinine, CBC with long-term drug use **NIPE:** Risk ↑ seizure activity

Diazoxide (Hyperstat, Proglycem)
Uses: Hypoglycemia due to hy-perinsulinism (Proglycem); hypertensive crisis (Hyperstat) **Action:** Inhibits pan-creatic insulin release; antihypertensive **Dose:** *Hypertensive crisis:* IV: 1–3 mg/kg (maximum: 150 mg in a single inj); repeat dose in 5–15 min until BP controlled; repeat every 4–24 h; monitor BP closely. *Adults & Peds.* 3–8 mg/kg/24 h PO ÷ q8–12h. *Neonates.* 8–15 mg/kg/24 h ÷ in 3 equal doses; maint 8–10 mg/kg/24 h PO in 2–3 equal doses **Caution/Contra:** [C, ?] Hypersensitivity to thiazides or other sulfonamide-containing products; HTN associated with aortic coarctation, ar-teriovenous shunt, or pheochromocytoma **Supplied:** Inj 15 mg/mL; caps 50 mg; oral susp 50 mg/mL **Notes/SE:** Hyperglycemia, hypotension, dizziness, Na and water retention; N/V, weakness **Interactions:** ↑ effects with carboplatin, cisplatin, diuretics, phenothiazines; ↑ effects of anticoagulants; ↓ effects with sulfonylureas; ↓ effects of phenytoin, sulfonylureas; **Labs:** ↑ serum uric acid, AST, alkaline phos-phatase, false-negative response to glucagon **NIPE:** Daily wts, ↑ reversible body hair growth

Dibucaine (Nupercainal)
Uses: Hemorrhoids and minor skin condi-tions **Action:** Topical anesthetic **Dose:** Insert PR with applicator bid and after each bowel movement; apply sparingly to skin **Caution/Contra:** [C, ?] **Supplied:** 1% oint with rectal applicator; 0.5% cream **Notes/SE:** Local irritation, rash **Interac-tions:** None noted

Diclofenac (Cataflam, Voltaren)
Uses: Arthritis and pain **Action:** NSAID **Dose:** 50–75 mg PO bid; take with food or milk **Caution/Contra:** [B (D 3rd trimester or near delivery), ?] Caution in CHF, HTN, renal/hepatic dysfunction, and Hx PUD. **Supplied:** Tabs 50 mg; tabs DR 25, 50, 75, 100 mg; XR tabs 100 mg; ophth soln 0.1% **Notes/SE:** Abdominal cramps, heartburn, GI ulceration, rash, interstitial nephritis **Interactions:** ↑ risk of bleeding with feverfew, garlic, ginger, ginkgo biloba; ↑ effects of digoxin, methotrexate, cyclosporine, lithium, insulin, sulfonylureas, K⁺-sparing diuretics, warfarin; ↓ effects with ASA; ↓ effects of thi-azide diuretics, furosemide, BBs **Labs:** ↑ LFTs, serum glucose & cortisol, ↓ serum uric acid; **NIPE:** Risk of photosensitivity, monitor LFTs, CBC, BUN, creatinine, take with food, do not crush tablets

Dicloxacillin (Dynapen, Dycill)
Uses: Infections due to susceptible strains of *S. aureus* and *Streptococcus* **Action:** Bactericidal; inhibits cell wall syn-thesis **Dose:** *Adults.* 250–500 mg qid. *Peds <40 kg.* 12.5–25 mg/kg/d ÷ qid; take on empty stomach **Caution/Contra:** [B, ?] **Supplied:** Caps 125, 250, 500 mg; soln

62.5 mg/5 mL **Notes/SE:** Diarrhea, nausea, abdominal pain **Interactions:** ↑ effects with disulfiram, probenecid; ↑ effects of methotrexate, ↓ effects with macrolides, tetracyclines, food; ↓ effects of oral contraceptives, warfarin **Labs:** False ↑ nafcillin level, urine & serum proteins, uric acid **NIPE:** Take with water

Dicyclomine (Bentyl) Uses: Functional irritable bowel syndromes **Action:** Smooth-muscle relaxant **Dose:** *Adults.* 20 mg PO qid; ↑ to a max dose of 160 mg/d or 20 mg IM q6h. *Peds. Infants >6 mon:* 5 mg/dose tid–qid. *Children:* 10 mg/dose tid–qid **Caution/Contra:** [B, –] Infants <6 mon, narrow-angle glaucoma, MyG, severe UC, obstructive uropathy **Supplied:** Caps 10, 20 mg; tabs 20 mg; syrup 10 mg/5 mL; inj 10 mg/mL **Notes/SE:** Anticholinergic side effects may limit dose **Interactions:** ↑ anticholinergic effects with anticholinergics, antihistamines, amantadine, MAOIs, TCAs, phenothiazines; ↑ effects of atenolol, digoxin; ↓ effects with antacids; ↓ effects of haloperidol, ketoconazole, levodopa, phenothiazines **NIPE:** ⊘ alcohol, CNS depressant; adequate hydration

Didanosine [ddI] (Videx) **WARNING:** Hypersensitivity manifested as fever, rash, fatigue, GI/respiratory symptoms reported; stop drug immediately and do not rechallenge; lactic acidosis and hepatomegaly/steatosis reported Uses: HIV infection in zidovudine-intolerant patients **Action:** Nucleoside antiretroviral agent **Dose:** *Adults. >60 kg:* 400 mg/d PO or 200 mg PO bid. *<60 kg:* 250 mg/d PO or 125 mg PO bid; adults should take 2 tabs/administration. *Peds.* Dose by following table; ↓ in renal impairment, thoroughly chew tablets, do not mix with fruit juice or other acidic beverages; reconstitute powder with water **Caution/Contra:** [B, –] CDC recommends HIV-infected mothers not breast-feed due to risk of transmission of HIV to their infant. **Supplied:** Chew tabs 25, 50, 100, 150, 200 mg; powder packets 100, 167, 250, 375 mg; powder for soln 2, 4 g **Notes/SE:** Pancreatitis, peripheral neuropathy, diarrhea, HA **Interactions:** ↑ effects with allopurinol, ganciclovir; ↓ effects with methadone, food; ↑ risk of pancreatitis with thiazide diuretics, IV pentamidine, alcohol; ↓ effects of azole antifungals, dapsone, delavirdine, ganciclovir, indinavir, quinolones, ranitidine, tetracyclines **Labs:** ↑ LFTs, uric acid, amylase, lipase, triglycerides **NIPE:** May cause hyperglycemia, take w/o food, chew or crush tabs

Diflunisal (Dolobid) Uses: Mild–moderate pain; osteoarthritis **Action:** NSAID **Dose:** *Pain:* 500 mg PO bid. *Osteoarthritis:* 500–1500 mg PO in 2–3 ÷ doses; ↓ in renal impairment, take with food/milk **Caution/Contra:** [C (D 3rd trimester or near delivery), ?] Caution in CHF, HTN, renal/hepatic dysfunction, and Hx PUD. **Supplied:** Tabs 250, 500 mg **Notes/SE:** May prolong bleeding time; HA, abdominal cramps, heartburn, GI ulceration, rash, interstitial nephritis, fluid retention **Interactions:** ↑ effects with probenecid; ↑ effects of acetaminophen, anticoagulants, digoxin, HCTZ, indomethacin, lithium, methotrexate, phenytoin, sulfonamides, sulfonylureas; ↓ effects with antacids, ASA; ↓ effects of furosemide **Labs:** ↑ salicylate levels, PT, ↓ uric acid, T3, T4; **NIPE:** Take with food, ⊘ chew or crush tabs

Digoxin (Lanoxin, Lanoxicaps) **Uses:** CHF, AF and flutter, and PAT **Action:** Positive inotrope; ↑ AV node refractory period **Dose:** *Adults. PO digitalization:* 0.50–0.75 mg PO, then 0.25 mg PO q6–8h to total 1.0–1.5 mg. *IV or IM digitalization:* 0.25–0.5 mg IM or IV, then 0.25 mg q4–6h to total ≅1 mg. *Daily maint:* 0.125–0.5 mg/d PO, IM, or IV (average daily dose 0.125–0.25 mg). *Peds. Preterm infants: Digitalization:* 30 μg/kg PO or 25 μg/kg IV; give 1/2 of dose initially, then 1/4 of dose at 8–12-h intervals for 2 doses. *Maint:* 5–7.5 μg/kg/24 h PO or 4–6 μg/kg/24 h IV ÷ q12h. *Term infants: Digitalization:* 25–35 μg/kg PO or 20–30 μg/kg IV; give 1/2 the dose initially, then 1/3 of the dose at 8–12 h. *Maint:* 6–10 μg/kg/24 h PO or 5–8 μg/kg/24 h ÷ q12h. *1 mon–2 y: Digitalization:* 35–60 μg/kg PO or 30–50 μg/kg IV; give 1/2 the dose initially, then 1/3 of the dose at 8–12-h intervals for 2 doses. *Maint:* 10–15 μg/kg/24 h PO or 7.5–15 μg/kg/24 h IV ÷ q12h. *2–10 y: Digitalization:* 30–40 μg/kg PO or 25 μg/kg IV; give 1/2 dose initially, then 1/3 of the dose at 8–12-h intervals for 2 doses. *Maint:* 8–10 μg/kg/24 h PO or 6–8 μg/ kg/24 h IV ÷ q12h. *7–10 y:* Same as for adults; ↓ in renal impairment, follow serum levels **Caution/Contra:** [C, +] Contra AV block **Supplied:** Caps 0.05, 0.1, 0.2 mg; tabs 0.125, 0.25, 0.5 mg; elixir 0.05 mg/mL; inj 0.1, 0.25 mg/mL **Notes/SE:** See Drug Levels, Table 2, page 245. IM inj painful and erratic absorption; can cause heart block; ↓ K⁺ potentiates toxicity; N/V, HA, fatigue, visual disturbances (yellow-green halos around lights), cardiac arrhythmias, multiple drug interactions **Interactions:** ↑ effects with alprazolam, amiodarone, azole antifungals, BBs, carvedilol, cyclosporine, corticosteroids, diltiazem, diuretics, erythromycin, NSAIDs, quinidine, spironolactone, tetracyclines, verapamil, goldenseal, hawthorn, licorice, quinine, Siberian ginseng; ↓ effects with charcoal, cholestyramine, cisapride, neomycin, rifampin, sucralfate, thyroid hormones, psyllium, St. John's Wort **Labs:** ↓ PT, monitor serum electrolytes, LFTs, BUN, creatinine **NIPE:** Different bioavailability in various brands

Digoxin Immune Fab (Digibind) **Uses:** Life-threatening digoxin intoxication **Action:** Antigen-binding fragments bind and inactivate digoxin **Dose:** *Adults & Peds.* Based on serum level and patient's weight; see charts provided with the drug **Caution/Contra:** [C, ?] Hypersensitivity to sheep products **Supplied:** Inj 38 mg/vial **Notes/SE:** Each vial binds ≅0.6 mg of digoxin; in renal failure may require redosing in several days because of breakdown of the immune complex; worsening of cardiac output or CHF, hypokalemia, facial swelling, redness **Interactions:** ↓ effects of cardiac glycosides **NIPE:** Will take up to 1 wk for accurate serum digoxin levels after use of digibind

Diltiazem (Cardizem, Cardizem CD, Cardizem SR, Cartia XT, Dilacor XR, Diltia XT, Tiamate, Tiazac) **Uses:** Angina, prevention of reinfarction, HTN, AF or flutter, and PAT **Action:** Ca channel blocker **Dose:** *Oral:* Initially, 30 mg PO qid; ↑ to 180–360 mg/d in 3–4 ÷ doses PRN. *SR:* 60–120 mg PO bid; ↑ to 360 mg/d max. *CD:* 120–360 mg/d (max 480 mg/d). *IV:* 0.25 mg/kg IV bolus over 2 min; may repeat in 15 min at 0.35 mg/kg; may begin inf of 5–15 mg/h **Caution/Contra:** [C, +] Sick sinus syndrome, AV block, hypotension, AMI, pulmonary congestion **Supplied:** *Cardizem CD:* caps 120, 180, 240, 300, 360 mg; *Cardizem SR:* caps 60, 90, 120 mg; *Cardizem:* Tabs 30, 60, 90, 120 mg; *Cartia XT:* Caps 120, 180, 240, 300 mg; *Dilacor XR:* Caps 180, 240 mg; *Diltia XT:* Caps 120, 180, 240 mg; *Tiazac:* Caps 120, 180, 240, 300, 360, 420 mg; *Tiamate (ER):* Tabs 120, 180, 240 mg; inj 5 mg/mL **Notes/SE:** Cardizem CD, Dilacor XR, and Tiazac not interchangeable; gingival hyperplasia, bradycardia, AV block, ECG abnormalities, peripheral edema, dizziness, HA **Interactions:** ↑ effects with α-blockers, azole antifungals, BBs, erythromycin, H_2 receptor antagonists, nitroprusside, quinidine, alcohol, grapefruit juice; ↑ effects of carbamazepine, cyclosporine, digitalis glycosides, quinidine, phenytoin, prazosin, theophylline, TCAs; ↓ effects with NSAIDs, phenobarbital, rifampin **Labs:** False ↑ urine ketones, ↑ LFTs, BUN, creatinine **NIPE:** ⊘ chew or crush SR or ER preparations, risk of photosensitivity

Dimenhydrinate (Dramamine, others)
Uses: Prevention and Rx of nausea, vomiting, dizziness, or vertigo of motion sickness **Action:** Antiemetic **Dose:** *Adults.* 50–100 mg PO q4–6h, max 400 mg/d; 50 mg IM/IV PRN. *Peds.* 5 mg/kg/24 h PO or IV ÷ qid (max 300 mg/d) **Caution/Contra:** [B, ?] **Supplied:** Tabs 50 mg; chew tabs 50 mg; liq 12.5 mg/4 mL, 12.5 mg/5 mL, 15.62 mg/5 mL; inj 50 mg/mL **Notes/SE:** Anticholinergic side effects **Interactions:** ↑ effects with CNS depressants, antihistamines, opioids, quinidine, MAOIs, TCAs, alcohol **Labs:** False ↓ allergy skin tests **NIPE:** ⊘ drug 72 h prior to allergy skin testing, take <motion sickness occurs

Dimethyl Sulfoxide [DMSO] (Rimso-50)
Uses: Interstitial cystitis **Action:** Unknown **Dose:** Intravesical, 50 mL, retain for 15 min; repeat q2wk until relief **Caution/Contra:** [C, ?] **Supplied:** 50% soln in 50 mL **Notes/SE:** Cystitis, eosinophilia, GI, taste disturbance **Interactions:** ↓ effects of sulindac **Labs:** monitor CBC, LFTs, BUN, creatinine levels **NIPE:** ↑ taste & smell of garlic

Dinoprostone (Cervidil Vaginal Insert, Prepidil Vaginal Gel)
Uses: Induces labor; terminates PRG (12–28 wk); evacuates uterus in missed abortion or fetal death; **Action:** prostaglandin; changes consistency, dilatation, and effacement of the cervix; induces uterine contraction. **Dose:** *Gel.* 0.5 mg; if no cervical/uterine response, repeat 0.5 mg q6 h (max 24 h dose 1.5 mg); *vaginal insert:* 1 insert (10 mg = 0.3 mg dinoprostone/h over 12h); remove with onset of labor or 12 h after insertion; *vaginal supp:* 20 mg repeated every 3–5 h; adjust PRN; Suppository: 1 high in vagina, repeat at 3–5-h intervals until abortion, (240 mg max); **Caution/Contra:** [X, ?] ruptured membranes, hypersensitivity to prostaglandins, placenta previa or unexplained vaginal bleeding during PRG, when oxytocic drugs contraindicated or if prolonged uterine contractions are inappropriate (Hx C-section or major uterine surgery, presence of cephalopelvic disproportion, etc) **Supplied:** Vaginal gel 0.5 mg/3 g; vaginal supp 20 mg; vaginal insert 0.3 mg/h **Notes:** N/V/D, dizziness, flushing, headache, fever **Interactions:** ↑ effects of

oxytocics, ↓ effects with large amts alcohol **NIPE:** Pt supine >insertion of supp or gel up to ½ h

Diphenhydramine (Benadryl)
Uses: Treats and prevents allergic reactions, motion sickness, potentiate narcotics, sedation, cough suppression, and treatment of extrapyramidal reactions **Action:** Antihistamine, antiemetic **Dose:** *Adults.* 25–50 mg PO, IV, or IM bid–tid. *Peds.* 5 mg/kg/24 h PO or IM ÷ q6h (max 300 mg/d); ↑ dosing interval in moderate/severe renal failure **Caution/Contra:** [B, –] **Supplied:** Tabs and caps 25, 50 mg; chew tabs 12.5 mg; elixir 12.5 mg/5 mL; syrup 12.5 mg/5 mL; liq 6.25 mg/5 mL, 12.5 mg/5 mL; inj 50 mg/mL **Notes/SE:** Anticholinergic side effects (xerostomia, urinary retention, sedation) **Interactions:** ↑ effects with CNS depressants, antihistamines, opioids, MAOIs, TCAs, alcohol; ↑ effects of metoprolol **Labs:** ↓ response to allergy skin testing **NIPE:** ↑ risk of photosensitivity

Diphenoxylate + Atropine (Lomotil) [C-V]
Uses: Diarrhea **Action:** Constipating meperidine congener **Dose:** *Adults.* Initially, 5 mg PO tid–qid until under control, then 2.5–5.0 mg PO bid. *Peds >2 y.* 0.3–0.4 mg/kg/24 h (of diphenoxylate) bid–qid **Caution/Contra:** [C, +] Contra obstructive jaundice, diarrhea due to bacterial infection **Supplied:** Tabs 2.5 mg of diphenoxylate/0.025 mg of atropine; liq 2.5 mg diphenoxylate/0.025 mg atropine/5 mL **Notes/SE:** Drowsiness, dizziness, xerostomia, blurred vision, urinary retention, constipation **Interactions:** ↑ effects with CNS depressants, opioids, alcohol, ↑ risk HTN crisis with MAOIs **NIPE:** ↓ effectiveness with diarrhea caused by antibiotics

Diphtheria and Tetanus Toxoids [DT and Td]
Uses: Vaccine against diphtheria, tetanus, when pertussis vaccination contraindicated **Action:** Active immunization **Dose:** *Adults and Peds >7 y.* (Use Td) two 0.5-mL doses IM @ 4–6-wk intervals, reinforcing dose 6–12 mon later, booster every 10 y; *Peds.* (use DT). *6 wk–1 y:* Three 0.5-mL doses IM @ 4-wk intervals, reinforcing dose @ 6–12 mon after 3rd inj. *1–6 y:* Two 0.5-mL doses IM @ 4-wk intervals, reinforcing dose 6–12 mon after 2nd dose (use adult formulation [Td] if last dose after 7th birthday) **Contra/Caution:** [C, ?] Immunosuppressed, Hx allergy to any component of the vaccine, previous neurologic reaction to dose **Supplied:** Single-dose vials, varying concs of diphtheria and tetanus toxoids: 0.5-mL DT for peds = 6 y; Td if >7 y and adults **Notes/SE:** DT contains higher conc of diphtheria toxoid than Td; DTaP preferred in children in U.S.; drowsiness, restlessness, fever, nodule redness, pain, and swelling at site **Interactions:** ↓ effects with immunosuppressants, corticosteroids **NIPE:** IM injection only, only 1 inj/site, shake vial <admin

Diphtheria, Tetanus Toxoids, and Acellular Pertussis Adsorbed [DTaP] (Tripedia, ACEL-IMUNE, Infanrix)
Uses: Vaccine against diphtheria, tetanus, and pertussis **Action:** Active immunization **Dose:** *Peds.* 0.5 mL IM @ 2, 4, 6, and 15–18 mon and 4–6 y; 5th dose not needed if 4th dose given on/after 4th birthday **Contra/Caution:** [C, ?] Immunosuppressed, Hx allergy to any component of the vaccine, previous neurologic reaction to dose, Hx

of seizures **Supplied:** Single-dose vials **Notes/SE:** Acellular pertussis is currently recommended over whole-cell pertussis vaccines due to lower incidence of side effects; local and febrile reactions, prolonged crying, rashes, hypotonic-hyporesponsive episodes, rare anaphylaxis and seizures **Interactions:** ↓ effects with immunosuppressants, corticosteroids **NIPE:** Not usually given to children >7 y, nodule may develop at inj site & take wks to resolve

Diphtheria, Tetanus Toxoids, and Acellular Pertussis Adsorbed, Hepatitis B (recombinant), and Inactivated Poliovirus Vaccine [IPV] Combined (Pediarix) **Uses:** Vaccine
against diphtheria, tetanus, pertussis, HBV, polio (types 1, 2, 3) as a three-dose primary series in infants and children younger than age 7, born to HB$_s$ Ag – mothers **Action:** Active immunization **Dose:** *Infants.* 3 0.5-mL doses IM at 6–8-wk intervals, start at 2 mon; child given 1 dose of hepatitis B vaccine, same; child previously vaccinated with one or more doses of Infanrix or IPV, use to complete series **Contra/Caution:** [C, N/A] Contra if HB$_s$ AG + mother, adults, children >7 y, immunosuppressed, in hypersensitivity to yeast, neomycin, or polymyxin B, Hx allergy to any component of the vaccine, encephalopathy, or progressive neurologic disorders; caution in bleeding disorders **Supplied:** Single-dose vials 0.5 mL **Notes:** drowsiness, restlessness, fever, fussiness, ↓ appetite; nodule redness, pain, and swelling at site **Interactions:** ↓ effects with immunosuppressants, corticosteroids

Dipivefrin (Propine) **Uses:** Open-angle glaucoma **Action:** α-Adrenergic
agonist **Dose:** 1 gt into eye q12h **Caution/Contra:** [B, ?] Contra closed-angle glaucoma **Supplied:** 0.1% soln **Notes/SE:** HA, local irritation, blurred vision, photophobia, HTN **Interactions:** ↑ effects with BBs, ophthalmic anhydrase inhibitors, osmotic drugs, sympathomimetics, ↑ risk of cardiac arrhythmias with digoxin, TCAs **NIPE:** Discard discolored solutions

Dipyridamole (Persantine) **Uses:** Prevents postoperative thromboembolic disorders, often in combination with ASA or warfarin (eg, CABG, vascular graft; with warfarin after artificial heart valve; chronic angina; with ASA to prevent coronary artery thrombosis); dipyridamole IV used in place of exercise stress test for CAD **Action:** Antiplatelet activity; coronary vasodilator **Dose:** *Adults.* 75–100 mg PO tid–qid; stress test 0.14 mg/kg/min (max 60 mg over 4 min). *Peds >12 y.* 3–6 mg/kg/d ÷ tid **Caution/Contra:** [B, ?/–] Caution with other drugs that affect coagulation **Supplied:** Tabs 25, 50, 75 mg; inj 5 mg/mL **Notes:** IV can worsen angina; HA, hypotension, nausea, abdominal distress, flushing, rash, dyspnea **Interactions:** ↑ effects with anticoagulants, heparin, evening primrose oil, feverfew, garlic, ginger, ginkgo biloba, ginseng, grapeseed extract; ↑ effects of adenosine; ↑ bradycardia with BBs; ↓ effects with aminophylline **NIPE:** ⊘ alcohol or tobacco because of vasoconstriction effect; + effects may take several mo

Dipyridamole and Aspirin (Aggrenox) **Uses:** Reduces rate of reinfarction after MI; prevents occlusion after CABG; ↓ risk of stroke **Action:** ↓ platelet aggregation (both agents) **Dose:** 1 cap PO bid **Caution/Contra:** [C, ?]

Contra in ulcers, bleed diathesis **Supplied:** Dipyridamole (ER) 200 mg/aspirin 25 mg **Notes/SE:** ASA component: allergic reactions, skin reactions, ulcers/GI bleed, bronchospasm; dipyridamole component: dizziness, HA, rash

Dirithromycin (Dynabac)   **Uses:** Bronchitis, community-acquired pneumonia, and skin and skin structure infections **Action:** Macrolide antibiotic **Dose:** 500 mg/d PO; take with food **Caution/Contra:** [C, M] **Supplied:** Tabs 250 mg **Notes/SE:** Abdominal discomfort, HA, rash, hyperkalemia **Interactions:** ↑ effects with antacids, H₂ antagonists, food; ↑ effects of theophylline; ↓ effects of penicillins **NIPE:** Take with food, ⊘ crush or chew

Disopyramide (Norpace, NAPAmide)   **Uses:** Suppression and prevention of VT **Action:** Class 1A antiarrhythmic **Dose:** *Adults.* 400–800 mg/d ÷ q6h for regular and q12h for SR. *Peds. <1 y:* 10–30 mg/kg/24 h PO (÷ qid). *1–4 y:* 10–20 mg/kg/24 h PO (÷ qid). *4–12 y:* 10–15 mg/kg/24 h PO (÷ qid). *12–18 y:* 6–15 mg/kg/24 h PO (÷ qid); ↓ in renal/hepatic impairment **Caution/Contra:** [C, +] AV block, cardiogenic shock **Supplied:** Caps 100, 150 mg; SR caps 100, 150 mg **Notes/SE:** See Drug Levels, Table 2, page 245. Anticholinergic side effects; negative inotropic properties may induce CHF **Interactions:** ↑ effects with cimetidine, clarithromycin, erythromycin, quinidine; ↑ effects of digoxin, hypoglycemics, insulin, warfarin; ↑ risk of arrhythmias with pimozide; ↓ effects with barbiturates, phenytoin, phenobarbital, rifampin **Labs:** ↑ LFTs, lipids, BUN, creatinine; ↓ serum glucose, HMG, HCT **NIPE:** Risk of photosensitivity, daily wts

Dobutamine (Dobutrex)   **Uses:** Short-term use in cardiac decompensation secondary to depressed contractility **Action:** Positive inotropic agent **Dose:** *Adults & Peds.* Cont IV inf of 2.5–15 μg/kg/min; rarely, 40 μg/kg/min may be required; titrate according to response **Caution/Contra:** [C, ?] **Supplied:** Inj 250 mg/20 mL **Notes/SE:** Monitor PWP and cardiac output if possible, check ECG for ↑ heart rate, ectopic activity, follow BP; chest pain, HTN, dyspnea **Interactions:** ↑ effects with furazolidone, methyldopa, MAOIs, TCAs; ↓ effects with BBs, sodium bicarbonate; ↓ effects of guanethidine **Labs:** ↓ K; **NIPE:** eval for adequate hydration; monitor I&O, cardiac output, ECG, BP during infusion

Docetaxel (Taxotere)   **Uses:** Breast (anthracycline-resistant), ovarian, lung, and prostate CAs **Action:** Antimitotic agent; promotes microtubular aggregation; semisynthetic taxoid **Dose:** 100 mg/m² over 1 h IV q3wk (refer to specific protocols); start dexamethasone 8 mg bid prior to docetaxel and continue for 3–4 d; ↓ dose with ↑ bilirubin levels **Caution/Contra:** [D, –] **Supplied:** Inj 20, 40, 80 mg/mL **Notes/SE:** Myelosuppression, neuropathy, N/V; fluid retention syndrome; cumulative doses of 300–400 mg/m² w/o steroid prep and posttreatment and 600–800 mg/m² with steroid prep; hypersensitivity reactions possible, but rare with steroid prep **Interactions:** ↑ effects with cyclosporine, ketoconazole, erythromycin, terfenidine **Labs:** ↑ AST, ALT, alkaline phosphatase **NIPE:** ↑ fluids to 2–3 L/d, ↑ risk of hair loss, ↑ susceptibility to infection, urine may become reddish-brown

Docusate Calcium (Surfak)/Docusate Potassium (Dialose)/ Docusate Sodium (DOSS, Colace) Uses: Constipation; adjunct to painful anorectal conditions (hemorrhoids) **Action:** Stool softener **Dose:** *Adults.* 5 ÷ qid–qid. *Peds. 3–6 y:* 20–60 mg/24 h ÷ qid–qid. *6–12 y:* 40–150 mg/24 h ÷ qid–qid **Caution/Contra:** [C, ?] **Supplied:** *Ca:* Caps 50, 240 mg. *K:* Caps 100, 240 mg. *Na:* Caps 50, 100 mg; syrup 50, 60 mg/15 mL; liq 150 mg/15 mL; soln 50 mg/mL **Notes/SE:** No significant side effects, rare abdominal cramping, diarrhea; no laxative action **Interactions:** ↑ absorption of mineral oil **Labs:** ↓ K⁺ chloride **NIPE:** Short-term use, take with juices or milk to mask bitter taste

Dofetilide (Tikosyn) **WARNING:** To minimize the risk of induced arrhythmia, patients initiated or reinitiated on Tikosyn should be placed for a minimum of 3 d in a facility that can provide calculations of CrCl, continuous ECG monitoring, and cardiac resuscitation **Uses:** Maintains NSR in AF/A flutter after conversion **Action:** Type III antiarrhythmic **Dose:** 125–500 μg PO bid based on CrCl and QTc (see insert) **Caution/Contra:** [C, +] Contra in prolonged QT interval, verapamil, cimetidine, trimethoprim, or ketoconazole **Supplied:** Caps 125, 250, 500 μg **Notes/SE:** Ventricular arrhythmias, HA, chest pain, dizziness **Interactions:** ↑ effects with amiloride, amiodarone, azole antifungals, cimetidine, diltiazem, macrolides, metformin, megestrol, nefazadone, norfloxacin, SSRIs, TCAs, triamterene, trimethoprim, verapamil, zafirlukast, quinine, grapefruit juice **NIPE:** Take w/o regard to food; monitor LFTs, CrCl, creatinine

Dolasetron (Anzemet) Uses: Prevents chemotherapy-associated N/V **Action:** 5-HT₃ receptor antagonist **Dose:** *Adults & Peds.* 1.8 mg/kg IV as single dose 30 min prior to chemotherapy. *Adults.* 100 mg PO as a single dose 1 h prior to chemotherapy. *Peds.* 1.8 mg/kg PO to max 100 mg as single dose **Caution/Contra:** [B, ?] **Supplied:** Tabs 50, 100 mg; inj 20 mg/mL **Notes/SE:** Prolongs QT interval, HTN, HA, abdominal pain, urinary retention, transient ↑ LFTs **Interactions:** ↑ effects with cimetidine; ↑ risk of arrhythmias with diuretics; ↓ effects with rifampin **Labs:** ↑ ALT, AST, alkaline phosphatase, PTT **NIPE:** Monitor LFTs, PTT, CBC, platelets, & alkaline phosphatase with prolonged use

Dopamine (Intropin) Uses: Short-term use in cardiac decompensation secondary to decreased contractility; increases organ perfusion (at low dose) **Action:** Positive inotropic agent with dose-related response; 2–10 μg/kg/min β-effects (increases cardiac output and renal perfusion); 10–20 μg/kg/min β-effects (peripheral vasoconstriction, pressor); >20 μg/kg/min peripheral and renal vasoconstriction **Dose:** *Adults & Peds.* 5 μg/kg/min by cont inf, ↑ increments of 5 μg/kg/min to 50 μg/kg/min max based on effect **Caution/Contra:** [C, ?] **Supplied:** Inj 40, 80, 160 mg/mL **Notes/SE:** Dosage >10 μg/kg/min may ↓ renal perfusion; monitor urinary output; monitor ECG for ↑ in heart rate, BP, and ectopic activity; monitor PCWP and cardiac output if possible **Interactions:** ↑ effects with α-blockers, diuretics, ergot alkaloids, MAOIs, BBs, anesthetics, phenytoin; ↓ effects with guanethidine **Labs:** False ↑ urine catecholamines, urine amino acids; false ↓ serum creatinine **NIPE:** Maintain adequate hydration

Dornase Alfa (Pulmozyme) **Uses:** ↓ Frequency of respiratory infections in patients with CF **Action:** Enzyme that selectively cleaves DNA **Dose:** Inhal 2.5 mg/d **Caution/Contra:** [B, ?] **Supplied:** Soln for inhal 1 mg/mL **Notes/SE:** Use with recommended neb; pharyngitis, voice alteration, chest pain, rash **Interactions:** none noted **NIPE:** ⊘ mix or dilute with other drugs

Dorzolamide (Trusopt) **Uses:** Glaucoma **Action:** Carbonic anhydrase inhibitor **Dose:** 1 gtt in eye(s) tid **Caution/Contra:** [C, ?] **Supplied:** 2% soln **Notes/SE:** Local irritation, bitter taste, superficial punctate keratitis, ocular allergic reaction **Interactions:** ↑ effects with oral carbonic anhydrase inhibitors, salicylates **NIPE:** ⊘ wear soft contact lenses

Dorzolamide and Timolol (Cosopt) **Uses:** Glaucoma **Action:** carbonic anhydrase inhibitor with β-adrenergic blocker **Dose:** 1 gt in eye(s) bid **Caution/Contra:** [C, ?] **Supplied:** Soln dorzolamide 2% and timolol 0.5% **Notes/SE:** See Dorzolamide

Doxazosin (Cardura) **Uses:** HTN and symptomatic BPH **Action:** α₁-Adrenergic blocker; relaxes vascular and bladder neck smooth muscle **Dose:** *HTN:* Initially 1 mg/d PO; may be ↑ to 16 mg/d PO. *BPH:* Initially 1 mg/d PO, may be ↑ to 8 mg/d PO **Caution/Contra:** [B, ?] **Supplied:** Tabs 1, 2, 4, 8 mg **Notes/SE:** Doses >4 mg ↑ likelihood of orthostatic hypotension, dizziness, HA, drowsiness, sexual dysfunction **Interactions:** ↑ effects with nitrates, antihypertensives, alcohol; ↓ effects with NSAIDs, butcher's broom; ↓ effects of clonidine **NIPE:** May take with food

Doxepin (Sinequan, Adapin) **Uses:** Depression, anxiety, chronic pain **Action:** TCA; increases the synaptic CNS concs of serotonin or norepinephrine **Dose:** 25–150 mg/d PO, usually hs but can be in ÷ doses; ↓ in hepatic impairment **Caution/Contra:** [C, ?/–] **Supplied:** Caps 10, 25, 50, 75, 100, 150 mg; oral conc 10 mg/mL **Notes/SE:** Anticholinergic side effects, hypotension, tachycardia, drowsiness, photosensitivity **Interactions:** ↑ effects with fluoxetine, MAOIs, albuterol, CNS depressants, anticholinergics, cimetidine, oral contraceptives, propoxyphene, quinidine, alcohol, grapefruit juice; ↑ effects of carbamazepine, anticoagulants, amphetamines, thyroid drugs, sympathomimetics; ↓ effects with ascorbic acid, cholestyramine, tobacco; ↓ effects of bretyllium, guanethidine, levodopa **Labs:** ↑ serum bilirubin, alkaline phosphatase, glucose **NIPE:** Risk of photosensitivity, urine may turn blue-green, may take 4–6 wk for full effect

Doxepin, Topical (Zonalon) **Uses:** Short-term Rx pruritus (atopic dermatitis or lichen simplex chronicus) **Action:** Antipruritic; H₁- and H₂-receptor antagonism **Dose:** Apply thin coating qid for max 8 d **Caution/Contra:** [C, ?/–] **Supplied:** 5% cream **Notes/SE:** Limited application area to avoid systemic toxicity (hypotension, tachycardia, drowsiness, photosensitivity) **NIPE:** Occlusive dressings will ↑ systemic absorption

Doxorubicin (Adriamycin, Rubex) **Uses:** Acute leukemias; Hodgkin's and NHLs; breast CA; soft tissue and osteosarcomas; Ewing's sarcoma; Wilms' tumor; neuroblastoma; bladder, ovarian, gastric, thyroid, and lung CAs **Action:** Intercalates DNA; inhibits DNA topoisomerases I and II **Dose:** 60–75 mg/m² q3wk; ↓ cardiotoxicity with weekly (20 mg/m²/wk) or cont inf (60–90 mg/m² over 96 h) (refer to specific protocols) **Caution/Contra:** [D, ?] **Supplied:** Inj 10, 20, 50, 75, 200 mg **Notes/SE:** Myelosuppression; extravasation leads to tissue damage; venous streaking and phlebitis, N/V/D, mucositis, radiation recall phenomenon. Cardiomyopathy rare but dose related; limit of 550 mg/m² cumulative dose (400 mg/m² if prior mediastinal irradiation); dexrazoxane may limit cardiac toxicity **Interactions:** ↑ effects with streptozocin, verapamil, green tea; ↑ bone-marrow depression with antineoplastic drugs and radiation; ↓ effects with phenobarbital; ↓ effects of digoxin, phenytoin, live virus vaccines **Labs:** ↑ urine and plasma uric acid levels **NIPE:** ⊘ PRG, use contraception at least 4 mon >drug treatment

Doxycycline (Vibramycin) **Uses:** Broad-spectrum antibiotic, activity against *Rickettsia* spp, *Chlamydia*, and *M. pneumoniae* **Action:** Tetracycline; interferes with protein synthesis **Dose:** *Adults.* 100 mg PO q12h on 1st day, then 100 mg PO qd–bid or 100 mg IV q12h. *Peds >8y.* 5 mg/kg/24 h PO, to a max of 200 mg/d ÷ qd–bid **Supplied:** Tabs 50, 100 mg; caps 20, 50, 100 mg; syrup 50 mg/5 mL; susp 25 mg/5 mL; inj 100, 200 mg/vial **Caution/Contra:** [D, +] **Notes/SE:** Useful for chronic bronchitis; tetracycline of choice in renal impairment; diarrhea, GI disturbance, photosensitivity **Interactions:** ↑ effects of digoxin, warfarin; ↓ effects with antacids, iron, barbiturates, carbamazepine, phenytoins, food; ↓ effects of penicillins **Labs:** False neg urine glucose, false ↑ urine catecholamines; false ↓ urine urobilinogen **NIPE:** ↑ risk of superinfection, ⊘ PRG, use barrier contraception

Dronabinol (Marinol) [C-II] **Uses:** N/V; appetite stimulation **Action:** Antiemetic; inhibits the vomiting center in the medulla **Dose:** *Adults & Peds.* *Antiemetic:* 5–15 mg/m²/dose q4–6h PRN. *Adults.* *Appetite:* 2.5 mg PO before lunch and dinner **Caution/Contra:** [C, ?] **Supplied:** Caps 2.5, 5, 10 mg **Notes/SE:** Principal psychoactive substance present in marijuana; drowsiness, dizziness, anxiety, mood change, hallucinations, depersonalization, orthostatic hypotension, tachycardia **Interactions:** ↑ effects with anticholinergics, CNS depressants, alcohol; ↓ effects of theophylline **Labs:** ↓ FSH, LH, growth hormone, testosterone

Droperidol (Inapsine) **Uses:** N/V; anesthetic premedication **Action:** Tranquilization, sedation, and antiemetic **Dose:** *Adults.* *Nausea:* 2.5–5 mg IV or IM q3–4h PRN. *Premed:* 2.5–10 mg IV, 30–60 min preop. *Peds.* *Premed:* 0.1–0.15 mg/kg/dose **Caution/Contra:** [C, ?] **Supplied:** Inj 2.5 mg/mL **Notes/SE:** Drowsiness, moderate hypotension, occasional tachycardia and extrapyramidal reactions, QT interval prolongation, arrhythmias **Interactions:** ↑ effects with CNS depressants, fentanyl, alcohol; ↑ hypotension with antihypertensives, nitrates

Drotrecogin Alfa (Xigris) **Uses:** Reduces mortality in adults with severe sepsis (associated with acute organ dysfunction) who have a high risk of death (eg, as determined by APACHE II) **Action:** Recombinant form of human activated protein C; exact mechanism unknown **Dose:** 24 μg/kg/h for a total of 96 h **Caution/Contra:** [C, ?] Contra in active bleeding, recent stroke or CNS surgery, head trauma, epidural catheter, CNS lesion at risk for herniation **Supplied:** 5-, 20-mg vials for reconstitution **Notes/SE:** Bleeding most common SE **Interactions:** ↑ risk of bleeding with platelet inhibitors, anticoagulants **Labs:** ↑ aPTT **NIPE:** d/c drug 2 h <invasive procedures

Dutasteride (Avodart) **Uses:** Symptomatic BPH **Action:** 5α-reductase inhibitor **Dose:** 0.5 mg PO qd **Caution/Contra:** [X, –] Women and children, caution in hepatic impairment, pregnant women should avoid handling pills **Supplied:** Caps 0.5 mg **Notes/SE:** Do not donate blood until 6 mon after discontinuation of this drug; ↓ PSA levels, impotence, ↓ libido, gynecomastia **Interactions:** ↑ effects with cimetidine, ciprofloxacin, diltiazem, ketoconazole, ritonavir, verapamil **Labs:** ↓ PSA levels **NIPE:** ⊘ handling by pregnant women, take w/o regard to food

Echothiophate Iodine (Phospholine Ophthalmic) **Uses:** Glaucoma **Action:** Cholinesterase inhibitor **Dose:** 1 gt eye(s) bid with one dose hs **Caution/Contra:** [C, ?] **Supplied:** Powder to reconstitute 1.5 mg/0.03%; 3 mg/ 0.06%; 6.25 mg/0.125%; 12.5 mg/0.25% **Notes/SE:** Local irritation, myopia, blurred vision, hypotension, bradycardia **Interactions:** ↑ effects with cholinesterase inhibitors, pilocarpine, succinylcholine, carbamate or organophosphate insecticides; ↑ effects of cocaine; ↓ effects with anticholinergics, atropine, cyclopentolate, ophthalmic adrenocorticoids **NIPE:** ⊘ drug 2 wk <surgery if succinylcholine to be administered, keep drug refrigerated, monitor for lens opacities

Econazole (Spectazole) **Uses:** Most tinea, cutaneous *Candida,* and tinea versicolor infections **Action:** Topical antifungal **Dose:** Apply to areas bid (qd for tinea versicolor) for 2–4 wk **Caution/Contra:** [C, ?] **Supplied:** Topical cream 1% **Notes/SE:** Symptom/clinical improvement seen early in treatment, must carry out course of therapy to avoid recurrence; local irritation, pruritus, erythema **Interactions:** ↓ effects with corticosteroids **NIPE:** Topical use only, avoid eye area

Edrophonium (Tensilon) **Uses:** Diagnosis of MyG; acute MyG crisis; curare antagonist **Action:** Anticholinesterase **Dose:** *Adults. Test for MyG:* 2 mg IV in 1 min; if tolerated, give 8 mg IV; positive test is a brief ↑ in strength. *Peds. Test for MyG:* Total dose of 0.2 mg/kg. Give 0.04 mg/kg as a test dose. If no response occurs, give the remainder of the dose in 1-mg increments to max of 10 mg; ↓ in renal impairment **Caution/Contra:** [C, ?] GI or GU obstruction; hypersensitivity to sulfite **Supplied:** Inj 10 mg/mL **Notes/SE:** Can cause severe cholinergic effects; keep atropine available **Interactions:** ↑ effects with tacrine; ↑ cardiac effects with digoxin; ↑ effects of neostigmine, pyridostigmine, succinylcholine, jaborandi tree, pill-bearing spurge; ↓ effects with corticosteroids, procainamide, quinidine **Labs:** ↑ AST, ALT, serum amylase **NIPE:** ↑ risk uterine irritability & premature labor in pregnant pts near term

Efavirenz (Sustiva) Uses: HIV infections Action: antiretroviral; nonnucleoside reverse transcriptase inhibitor Dose: *Adults.* 600 mg/d PO. *Peds.* refer to product information; take hs, avoid high-fat meals Caution/Contra: [C, ?] CDC recommends HIV-infected mothers not breast-feed due to risk of transmission of HIV to infant. Supplied: Caps 50, 100, 200 mg Notes/SE: Somnolence, vivid dreams, dizziness, rash, N/V/D Interactions: ↑ effects with ritonavir; ↑ effects of CNS depressants, ergot derivatives, midazolam, ritonavir, simvastatin, triazolam, warfarin; ↓ effects with carbamazepine, phenobarbital, rifabutin, rifampin, saquinavir, St. John's Wort; ↓ effects of amprenavir, carbamazepine, clarithromycin, indinavir, phenobarbital, saquinavir, warfarin; may alter effectiveness of oral contraceptive Labs: ↑ AST, ALT, amylase, total cholesterol, triglycerides; false + urine cannabinoid test NIPE: ⊘ high–fat foods, take w/o regard to food, use barrier contraception

Eletriptan (Relpax) Uses: Acute Rx of migraine Action: Selective serotonin (5-HT$_{1B/1D}$)-receptor agonist Dose: 20–40 mg PO, repeat after 2 h PRN (max 80 mg/d) Caution: [C,+/-]; ⊘ use w/n 72 h with potent CYP3A4 inhibitors Contra: Avoid in pts with ischemic heart disease, cerebrovascular disease, PVD, uncontrolled HTN, hemiplegic or basilar migraine, w/n 24 h of treatment with another serotonin agonist or ergot, severe hepatic impairment Supplied: Tabs 20, 40 mg SE: Dizziness, nausea, paresthesias, chest pain, HTN Interactions: ↑ effects with clarithromycin, erythromycin, fluconazole, ketoconazole, itraconazole, nefazodone, nelfinavir, propranolol, ritonavir, troleandomycin, verapamil; ↑ risk of weakness, hyperreflexia and incoordination with fluoxetine, fluvoxamine, paroxetine, sertraline; ↑ risk of vasospastic reactions with dihydroergotamine, ergots, methysergide NIPE: ⊘ take with CAD or risk factors for CAD; drug excreted in breast milk

Emedastine (Emadine) Uses: Allergic conjunctivitis Action: Antihistamine; selective H₁-antagonist Dose: 1 gt in eye(s) up to qid Caution/Contra: [B, ?] Supplied: 0.5% soln Notes/SE: Blurred vision, burning, corneal infiltrates and staining, dry eyes, foreign body sensation, hyperemia, keratitis, tearing, HA, pruritus, rhinitis, sinusitis, asthenia, bad taste, dermatitis, discomfort NIPE: ⊘ wear soft contact lens for 15 min >use

Emtricitabine (Emtriva) WARNING: Class warning for lipodystrophy, lactic acidosis, and severe hepatomegaly Uses: HIV-1 infection Action: Nucleoside reverse transcriptase inhibitor (NRTI) Dose: *Adults.* 200 mg PO QD; ?dose for renal dysfunction. *Peds.* Caution: [B,–] Contra: N/A Supplied: 200 mg caps SE: HA, diarrhea, nausea, rash Notes: Rare hyperpigmentation of feet/hands; post-treatment exacerbation of hepatitis; first NRTI with QD dosing Interactions: None noted with additional NRTIs NIPE: Take w/o regard to food, causes redistribution and accumulation of body fat; take with other antiretrovirals; not a cure for HIV or prevention of opportunistic infections

Enalapril (Vasotec) Uses: HTN, CHF, DN, and asymptomatic LVD Action: ACE inhibitor Dose: *Adults.* 2.5–5 mg/d PO; ↑ by effect to 10–40 mg/d as

1–2 ÷ doses, or 1.25 mg IV q6h. *Peds.* 0.05–0.08 mg/kg/dose PO q12–24h; ↓ in renal impairment **Caution/Contra:** [C (1st trimester; D 2nd and 3rd trimesters), +] **Supplied:** Tabs 2.5, 5, 10, 20 mg; inj 1.25 mg/mL **Notes/SE:** Symptomatic hypotension with initial dose, especially with concomitant diuretics; DC diuretic for 2–3 d prior to initiation; monitor for ↑ in K; may cause a nonproductive cough, angioedema **Interactions:** ↑ effects with loop diuretics; ↑ risk of cough with capsaicin; ↑ effects of α-blockers, insulin, lithium; ↑ risk of hyperkalemia with K⁺, K⁺-sparing diuretics, salt substitutes, trimethoprim; ↓ effects with ASA, NSAIDs, rifampin **Labs:** May cause ↑ serum K⁺, direct Coombs test, false ↑ urine acetone **NIPE:** Several wk for full hypotensive effect

Enfuvirtide (Fuzeon)   WARNING: Rarely causes hypersensitivity, never rechallenge patient **Uses:** Combination with antiretroviral agents for HIV-1 with evidence of viral replication despite therapy **Action:** Fusion inhibitor **Dose:** *Adults.* 90 mg (1 mL) sq BID in upper arm, anterior thigh, or abdomen *Peds.* 6–16 y: 2 mg/kg sq BID, 90 mg max **Caution:** [B,–] **Contra:** Previous hypersensitivity to drug **Supplied:** 90 mg/mL (reconstituted); dispensed as patient convenience kit (1 mon supply of drug syringes, swabs, educational materials, etc) **SE:** Injection-site reactions (common); pneumonia, diarrhea, nausea, fatigue, insomnia, peripheral neuropathy **Notes:** Rotate injection site; restricted drug distribution system; immediately administer upon reconstitution or refrigerate for up to 24 h before use **Interactions:** None noted with other antiretrovirals **NIPE:** Does not cure HIV; does not ↓ risk of transmission or prevent opportunistic infections; take w/o regard to food

Enoxaparin (Lovenox)   **Uses:** Prevention and Rx of DVT; Rx PE; unstable angina and non-Q-wave MI **Action:** LMW heparin **Dose:** *Prevention:* 30 mg bid SC or 40 mg SC q24h. *DVT/PE:* 1 mg/kg SC q12h or 1.5 mg/kg SC q24h. *Angina:* 1 mg/kg SC q12h; ↓ or avoid with severe renal impairment **Caution/Contra:** [B, ?] Active bleeding; not recommended for thromboprophylaxis in prosthetic heart valves **Supplied:** Inj 10 mg/0.1 mL (30-, 40-, 60-, 80-, 100-mg syringes) **Notes/ SE:** Does not significantly affect bleeding time, platelet function, PT, or aPTT; bleeding, bruising, thrombocytopenia, pain at inj site; ↑ serum transaminases **Interactions:** ↑ bleeding effects with ASA, anticoagulants, cephalosporins, NSAIDS, penicillin, chamomile, garlic, ginger, ginkgo biloba, feverfew, horse chestnut **Labs:** ↑ AST, ALT **NIPE:** No need to monitor aPTT, admin deep SQ NOT MI

Entacapone (Comtan)   **Uses:** Parkinson's disease **Action:** Selective reversible COMT inhibitor **Dose:** 200 mg concurrently with each levodopa/carbidopa dose to a max of 8×/d **Caution/Contra:** [C, ?] Hepatic impairment **Supplied:** Tabs 200 mg **Notes/SE:** Dyskinesia, hyperkinesia, nausea, dizziness, hallucinations, orthostatic hypotension, brown-orange urine **Interactions:** ↑ effects with ampicillin, choramphenicol, cholestyramine, erythromycin, MAOIs, probenecid, rifampin; ↑ risk of arrhythmias & HTN with bitolterol, dopamine, dobutamine, epinephrine, isoetherine, methyldopa, norepinephine **NIPE:** ⊘ d/c abruptly, breast-feed

Ephedrine **Uses:** Acute bronchospasm, nasal congestion, hypotension, narcolepsy, enuresis, and MyG **Action:** Sympathomimetic; stimulates both α- and β-receptors **Dose:** *Adults.* 25–50 mg IM or IV q10min to a max of 150 mg/d or 25–50 mg PO q3–4h PRN. *Peds.* 0.2–0.3 mg/kg/dose IM or IV q4–6h PRN **Caution/Contra:** [C, ?/–] **Supplied:** Inj 25, 50 mg/mL; caps 25, 50 mg; syrup 11, 20 mg/5 mL **Notes/SE:** CNS stimulation, nervousness, anxiety, trembling, HTN, tachycardia **Interactions:** ↑ effects with acetazolamide, antacids, MAOIs, TCAs, urinary alkalinizers; ↑ effects of sympathomimetics; ↓ response with diuretics, methyldopa, reserpine, urinary acidifiers; ↓ effects of antihypertensives, BBs, dexamethasone, guanethidine **Labs:** false ↑ urine amino acids **NIPE:** ⊘ alcohol, store away from light/heat

Epinephrine (Adrenalin, Sus-Phrine) **Uses:** Cardiac arrest, anaphylactic reactions, acute asthma **Action:** β-Adrenergic agonist with some α-effects **Dose:** *Adults.* *Emergency cardiac care:* 0.5–1.0 mg (5–10 mL of 1:10,000) IV q5min to response. *Anaphylaxis:* 0.3–0.5 mL of 1:1000 dilution SC; may repeat q10–15min to a max of 1 mg/dose and 5 mg/d. *Asthma:* 0.3–0.5 mL of 1:1000 dilution SC, repeated at 20-min–4-h intervals or 1 inhal (met-dose) repeat in 1–2 min or susp 0.1–0.3 mL SC for extended effect. *Peds.* *Emergency cardiac care:* 0.1 mL/kg of 1:10,000 dilution IV q3–5min to response **Caution/Contra:** [C, ?] **Supplied:** Inj 1:1000, 1:2000, 1:10,000, 1:100,000; susp for inj 1:200; aerosol; soln for inhal **Notes/SE:** Sus-Phrine offers sustained action. In acute cardiac settings, can give via ET tube if no central line; tachycardia, HTN, CNS stimulation, nervousness, anxiety, trembling **Interactions:** ↑ HTN effects with α-blockers, BBs, ergot alkaloids, furazolidone, MAOIs; ↑ cardiac effects with antihistamines, cardiac glycosides, levodopa, thyroid hormones, TCAs; ↑ effects of sympathomimetics; ↓ effects of diuretics, guanethidine, hypoglycemics, methyldopa **Labs:** ↑ serum bilirubin, glucose, & uric acid, urine catecholamines **NIPE:** ⊘ OTC inhalation drugs

Eplerenone (Inspra) **Uses:** HTN **Action:** Aldosterone antagonist **Dose:** *Adults.* 50 mg PO qd; max dose 50 mg PO bid; ↓ dose to 25 mg PO if used with weak inhibitors of CYP3A4 (eg, erythromycin, fluconazole, verapamil, saquinavir) **Caution/Contra:** [B, +/–] K⁺ > 5.5 mEq/L, type 2 DM with microalbuminuria, SCr > 2.0 mg/dL in males or > 1.8 mg/dL in females, CrCl < 50 mL/min, use of K⁺ supplements or K⁺-sparing diuretics, use of strong inhibitors of CYP3A4 **Supplied:** Tabs 25 mg **Notes/SE:** Hyperkalemia, HA, dizziness, gynecomastia, hypercholesterolemia, hypertriglyceridemia **Interactions:** ↑ risk hyperkalemia with ACEIs; ↑ risk of toxic effects with azole antifungals, erythromycin, saquinavir, verapamil, ↑ effects of lithium; ↓ effects with NSAIDs **NIPE:** ⊘ high-K⁺ foods, may cause reversible breast pain or enlargement with use

Epoetin Alfa [Erythropoietin, EPO] (Epogen, Procrit) **Uses:** Anemia associated with CRF, zidovudine treatment in HIV-infected patients, CA chemotherapy; reduction in transfusions associated with surgery **Action:** Erythropoietin supplementation **Dose:** *Adults & Peds.* 50–150 U/kg 3×/wk; adjust the dose q4–6wk as needed. *Surgery:* 300 U/kg/d for 10 d prior to surgery **Caution/Contra:** [C, +] Uncontrolled HTN **Supplied:** Inj 2000, 3000, 4000, 10,000, 20,000 U/mL **Notes/SE:** HTN, HA, tachycardia, N/V; store in refrigerator **Interactions:** None noted **Labs:** ↑ WBCs, platelets **NIPE:** Monitor for access line clotting, ⊘ shake vial

Epoprostenol (Flolan) **Uses:** Pulmonary HTN **Action:** Dilates the pulmonary and systemic arterial vascular beds; inhibits platelet aggregation **Dose:** 4 ng/kg/min IV cont inf; adjustments based on response and package insert guidelines **Caution/Contra:** [B, ?] Chronic use in CHF **Supplied:** Inj 0.5, 1.5 mg **Notes/SE:** Flushing, tachycardia, CHF, fever, chills, nervousness, HA, jaw pain, flu-like symptoms **Interactions:** ↑ risk of bleeding with anticoagulants, antiplatelets; ↑ effects of digoxin; ↓ BP with antihypertensives, diuretics, vasodilators **NIPE:** ⊘ mix or administer with other drugs

Eprosartan (Teveten) **Uses:** HTN, DN, CHF **Action:** Angiotensin II receptor antagonist **Dose:** 400–800 mg/d single dose or bid **Caution/Contra:** [C (1st trimester; D 2nd and 3rd trimesters), ?] **Supplied:** Tabs 400, 600 mg **Notes/SE:** Fatigue, depression, hypertriglyceridemia, URI, UTI **Interactions:** ↑ risk of hyperkalemia with K+-sparing diuretics, K+ supplements, trimethoprim; ↑ effects of lithium **Labs:** ↑ ALT, AST, alkaline phosphatase, BUN, creatinine; ↓ HMG **NIPE:** Monitor LFTs, CBC & differential, renal function; ⊘ PRG, breast-feeding

Eptifibatide (Integrilin) **Uses:** Acute coronary syndrome **Action:** Glycoprotein IIb/IIIa inhibitor **Dose:** 180-μg/kg IV bolus, then 2-μg/kg/min inf; ↓ adjust in renal impairment (SCr = 2 mg/dL and = 4 mg/dL: 135-μg/kg bolus and 0.5-μg/kg/min inf) **Caution/Contra:** [B, ?] Hx abnormal bleeding or stroke (w/n 30 d), any hemorrhagic stroke, severe HTN, major surgery (w/n 6 wk), platelet count <100,000 cells/mm³, renal dialysis **Supplied:** Inj 0.75, 2 mg/mL **Notes/SE:** Bleeding, hypotension, inj site reaction **Interactions:** ↑ bleeding with ASA, cephalosporins, clopidogrel, heparin, NSAIDs, thrombolytics, ticlopidine, warfarin, evening primrose oil, feverfew, garlic, ginger, ginkgo biloba, ginseng, grapeseed extract

Ertapenem (Invanz) **Uses:** Complicated intraabdominal, urinary, and skin infections, acute pelvic infections, community-acquired pneumonia **Action:** A carbapenem; β-lactam antibiotic, inhibits cell wall synthesis; active against gram –/+ anaerobes, but not *Pseudomonas,* penicillin-resistant pneumococci, MRSA, *Mycoplasma, Chlamydia* **Dose:** 1 g IM/IV once daily; reduce dose by 50% if CrCl <30 mL/min **Caution/Contra:** [C, ?/–] Contra in <18 y, caution in penicillin allergy **Supplied:** Inj 1 g/vial **Notes/SE:** N/V/D, inj site reactions, ↑ LFTs **Interactions:** ↑ effects with probenecid; **Labs:** ↑ AST, ALT, serum alkaline phosphatase, bilirubin, glucose, creatinine, PT, RBCs, urine WBCs **NIPE:** Monitor for superinfection

Erythromycin (E-Mycin, Ilosone, Erythrocin) Uses: Infections caused by group A streptococci (*S. pyogenes*), α-hemolytic streptococci, and *N. gonorrhoeae* in penicillin-allergic patients; *S. pneumoniae*, *M. pneumoniae*, and *Legionella* infections Action: Bacteriostatic; interferes with protein synthesis Dose: Adults: 250–500 mg PO qid or 500 mg–1 g IV qid Peds: 30–50 mg/kg/24 h PO or IV ÷ q6h, to a max of 2 g/d; take with food to minimize GI upset Caution/Contra: [B, +] Supplied: *Powder for inj as lactobionate and gluceptate salts:* 500 mg, 1 g. *Base:* Tabs 250, 333, 500 mg; caps 250 mg. *Estolate:* Tabs 500 mg; caps 250 mg; susp 125, 250 mg/5 mL. *Stearate:* Tabs 250, 500 mg. *Ethylsuccinate:* Chew tabs 200 mg; tabs 400 mg; susp 200, 400 mg/5 mL Notes/SE: Mild GI disturbances; cholestatic jaundice (estolate); erythromycin base not well absorbed from the GI tract; some forms better tolerated with respect to GI irritation; lactobionate salt contains benzyl alcohol (caution in neonates); part of the Condon bowel prep Interactions: ↑ effects with amprenavir, indinavir, ritonavir, saquinavir, grapefruit juice; ↑ effects of alprazolam, benzodiazepines, buspirone, carbamazepine, clozapine, colchicines, cyclosporine, digoxin, felodipine, lovastatin, midazolam, quinidine, sildenafil, simvastatin, tacrolimus, theophylline, triazolam, valproic acid; ↑ QT with astemizole, cisapride; ↓ effects of penicillin, zafirlukast Labs: False ↑ AST, ALT, serum bilirubin, urine amino acids, false ↓ folate assay NIPE: Take with food if GI upset, monitor for superinfection & ototoxicity

Erythromycin and Benzoyl Peroxide (Benzamycin) Uses: Topical Rx of acne vulgaris Action: Macrolide antibiotic with keratolytic Dose: Apply bid (AM & PM) Caution/Contra: [C, ?] Supplied: Gel erythromycin 30 mg/ benzoyl peroxide 50 mg/g Notes/SE: Local irritation

Erythromycin and Sulfisoxazole (Eryzole, Pediazole) Uses: Upper and lower respiratory tract; bacterial infections; otitis media in children due to *H. influenzae*; infections in penicillin-allergic patients Action: Macrolide antibiotic with sulfonamide Dose: Based on erythromycin content. Adults: 400 mg erythromycin/1200 mg sulfisoxazole PO q6h. Peds >2 mon. 40–50 mg/kg/d of erythromycin PO ÷ tid–qid; max 2 g erythromycin or 6 g sulfisoxazole/d or estimated dose of 1.25 mL/kg/d ÷ tid–qid; ↓ ? in renal impairment Caution/Contra: (D if given near term), +] Infants <2 mon Supplied: Susp erythromycin ethylsuccinate 200 mg/sulfisoxazole 600 mg/5 mL Notes/SE: GI disturbance; see Erythromycin. Additional Interactions: ↑ effects of sulfonamides with ASA, diuretics, NSAIDs, probenecid Labs: False + urine protein NIPE: ↑ risk of photosensitivity, ↑ fluid intake

Erythromycin, Ophthalmic (Ilotycin Ophthalmic) Uses: Conjunctival infections Action: Macrolide antibiotic Dose: Apply q6h Caution/Contra: [B, +] Supplied: 0.5% oint Notes/SE: Local irritation NIPE: May cause burning, stinging, blurred vision

Erythromycin, Topical (Akne-Mycin Topical, Del-Mycin Topical, Emgel Topical, Staticin Topical) Uses: Acne Action: Macrolide antibiotic **Dose:** Wash and dry area, apply 2% product over area bid **Caution/Contra:** [B, +] **Supplied:** Soln 1.5, 2%; gel; impregnated pads and swabs 2% **Notes/SE:** Local irritation

Escitalopram (Lexapro)   **Uses:** Rx depression **Action:** Selective serotonin reuptake inhibitor **Dose:** 10 mg-20 mg PO daily; 10 mg PO daily with hepatic impairment **Caution:** [C,?/-] **Contra:** Use with or w/n 14 d of MAOI **Supplied:** Tab 10, 20 mg; solution 5mg/5ml **SE:** Nausea, diarrhea, dry mouth, insomnia, dizziness, sweating, fatigue **Notes:** N/A **Interactions:** ↑ risk of serotonin syndrome with linezolid; ↑ risk of bleeding with anticoagulants, ASA, NSAIDs; may ↑ CNS effects with CNS depressants **NIPE:** ⊘ d/c abruptly; may take up to 2–4 wk for full effects; take w/o regard to food

Esmolol (Brevibloc)   **Uses:** SVT and noncompensatory sinus tachycardia **Action:** β-Adrenergic blocking agent; class II antiarrhythmic **Dose:** *Adults & Peds.* Initiate treatment with 500 μg/kg load over 1 min, then 50 μg/kg/min for 4 min; if inadequate response, repeat the loading dose and follow with maint inf of 100 μg/kg/min for 4 min; titrate by repeating loading, then incremental ↑ in the maint dose of 50 μg/kg/min for 4 min until desired heart rate reached or BP decreases; average dose 100 μg/kg/min **Caution/Contra:** [C (1st trimester; D 2nd or 3rd trimester), ?] Sinus bradycardia, heart block, uncompensated CHF, cardiogenic shock **Supplied:** Inj 10, 250 mg/mL **Notes/SE:** Monitor for hypotension; ↓ or discontinuing inf reverses hypotension in ~30 min; bradycardia, diaphoresis, dizziness, pain on inj **Interaction:** ↑ effects with verapamil; ↑ effects of digoxin, antihypertensives, nitrates; ↑ HTN with amphetamines, cocaine, ephedrine, epinephrine, MAOIs, norepinephrine, phenylephrine, pseudoephedrine; ↓ effects of glucagons, insulin, hypoglycemics, theophylline; ↓ effects with NSAIDs, thyroid hormones **Labs:** ↑ glucose, cholesterol **NIPE:** Monitor BS of pts with DM

Esomeprazole (Nexium)   **Uses:** Short-term (4–8 wk) Rx confirmed erosive esophagitis/GERD; Rx of *H. pylori* infection in combination with antibiotics to reduce risk of duodenal ulcer **Action:** Proton pump inhibitor, ↓ acid production **Dose:** *GERD/erosive gastritis:* 20–40 mg/d PO 4–8 wk; repeat PRN ×4–8 wk; maint 20 mg/d PO; can open capsule and sprinkle on applesauce. *H. pylori infection:* 40 mg/d PO, plus clarithromycin 500 mg PO bid and amoxicillin 1000 mg/d for 10 d **Caution/Contra:** [B, ?/–] **Supplied:** Caps, 20, 40 mg **Notes/SE:** Related to omeprazole; HA, diarrhea, abdominal pain **Interactions:** ↑ effects with amoxicillin, clarithromycin; ↑ effects of diazepam, phenytoin, warfarin; ↓ effects with food; ↑ effects of azole antifungals, digoxin **Labs:** ↑ LFTs, bilirubin, serum creatinine, uric acid, TSH; ↓ Hgb, WBC, platelets, K⁺, sodium, thyroxine **NIPE:** Take at least 1 h <meals

Estazolam (ProSom) [C-IV]   **Uses:** Insomnia **Action:** Benzodiazepine **Dose:** 1–2 mg PO hs PRN; ↓ in hepatic impairment; avoid abrupt withdrawal **Caution/Contra:** [X, –] **Supplied:** Tabs 1, 2 mg **Notes/SE:** Somnolence, weakness, alpitations **Interactions:** ↑ effects with azole antifungals, cimetidine, ciprofloxin, larithromycin, clozapine, CNS depressants, diltiazem, disulfiram, digoxin, erythromycin, isoniazid, labetalol, levodopa, oral contraceptives, phenytoin, probenecid, valporic acid, verapamil, alcohol, kava kava, valerian; ↑ effects of digoxin, phenytoin; ↓ effects with carbamazepine, rifampin, ritabutin, theophylline, aminophylline, dyphylline, tobacco, oxitriphylline **NIPE:** ⊘ PRG, breast-feeding, alcohol

sterified Estrogens (Estratab, Menest) **Uses:** Vasomotor symptoms, atrophic vaginitis, or kraurosis vulvae associated with menopause; osteoporosis, female hypogonadism **Action:** Estrogen supplementation **Dose:** *Menopause:* 0.3–1.25 mg/d, administered cyclically 3 wk on and 1 wk off. *Hypogonadism:* 2.5 mg PO qd–tid; not recommended in severe hepatic impairment **Caution/Contra:** [X, –] Genital bleeding of unknown cause, breast CA, estrogen-dependent tumors, thromboembolic disorders, thrombosis, thrombophlebitis, recent MI **Supplied:** Tabs 0.3, 0.625, 1.25, 2.5 mg **Notes/SE:** Nausea, bloating, breast enlargement/tenderness, edema, HA, hypertriglyceridemia, gallbladder disease **Interactions:** ↑ effects of corticosteroids, cyclosporine, TCAs, theophylline, caffeine, tobacco; ↓ effects with barbiturates, phenytoin, rifampin; ↓ effects of anticoagulants, clibrate, hypoglycemics, insulin, tamoxifen **Labs:** ↑ prothrombin & factors VII, VIII, IX, X, platelet aggregability, thyroid-binding globulin, T4, triglycerides; ↓ antithrombin III, folate **NIPE:** ⊘ PRG, breast-feeding

Esterified Estrogens + Methyltestosterone (Estratest) **Uses:** Moderate/severe menopausal vasomotor symptoms; postpartum breast engorgement **Action:** Estrogen and androgen supplementation **Dose:** 1 tab/d for 3 wk, then 1 wk off **Caution/Contra:** [X, –] Genital bleeding of unknown cause, breast CA, estrogen-dependent tumors, thromboembolic disorders, thrombosis, thrombophlebitis, recent MI **Supplied:** Tabs (estrogen/methyltestosterone) 0.625 mg/1.25 mg, 1.25 mg/2.5 mg **Notes/SE:** Nausea, bloating, breast enlargement/tenderness, edema, HA, hypertriglyceridemia, gallbladder disease; **see Esterified Estrogens. Additional Interactions:** ↑ effects of insulin; ↓ effects of oral anticoagulants

Estradiol (Estrace) **Uses:** Atrophic vaginitis, kraurosis vulvae vasomotor symptoms associated with menopause, osteoporosis **Action:** Estrogen supplementation **Dose:** *Oral:* 1–2 mg/d, adjust PRN to control symptoms. *Vaginal cream:* 2–4 g/d for 2 wk, then 1 g 1–3×/wk **Caution/Contra:** [X, –] Genital bleeding of unknown cause, breast CA, estrogen-dependent tumors, thromboembolic disorders, thrombosis, thrombophlebitis; recent MI; not recommended in severe hepatic impairment **Supplied:** Tabs 0.5, 1, 2 mg; vaginal cream **Notes/SE:** Nausea, bloating, breast enlargement/tenderness, edema, HA, hypertriglyceridemia, gallbladder disease **Interactions:** ↑ effects with grapefruit juice; ↑ effects of corticosteroids, cyclosporine, TCAs, theophylline, caffeine, tobacco; ↓ effects with barbiturates, carbamazepine, phenytoin, primidone, rifampin; ↓ effects of clofibrate, hypoglycemics, insulin, tamoxifen, warfarin **Labs:** ↑ prothrombin & factors VII, VIII, IX, X, platelet aggregability, thyroid-binding globulin, T4, triglycerides; ↓ antithrombin III, folate **NIPE:** ⊘ PRG, breast-feeding

Estradiol Cypionate and Medroxyprogesterone Acetate (Lunelle)
WARNING: Cigarette smoking ↑ risk of serious cardiovascular SE from contraceptives containing estrogen. This risk ↑ with age and with heavy smoking (>15 cigarettes/day) and is quite marked in women >35 y. Women who use Lunelle should be strongly advised not to smoke **Uses:** contraceptive **Action:** estrogen and progestin **Dose:** 0.5 mL IM (deltoid, and thigh, buttock) monthly, do not exceed 33 d **Caution/Contra:** [X, M] Contra PRG, heavy smokers >35 y, DVT, PE, cerebro/cardiovascular disease, estrogen-dependent neoplasm, undiagnosed abnormal uterine bleeding, hepatic tumors, cholestatic jaundice. Caution HTN, gallbladder disease, ↑ lipids, migraines, sudden HA, valvular heart disease with complications **Supplied:** Estradiol cypionate (5 mg), medroxyprogesterone acetate (25 mg) single-dose vial or prefilled syringe (0.5 mL) **Notes/SE:** Start w/in 5 d of menstruation; arterial thromboembolism, HTN, cerebral hemorrhage, MI, amenorrhea, acne, breast tenderness; **see Estradiol. Additional Interactions:** ↓ effects with aminoglutethimide

Estradiol, Transdermal (Estraderm)
Uses: Severe menopausal vasomotor symptoms; female hypogonadism **Action:** Estrogen supplementation **Dose:** 0.1 mg/d patch 1–2×/wk depending on product; adjust PRN to control symptoms **Caution/Contra:** [X, −] (See Estradiol Cypionate) **Supplied:** TD patches (delivers mg/24 h) 0.025, 0.0375, 0.05, 0.075, 0.1 **Notes/SE:** Nausea, bloating, breast enlargement/tenderness, edema, HA, hypertriglyceridemia, gallbladder disease; **see Estradiol. Additional NIPE:** Rotate application sites

Estramustine Phosphate (Estracyt, Emcyt)
Uses: Advanced prostate CA **Action:** Antimicrotubule agent; weak estrogenic and antiandrogenic activity **Dose:** 14 mg/kg/d in 3–4 ÷ doses; preferable to take on empty stomach, do not take with milk or milk products **Caution/Contra:** [NA, not used in females] Active thrombophlebitis or thromboembolic disorders **Supplied:** Caps 140 mg **Notes/SE:** N/V, exacerbation of preexisting CHF, thrombophlebitis, MI, PE; gynecomastia in 20–100% **Interactions:** ↓ effects with antacids, calcium supplements, calcium-containing foods; ↓ effects of anticoagulants **NIPE:** Take on empty stomach, may take several wk for full effects, store in refrig

Estrogen, Conjugated (Premarin)
WARNING: Should not be used for the prevention of cardiovascular disease. The WHI reported ↑ risk of MI, stroke, breast CA, PE, and DVT when combined with methoxyprogesterone over 5 y of treatment; ↑ risk of endometrial CA. **Uses:** Moderate–severe menopausal vasomotor symptoms; atrophic vaginitis; palliative therapy of advanced prostatic carcinoma; prevention and treatment of estrogen deficiency–induced osteoporosis **Action:** Hormonal replacement **Dose:** 0.3–1.25 mg/d PO cyclically; prostatic carcinoma requires 1.25–2.5 mg PO tid; **Caution/Contra:** [X, −] Not recommended

in severe hepatic impairment, genital bleeding of unknown cause, breast CA, estrogen-dependent tumors, thromboembolic disorders, thrombosis, thrombophlebitis, recent MI **Supplied:** Tabs 0.3, 0.625, 0.9, 1.25, 2.5 mg; inj 25 mg/mL **Notes/SE:** ↑ Risk of endometrial carcinoma, gallbladder disease, thromboembolism, HA, and possibly breast CA; generic products not equivalent **Interactions:** ↑ effects of corticosteroids, cyclosporine, TCAs, theophylline, tobacco; ↓ effects of anticoagulants, clofibrate; ↓ effects with barbiturates, carbamazepine, phenytoin, rifampin **Labs:** ↑ prothrombin & factors VII, VIII, IX, X, platelet aggregability, thyroid-binding globulin, T4, triglycerides; ↓ antithrombin III, folate **NIPE:** ⊘ PRG, breast-feeding

Estrogen, Conjugated-Synthetic (Cenestin)   **Uses:** Treatment of moderate–severe vasomotor symptoms associated with menopause **Action:** Hormonal replacement **Dose:** 0.625–1.25 mg/d PO **Caution/Contra:** [X,–]; see Estrogen, Conjugated (Premarin) **Supplied:** Tabs 0.625, 0.9, 1.25 mg **Notes:** Do not use in PRG; associated with an ↑ risk of endometrial CA, gallbladder disease, thromboembolism, and possibly breast CA; **see Estrogen, Conjugated**

Estrogen, ConjugatedEstrogen, Conjugated + Medroxyprogesterone (Prempro, Premphase)   **WARNING:** Should not be used for the prevention of cardiovascular disease; the WHI study reported ↑ risk of MI, stroke, breast CA, PE, and DVT over 5 y of treatment **Uses:** Moderate–severe menopausal vasomotor symptoms; atrophic vaginitis; prevention of postmenopausal osteoporosis **Action:** Hormonal replacement **Dose:** *Prempro:* 1 tab PO qd; *Premphase:* 1 tab PO qd **Caution/Contra:** [X,–] Not recommended in severe hepatic impairment, genital bleeding of unknown cause, breast CA, estrogen-dependent tumors, thromboembolic disorders, thrombosis, thrombophlebitis **Supplied:** Tabs (expressed as estrogen/medroxyprogesterone) *Prempro:* 0.625/2.5, 0.625/5 mg; *Premphase:* 0.625/0 (days 1–14) & 0.625/5 mg (days 15–28) **Notes/SE:** See Warning; gallbladder disease, thromboembolism, HA, breast tenderness; **see Estrogen, Conjugated. Additional Interactions:** ↓ effects with aminoglutethimide

Estrogen, Conjugated + Methylprogesterone (Premarin + Methylprogesterone)   **Uses:** Menopausal vasomotor symptoms; osteoporosis **Action:** Estrogen and androgen combination **Dose:** 1 tab/d; not recommended in severe hepatic impairment **Caution/Contra:** [X, –] Genital bleeding of unknown cause, breast CA, estrogen-dependent tumors, thromboembolic disorders, thrombosis, thrombophlebitis **Supplied:** Tabs containing 0.625 mg of estrogen, conjugated, and 2.5 or 5 mg of methylprogesterone **Notes/SE:** Nausea, bloating, breast enlargement/tenderness, edema, HA, hypertriglyceridemia, gallbladder disease; **see Estrogen, Conjugated**

Estrogen, Conjugated + Methyltestosterone (Premarin + Methyltestosterone)   **Uses:** Moderate–severe menopausal vasomotor symptoms; postpartum breast engorgement **Action:** Estrogen and androgen combination **Dose:** 1 tab/d for 3 wk, then 1 wk off **Caution/Contra:** [X, –] Not recommended in severe hepatic impairment, genital bleeding of unknown cause, breast CA, estrogen-dependent tumors, thromboembolic disorders, thrombosis, thrombophlebitis **Supplied:** Tabs (estrogen/methyltestosterone) 0.625 mg/5 mg, 1.25 mg/10 mg **Notes/SE:** Nausea, bloating, breast enlargement/tenderness, edema, HA, hypertriglyceridemia, gallbladder disease; **see Estrogen, Conjugated. Additional Interactions:** ↑ effects of insulin

Etanercept (Enbrel)   **Uses:** Reduces signs and symptoms in cases of refractory RA **Action:** Binds TNF (disease-modifying antirheumatic drug) **Dose:** *Adults.* 25 mg SC 2× wk; *Peds 4–17 y.* 0.4 mg/kg SC 2× wk, max 25 mg **Caution/Contra:** [B, ?] Contra with active infection; caution in conditions that predispose to infection (ie, DM) **Supplied:** Inj 25 mg/vial **Notes/SE:** HA, rhinitis, inj site reaction **Interactions:** ↓ response to live virus vaccine **NIPE:** Rotate injection sites, ⊘ live vaccines

Ethambutol (Myambutol)   **Uses:** Pulmonary TB and other mycobacterial infections **Action:** Inhibits cellular metabolism **Dose:** *Adults & Peds >12 y.* 15–25 mg/kg/d PO as a single dose **Caution/Contra:** [B, +] Optic neuritis; ↓ in renal impairment, take with food, avoid antacids **Supplied:** Tabs 100, 400 mg; **Notes/SE:** HA, hyperuricemia, acute gout, abdominal pain, ↑ LFTs, optic neuritis, GI upset **Interactions:** ↑ neurotoxicity with neurotoxic drugs; ↓ effects with aluminum salts **NIPE:** Monitor visual acuity

Ethinyl Estradiol (Estinyl, Feminone)   **Uses:** Menopausal vasomotor symptoms; female hypogonadism **Action:** Estrogen supplement **Dose:** 0.02–1.5 mg/d ÷ qd–tid; **Caution/Contra:** [X, –] Not recommended in severe hepatic impairment; genital bleeding of unknown cause, breast CA, estrogen-dependent tumors, thromboembolic disorders, thrombosis, thrombophlebitis **Supplied:** Tabs 0.02, 0.05, 0.5 mg **Notes/SE:** Nausea, bloating, breast enlargement/tenderness, edema, HA, hypertriglyceridemia, gallbladder disease **Interactions:** ↑ effects of corticosteroids; ↓ effects with barbiturates, carbamazepine, hypoglycemics, insulin, phenytoin, primidone, rifampin, ↓ effects of anticoagulants, tamoxifen; **Labs:** ↑ prothrombin & factors VII, VIII, IX, X, platelet aggregability, thyroid-binding globulin, T4, triglycerides; ↓ antithrombin III, folate **NIPE:** ⊘ PRG, breast-feeding

Ethinyl Estradiol and Levonorgestrel (Preven)   **Uses:** Emergency contraception ("morning-after pill"); prevents PRG after contraceptive failure or unprotected intercourse **Actions:** estrogen and progestin; interferes with implantation **Dose:** 4 tabs, take 2 tab q12 h × 2 (w/in 72 h of intercourse) **Supplied:** Kit ethinyl estradiol (0.05 mg), levonorgestrel (0.25 mg) blister pack with 4 pills and urine PRG test **Contra/Caution** [X, M] Known/suspected PRG, abnormal uterine bleeding **Notes:** Will not induce abortion; may increase risk of ectopic PRG; N/V, abdominal pain, fatigue HA, menstrual changes; **see Ethinyl Estradiol. Additional Interactions:** ↑ effects of ASA, benzodiazepines, metoprolol, TCAs **NIPE:** Monitor for vision changes or ↓ tolerance of contact lens

Ethinyl Estradiol and Norelgestromin (Ortho Evra) Uses: Contraceptive patch Action: estrogen and progestin Dose: Apply patch to abdomen, buttocks, upper torso (not breasts), or upper outer arm at the beginning of the menstrual cycle; new patch is applied weekly for 3 wk; wk 4 is patch-free. Caution/Contra: [X, M] Supplied: 20-cm² patch [6 mg norelgestromin (active metabolite norgestimate) and 0.75 mg of ethinyl estradiol] Notes/SE: Less effective in women > 90 kg; breast discomfort, HA, application site reactions, nausea, menstrual cramps; thrombosis risks similar to OCP; see Ethinyl Estradiol. Additional Labs: ↑ serum amylase, sodium, calcium, protein

Ethosuximide (Zarontin) Uses: Seizures Action: Anticonvulsant; increases the seizure threshold Dose: Adults. Initially, 500 mg PO ÷ bid; ↑ by 250 mg/d q4–7d PRN (max 1500 mg/d) Peds. 20–40 mg/kg/24 h PO ÷ bid to a max of 1500 mg/d; use with caution in renal/hepatic impairment Caution/Contra: [C, +] Supplied: Caps 250 mg; syrup 250 mg/5 mL Notes/SE: Blood dyscrasias, GI upset, drowsiness, dizziness, irritability Interactions: ↑ effects with isoniazid, phenobarbital, alcohol; ↑ effects of CNS depressants, phenytoin; ↓ effects with carbamazepine, valproic acid, ginkgo biloba; ↓ effects of phenobarbital NIPE: Take with food, ⊘ alcohol

Etidronate Disodium (Didronel) Uses: Hypercalcemia of malignancy, Paget's disease, and hypertropic ossification Action: Inhibition of normal and abnormal bone resorption Dose: 5–20 mg/kg/d, may be given in ÷ doses (duration 3–6 mon); 7.5 mg/kg/d IV inf over 2 h Caution/Contra: [B oral (C parenteral), ?] SCr >5 mg/dL Supplied: Tabs 200, 400 mg; inj 50 mg/mL Notes/SE: GI intolerance ↓ by ÷ oral daily doses; hypophosphatemia, hypomagnesemia, bone pain, abnormal taste, fever, convulsions, nephrotoxicity Interactions: ↓ effects with antacids, foods that contain calcium NIPE: ⊘ take with food, improvement may take 3 mo

Etodolac (Lodine) Uses: Arthritis and pain Action: NSAID Dose: 200–400 mg PO bid–qid (max 1200 mg/d) Caution/Contra: [C (D 3rd trimester), ?] Caution in CHF, HTN, renal/hepatic impairment, Hx PUD Supplied: Tabs 400, 500 mg; ER tabs 400, 500, 600 mg; caps 200, 300 mg Notes/SE: GI disturbance, dizziness, HA, rash, edema, renal impairment, hepatitis Interactions: ↑ risk of bleeding with anticoagulants, antiplatelets; ↑ effects of lithium, methotrexate, digoxin, cyclosporine; ↓ effects with ASA; ↓ effects of antihypertensives Labs: False + of urine ketones & bilirubin NIPE: Take with food

Etonogestrel/Ethinyl Estradiol (NuvaRing) Uses: Contraceptive Action: Estrogen and progestin combination Dose: Adults. Rule out PRG first; insert ring vaginally for 3 wk, remove for 1 wk; insert new ring 7 d after last removed (even if still bleeding) at same time of day ring removed. First day of menses is day 1; insert prior to day 5 even if still bleeding. Use other contraception for first 7 d of starting therapy. See insert if converting from other forms of contraception. Following delivery or 2nd trimester abortion, insert ring 4 wk postpartum (if not breast-feeding) **Caution/Contra:** [X, ?/–] Contra PRG, heavy smokers >35 y, DVT, PE, cerebro/cardiovascular disease, estrogen-dependent neoplasm, undiagnosed abnormal genital bleeding, hepatic tumors, cholestatic jaundice. Caution HTN, gallbladder disease, ↑ lipids, migraines, sudden HA **Supplied:** intravaginal ring: ethinyl estradiol 0.015 mg/d and etonogestrel 0.12 mg/d **Note:** If ring accidentally removed, rinse with cool/lukewarm water (not hot) and reinsert ASAP; if not reinserted w/n 3 h, effectiveness decreased. Do not use with diaphragm; **see Ethinyl Estradiol**

Etoposide [VP-16] (VePesid, Toposar)   **Uses:** Testicular CA, non-small-cell lung CAs, Hodgkin's and NHLs, pediatric ALL, and allogeneic/autologous BMT in high doses **Action:** Topoisomerase II inhibitor **Dose:** 50 mg/m²/d IV for 3–5 d; 50 mg/m²/d PO for 21 d (oral bioavailability = 50% of the IV form); 2–6 g/m² or 25–70 mg/kg used in BMT (refer to specific protocols); ↓ in renal/hepatic impairment **Caution/Contra:** [D, –] IT administration **Supplied:** Caps 50 mg; inj 20 mg/mL **Notes/SE:** Myelosuppression, N/V, and alopecia; hypotension if infused too rapidly; anaphylaxis or lesser hypersensitivity reactions (wheezing) rare; potential for secondary leukemias **Interactions:** ↑ bleeding with ASA, NSAIDs, warfarin; ↑ bone marrow suppression with antineoplastics & radiation; ↑ effects of cisplatin; ↓ effects of live vaccines **Labs:** ↑ uric acid **NIPE:** ⊘ alcohol, immunizations, PRG, breast-feeding; use contraception, 2–3 L/d fluids

Ezitimibe (Zetia)   **Uses:** Primary hypercholesterolemia alone or in combination with an HMG-CoA reductase inhibitor **Action:** Inhibits intestinal absorption of cholesterol and phytosterols **Dose:** 10 mg/d PO **Caution/Contra:** [C, +/–] Hepatic impairment **Supplied:** Tabs 10 mg **Notes/SE:** Diarrhea, abdominal pain, ↑ transaminases when used in combination with an HMG-CoA reductase inhibitor **Interactions:** ↑ effects with cyclosporine; ↓ effects with cholestryamine, fenofibrate, gemfibrozil **NIPE:** If used with fibrates ↑ risk of cholethiasis

Famciclovir (Famvir)   **Uses:** Acute herpes zoster (shingles) and genital herpes **Action:** Inhibits viral DNA synthesis **Dose:** *Zoster:* 500 mg PO q8h. *Simplex:* 125–250 mg PO bid; ↓ in renal impairment **Caution/Contra:** [B, –] **Supplied:** Tabs 125, 250, 500 mg **Notes/SE:** Fatigue, dizziness, HA, pruritus, nausea, diarrhea, paresthesia **Interactions:** ↑ effects with cimetidine, probenecid, theophylline; ↑ effects of digoxin **NIPE:** Not affected by food, therapy most effective if taken w/n 72 h of rash

Famotidine (Pepcid)   **Uses:** Short-term Rx of active duodenal ulcer and benign gastric ulcer; maint Rx for duodenal ulcer, hypersecretory conditions, GERD, and heartburn **Action:** H₂-antagonist; inhibits gastric acid secretion **Dose:** *Adults. Ulcer:* 20–40 mg PO hs or 20 mg IV q12h. *Hypersecretion:* 20–160 mg PO q6h. *GERD:* 20 mg PO bid; maint 20 mg PO hs. *Heartburn:* 10 mg PO PRN. *Peds.* 1–2 mg/kg/d; ↓ dose in severe renal insufficiency **Caution/Contra:** [B, M] **Supplied:** Tabs 10, 20, 40 mg; chew tabs 10 mg; susp 40 mg/5 mL; inj 10 mg/mL **Notes/SE:** Dizziness, HA, constipation, diarrhea, acne, thrombocytopenia, neutropenia, ↑ serum transaminases **Interactions:** ↑ effects of glipizide, glyburide, nifedipine, nitrendipine, nisoldipine, tolbutamide; ↓ effects with antacids; ↓ effects of azole antifungals, cefuroxime, enoxacin, diazepam **NIPE:** ⊘ ASA, alcohol, tobacco, caffeine; take at bedtime

Felodipine (Plendil) **Uses:** HTN and CHF **Action:** Ca channel blocker **Dose:** 5–20 mg PO qd; ↓ in hepatic impairment **Caution/Contra:** [C, ?] **Supplied:** ER tabs 2.5, 5, 10 mg **Notes/SE:** Follow BP in elderly and in impaired hepatic function; do not use doses >10 mg in these patients; bioavailability ↑ when administered with grapefruit juice; peripheral edema, flushing, tachycardia, HA, gingival hyperplasia **Interactions;** ↑ effects with azole antifungals, cimetidine, cyclosporine, ranitidine, propranolol, alcohol, grapefruit juice; ↑ effects of digoxin, erythromycin; ↓ effects with barbiturates, carbamazepine, nafcillin, oxcarbazepine, phenytoin; rifampin; ↓ effects of theophylline **NIPE:** ⊘ d/c abruptly

Fenofibrate (Tricor) **Uses:** Hypertriglyceridemia **Action:** Inhibits triglyceride synthesis **Dose:** 54–160 mg/d ↓ in renal impairment, take with meals **Caution/Contra:** [C, ?] **Supplied:** Tabs 54–160 mg **Notes/SE:** Take with meals to ↑ bioavailability; monitor LFTs; GI disturbances, cholecystitis, rash, arthralgia, myalgia, dizziness **Interactions;** ↑ effects of anticoagulants; ↓ effects with BBs, cholestyramine, colestipol, estrogens, resins, rifampin, thiazide diuretics **Labs:** ↑ LFTs, BUN, creatinine; ↓ Hgb, HCT, WBCs, uric acid

Fenoldopam (Corlopam) **Uses:** HTN emergency **Action:** Rapid vasodilator **Dose:** Initial dose 0.03–0.1 µg/kg/min IV cont inf, titrate to effect q15min with 0.05–0.1-µg/kg/min increments **Caution/Contra:** [B, ?] **Supplied:** Inj 10 mg/mL **Notes/SE:** Avoid concurrent use with β-blockers; hypotension, edema, facial flushing, N/V/D, atrial flutter/fibrillation, ↑ intraocular pressure, ↑ portal pressure in cirrhotic patients **Interactions:** ↑ effects with acetaminophen ↑ hypotension with BBs **Labs:** ↑ serum urea nitrogen, creatinine, LFTs, LDH; ↑ K+

Fenoprofen (Nalfon) **Uses:** Arthritis and pain **Action:** NSAID **Dose:** 200–600 mg q4–8h, to 3200 mg/d max; take with food **Caution/Contra:** [B (D 3rd trimester), +/–] Caution in patients with CHF, HTN, renal/hepatic impairment, Hx PUD **Supplied:** Caps 200, 300 mg; tabs 600 mg **Notes/SE:** GI disturbance, dizziness, HA, rash, edema, renal impairment, hepatitis **Interactions:** ↑ effects with ASA, anticoagulants; ↑ hyperkalemia with K+-sparing diuretics; ↑ effects of aminoglycoside, anticoagulants, lithium, methotrexate, phenytoin, sulfonamides, sulfonylureas; ↓ effects with phenobarbital; ↓ effects of antihypertensives **Labs:** False ↑ free and total triiodothyronine levels, false + urine barbiturates & benzodiazepines; ↑ serum sodium & chloride **NIPE:** ⊘ ASA, alcohol, OTC drugs

Fentanyl (Sublimaze) [C-II] **Uses:** Short-acting analgesic used in conjunction with anesthesia **Action:** Narcotic **Dose:** *Adults & Peds.* 0.025–0.15 mg/kg IV/IM titrated to effect; ↓ in renal impairment **Caution/Contra:** [B, +] ↑ ICP, respiratory depression, severe renal/hepatic impairment **Supplied:** Inj 0.05 mg/mL **Notes/SE:** 0.1 mg of fentanyl = 10 mg of morphine IM; sedation, hypotension, bradycardia, constipation, nausea, respiratory depression, rash, miosis **Interactions:** ↑ effects with CNS depressants, cimetidine, phenothiazines, ritonavir, TCAs, alcohol, grapefruit juice; ↑ risks of HTN crisis with MAOIs; ↓ effects with buprenorphine, dezocine, nalbuphine, pentazocine **Labs:** False ↑ serum amylase, lipase

Fentanyl, Transdermal (Duragesic) [C-II]   **Uses:** Chronic pain **Action:** Narcotic **Dose:** Apply patch to upper torso q72h. Dose calculated from narcotic requirements in previous 24 h; ↓ in renal impairment **Caution/Contra:** [B, +] ↑ ICP, respiratory depression, severe renal/hepatic impairment **Supplied:** TD patches deliver 25, 50, 75, 100 μg/h **Notes/SE:** 0.1 mg of fentanyl = 10 mg of morphine IM; sedation, ↓ BP, bradycardia, constipation, nausea, respiratory depression, rash, miosis; **see Fentanyl. NIPE:** ↑ risk of ↑ absorption with elevated temperature; cleanse skin ONLY with water, as soap, lotions, alcohol may ↑ absorption; ⊘ use in children <110 lb

Fentanyl, Transmucosal System (Actiq, Fentanyl Oralet) [C-II]
Uses: Induction of anesthesia; breakthrough CA pain **Action:** Narcotic **Dose:** *Adults & Peds. Anesthesia:* 5–15 μg/kg. *Pain:* 200 μg consumed over 15 min, titrate to effect; ↓ in renal impairment **Caution/Contra:** [B, +] ↑ ICP, respiratory depression, severe renal/hepatic impairment **Supplied:** Lozenges 100, 200, 300, 400 μg; lozenges on stick 200, 400, 600, 800, 1200, 1600 μg **Notes/SE:** Sedation, ↓ BP, bradycardia, constipation, nausea, respiratory depression, rash, miosis; **see Fentanyl. Additional NIPE:** ⊘ use for children <33 lb and <2 y old

Ferrous Gluconate (Fergon)   **Uses:** Iron deficiency anemia and iron supplementation **Action:** Dietary supplementation **Dose:** *Adults.* 100–200 mg Fe/d in ÷ doses; take on empty stomach (may take with meals if GI upset occurs); avoid antacids **Caution/Contra:** [A, ?] Hemochromatosis, hemolytic anemia **Supplied:** Tabs 240 (27 mg Fe), 325 mg (36 mg Fe) **Notes/SE:** 12% Fe; GI upset, constipation, dark stools, discoloration of urine **Interactions:** ↑ effects with chloramphenicol, citrus fruits or juices; ↓ effects with antacids, cimetidine, black cohosh, chamomile, feverfew, gossypol, hawthorn, nettle, plantain, St. John's Wort, whole grain breads, cheese, eggs, milk, coffee, tea, yogurt; ↓ effects of floroquinolones, levodopa **Labs:** False + guaiac test **NIPE:** ⊘ antacids, tetracyclines, take liquid form in liquids and through a straw to prevent teeth staining

Ferrous Gluconate Complex (Ferrlecit)   **Uses:** Iron deficiency anemia or supplement to erythropoietin therapy **Action:** Supplemental iron **Dose:** Test dose: 2 mL (25 mg Fe) infused over 1 h. If no reaction, 125 mg (10 mL) IV over 1 h until favorable hematocrit achieved. Usual cumulative dose 1 g Fe administered over 8 sessions **Caution/Contra:** [B, ?] **Supplied:** Inj 12.5 mg/mL Fe **Notes/SE:** Dosage expressed as mg Fe; may be infused during dialysis; hypotension, serious hypersensitivity reactions, GI disturbance, inj site reaction; **see Ferrous Gluconate**

Ferrous Sulfate   **Uses:** Iron deficiency anemia and iron Fe supplementation **Action:** Dietary supplementation **Dose:** *Adults.* 100–200 mg Fe in ÷ doses. *Peds.*

1–4 mg/kg/24 h ÷ qd–bid; take on empty stomach (take with meals if GI upset occurs); avoid antacids **Caution/Contra:** [A, ?] Hemochromatosis, hemolytic anemia **Supplied:** Tabs 187 (60 mg Fe), 200 (65 mg Fe), 324 (65 mg Fe), 325 mg (65 mg Fe); SR caplets and tabs 160 mg (50 mg Fe); gtt 75 mg/0.6 mL (15 mg Fe/0.6 mL); elixir 220 mg/5 mL (44 mg Fe/5 mL); syrup 90 mg/5 mL (18 mg Fe/5 mL) **Notes/SE:** Vitamin C taken with ferrous sulfate ↑ absorption of Fe; GI upset, constipation, dark stools, discolored urine; **see Ferrous Gluconate**

Fexofenadine (Allegra) **Uses:** Allergic rhinitis **Action:** Antihistamine **Dose:** *Adults & Peds >12 y.* 60 mg bid or 180 mg/d; adjust in renal impairment **Caution/Contra:** [C, ?] **Supplied:** Caps 60 mg, tabs 180 mg; also in combination with pseudoephedrine (60 mg fexofenadine/120 mg pseudoephedrine) **Notes/SE:** Drowsiness (uncommon) **Interactions:** ↑ effects with erythromycin, ketoconazole; ↓ effects with antacids **NIPE:** ⊘ alcohol or CNS depressants

Filgrastim [G-CSF] (Neupogen) **Uses:** Decrease incidence of infection in febrile neutropenic patients; Rx chronic neutropenia **Action:** Recombinant G-CSF **Dose:** *Adults & Peds.* 5 µg/kg/d SC or IV single daily dose; DC therapy when ANC >10,000 **Caution/Contra:** [C, ?] **Supplied:** Inj 300 µg/mL **Notes/SE:** Fever, alopecia, N/V/D, splenomegaly, bone pain, HA, rash **Interactions:** ↑ interference with cytotoxic drugs; ↑ release of neutrophils with lithium **NIPE:** Monitor CBC & platelets

Finasteride (Proscar, Propecia) **Uses:** BPH and androgenetic alopecia **Action:** Inhibits 5α-reductase **Dose:** *BPH:* 5 mg/d PO. *Alopecia:* 1 mg/d PO **Caution/Contra:** [X, –] Caution in hepatic impairment; pregnant women should avoid handling pills **Supplied:** Tabs 1 (Propecia), 5 (Proscar) mg **Notes/SE:** ↓ PSA levels; reestablish PSA baseline at 6 mon; 3–6 mon for effect on urinary symptoms; to maintain new hair must continue therapy; ↓ libido, impotence (rare) **Interactions:** ↑ effects with saw palmetto; ↓ effects with anticholinergics, adrenergic bronchodilators, theophylline

Flavoxate (Urispas) **Uses:** Symptomatic relief of dysuria, urgency, nocturia, suprapubic pain, urinary frequency, and incontinence **Action:** Antispasmodic **Dose:** 100–200 mg PO tid–qid **Caution/Contra:** [B, ?] Pyloric or duodenal obstruction, GI hemorrhage, GI obstruction, ileus, achalasia, BPH **Supplied:** Tabs 100 mg **Notes/SE:** Drowsiness, blurred vision, xerostomia **Interactions:** ↑ effects of CNS depressants **NIPE:** ↑ risk of heat stroke with exercise and in hot weather

Flecainide (Tambocor) **Uses:** Prevent AF/flutter and PSVT, Rx life-threatening ventricular arrhythmias **Action:** Class 1C antiarrhythmic **Dose:** *Adults.* 100 mg PO q12h; ↑ in increments of 50 mg q12h q4d to a max of 400 mg/d. *Peds.* 3–6 mg/kg/d in 3 ÷ doses; ↓ in renal impairment, monitor closely in hepatic impairment **Caution/Contra:** [C, +] 2nd- or 3rd-degree AV block, bifascicular or trifascicular block, cardiogenic shock **Supplied:** Tabs 50, 100, 150 mg **Notes/SE:** May cause new/worsened arrhythmias; initiate Rx in hospital; may dose q8h if the patient is intolerant or condition is uncontrolled at 12-h intervals; dizziness, visual disturbances, dyspnea, palpitations, edema, tachycardia, CHF, HA, fatigue, rash, nausea **Interactions:** ↑ effects with alkalinizing drugs, amiodarone, cimetidine, propranolol, quinidine; ↑ effects of digoxin; ↑ risk of arrhythmias with CCBs, antiarrhythmics, disopyramide; ↓ effects with acidifying drugs, tobacco **Labs:** ↑ alkaline phosphatase **NIPE:** Full effects may take 3–5 d

Floxuridine (FUDR) Uses: Colon, pancreatic, liver CAs; adenocarcinoma of the GI tract metastatic to the liver **Action:** Inhibitor of thymidylate synthase; interferes with DNA synthesis (S-phase specific) **Dose:** 0.1–0.6 mg/kg/d for 1–6 wk **Caution/Contra:** [D, –] **Supplied:** Inj 500 mg **Notes/SE:** Myelosuppression, anorexia, abdominal cramps, N/V/D, mucositis, alopecia, skin rash, and hyperpigmentation; rare neurotoxicity (blurred vision, depression, nystagmus, vertigo, and lethargy); intraarterial catheter-related problems (ischemia, thrombosis, bleeding, and infection) **Interactions:** ↑ effects with metronidazole **Labs:** ↑ LFTs, 5-HIAA urine excretion; ↓ plasma albumin **NIPE:** ↑ risk of photosensitivity - use sunscreen

Fluconazole (Diflucan) Uses: Oropharyngeal and esophageal candidiasis; cryptococcal meningitis; *Candida* infections of the lungs, peritoneum, and urinary tract; prevention of candidiasis in BMT patients on chemotherapy or radiation; candidal vaginitis **Action:** Antifungal; inhibits fungal cytochrome P-450 sterol demethylation **Dose:** *Adults.* 100–400 mg/d PO or IV. *Vaginitis:* 150 mg PO as a single dose. *Peds.* 3–6 mg/kg/d PO or IV; ↓ in renal impairment **Caution/Contra:** [C, –] **Supplied:** Tabs 50, 100, 150, 200 mg; susp 10, 40 mg/mL; inj 2 mg/mL **Notes/SE:** PO same blood levels as IV; PO preferred when possible; HA, rash, GI upset, hypokalemia, **Interactions:** ↑ effects with HCTZ, benzodiazepines, anticoagulants; ↑ effects of amitriptyline, carbamazepine, cyclosporine, hypoglycemics, losartan, methadone, phenytoin, quinidine, tacrolimus, TCAs, theophylline, caffeine, zidovudine; ↓ effects with cimetidine, rifampin **Labs:** ↑ LFTs

Fludarabine Phosphate (Flamp, Fludara) Uses: CLL, low-grade lymphoma, mycosis fungoides **Action:** Inhibits ribonucleotide reductase; blocks DNA polymerase-induced DNA repair **Dose:** 18–30 mg/m^2/d for 5 d, as a 30-min inf (refer to specific protocols) **Caution/Contra:** [D, –] **Supplied:** Inj 50 mg **Notes/SE:** Myelosuppression, N/V/D, and LFT elevations; edema, CHF, fever, chills, fatigue, dyspnea, nonproductive cough, pneumonitis; severe CNS toxicity rare in leukemia **Interactions:** ↑ effects with other myelosuppressive drugs; ↑ risk of pulmonary effects with pentostatin **NIPE:** may take several wk for full effect, use barrier contraception

Fludrocortisone Acetate (Florinef) Uses: Partial treatment for adrenocortical insufficiency **Action:** Mineralocorticoid replacement **Dose:** *Adults.* 0.05–0.2 mg/d PO. *Peds.* 0.05–0.1 mg/d PO **Caution/Contra:** [C, ?] **Supplied:** Tabs 0.1 mg **Notes/SE:** For adrenal insufficiency, must use with glucocorticoid supplement; dosage changes based on plasma renin activity; HTN, edema, CHF, HA, dizziness, convulsions, acne, rash, bruising, hyperglycemia, cataracts **Interac-**

tions: ↑ risk of hypokalemia with amphotericin B, thiazide diuretics, loop diuretics; ↓ effects with rifampin, barbiturates, hydantoins; ↓ effects of ASA, isoniazid **Labs:** ↓ serum K$^+$ **NIPE:** Eval for fluid retention

Flumazenil (Romazicon) Uses:
Reversal of the sedative effects of benzodiazepines (diazepam, etc) **Action:** Benzodiazepine receptor antagonist **Dose: Adults.** 0.2 mg IV over 15 s; repeat dose if desired level of consciousness not obtained, to 1 mg max. **Peds.** 0.01 mg/kg to max of 0.2 mg IV over 15 s. Repeat doses 0.005 mg/kg at 1-min intervals; ↓ in hepatic impairment **Caution/Contra:** [C, ?] **Supplied:** Inj 0.1 mg/mL **Notes/SE:** Does not reverse narcotic symptoms; N/V, palpitations, HA, anxiety, nervousness, hot flashes, tremor, blurred vision, dyspnea, hyperventilation, withdrawal syndrome **Interactions:** ↑ risk of seizures and arrhythmias when benzodiazepine action is reduced **NIPE:** Food given during IV administration will reduce drug serum level

Flunisolide (AeroBid, Nasalide) Uses:
Control of bronchial asthma in patients requiring chronic steroid therapy; relief of seasonal/perennial allergic rhinitis **Action:** Topical steroid **Dose: Adults.** 2–4 inhal bid. **Nasal:** 2 sprays/nostril bid. **Peds >6 y.** 2 inhal bid. **Nasal:** 1–2 sprays/nostril bid **Caution/Contra:** [C, ?] **Supplied:** Met-dose aerosol 250 mg; nasal spray 0.025% **Notes/SE:** Not for acute asthma attack; tachycardia, bitter taste, local effects, oral candidiasis **NIPE:** Shake well before use

Fluorouracil [5-FU] (Adrucil) Uses:
Colorectal, bladder, gastric, pancreatic, anal, head, neck, and breast CAs **Action:** Inhibitor of thymidylate synthetase (interferes with DNA synthesis, S-phase specific) **Dose:** 370–1000 mg/m^2/d push to 5–1 d IV push to 24-h cont inf; protracted venous inf of 200–300 mg/m^2/d (see specific protocol) **Caution/Contra:** [D, ?] Bilirubin >5 mg/dL **Supplied:** Inj 50 mg/mL **Notes/SE:** Stomatitis, esophagopharyngitis, N/V/D, anorexia; myelosuppression (leukocytopenia, thrombocytopenia, and anemia); rash, dry skin, and photosensitivity frequent; tingling in hands/feet followed by pain (palmar–plantar erythrodysesthesia); phlebitis and discoloration at inj sites **Interactions:** ↑ effects with leucovorin, calcium **Labs:** ↑ LFTs **NIPE:** ⊘ alcohol, ↑ risk of photosensitivity, ↑ fluids 2–3 L/d, use barrier contraception

Fluorouracil, Topical [5-FU] (Efudex) Uses:
Basal cell carcinoma of the skin, actinic and solar keratosis **Action:** Inhibitor of thymidylate synthetase (interferes with DNA synthesis, S-phase specific) **Dose:** Apply 5% cream bid for 4–6 wk **Caution/Contra:** [D, ?] **Supplied:** Cream 1, 5%; soln 1, 2, 5% **Notes/SE:** Rash, dry skin, photosensitivity; see Fluorouracil. **Additional NIPE:** ⊘ use occlusive dressing; wash hands immediately after application

Fluoxetine (Prozac, Sarafem) Uses:
Depression, OCD, bulimia, PMDD (Sarafem) **Action:** SSRI **Dose:** Initially, 20 mg/d PO; ↑ to a max of 80 mg/ 24 h; ÷ doses of 20 mg/d. Weekly regimen 90 mg/wk after 1–2 wk of standard dose. **Bulimia:** 60 mg/d in AM. **PMDD:** 20 mg/d or 20 mg intermittently starting 14 d prior to menses, repeat each cycle; ↓ in hepatic failure **Caution/Contra:**

[B, ?/–] Serious reactions with MAOI and thioridazine; wait 5 wk after DC before starting MAOI **Supplied:** *Prozac:* Caps 10, 20, 40 mg; scored tabs 10 mg; SR cap 90 mg; soln 20 mg/5 mL. *Sarafem:* 10, 20 mg caps **Notes/SE:** Nausea, nervousness, weight loss, HA, insomnia **Interactions:** ↑ effects with CNS depressants, MAOIs, alcohol, St. John's Wort; ↑ effects of alprazolam, BBs, carbamazepine, clozapine, cardiac glycosides, diazepam, dextromethorphan, loop diuretics, haloperidol, phenytoin, lithium, ritonavir, thioridazine, tryptophan, warfarin, sympathomimetic drugs; ↓ effects with cyproheptadine; ↓ effects of buspirone, statins **Labs:** ↑ LFTs, BUN, creatinine, urine albumin **NIPE:** Stop MAOIs 14 d <start of this drug

Fluoxymesterone (Halotestin)   Uses: Androgen-responsive metastatic breast CA **Action:** Inhibition of secretion of LH and FSH by feedback inhibition **Dose:** 10–40 mg/d **Caution/Contra:** [X, ?/–] Serious cardiac, liver, or kidney disease **Supplied:** Tabs 2, 5, 10 mg **Notes/SE:** Virilization, amenorrhea and menstrual irregularities, hirsutism, alopecia and acne, nausea, and cholestasis. *Hematologic toxicity symptoms:* Suppression of clotting factors II, V, VII, and X and polycythemia; ↑ libido, HA, anxiety **Interactions:** ↑ effects with narcotics, alcohol, echinacea; ↑ effects of anticoagulants, cyclosporine, insulin, hypoglycemics, tacrolimus; ↓ effects with anticholinergics, barbiturates **Labs:** ↑ creatinine, creatinine clearance; ↓ thyroxine-binding globulin, serum total T4 **NIPE:** Radiographic studies of skeletal maturation q6mon in children, monitor fluid retention

Fluphenazine (Prolixin, Permitil)   Uses: Psychotic disorders **Action:** Phenothiazine antipsychotic; blocks postsynaptic mesolimbic dopaminergic receptors in the brain **Dose:** 0.5–10 mg/d in ÷ doses PO q6–8h; average maint 5.0 mg/d or 1.25 mg IM initially, then 2.5–10 mg/d in ÷ doses q6–8h PRN; ↓ dose in elderly **Caution/Contra:** [C, ?/–] Narrow-angle glaucoma **Supplied:** Tabs 1, 2.5, 5, 10 mg; conc 5 mg/mL; elixir 2.5 mg/5 mL; inj 2.5 mg/mL; depot inj 25 mg/mL **Notes/SE:** Monitor LFT; may cause drowsiness; do not administer conc with caffeine, tannic acid, or pectin-containing products; extrapyramidal effects **Interactions:** ↑ effects with antimalarials, BBs, CNS depressants, alcohol, kava kava; ↑ effects of anticholinergics, BBs, nitrates; ↓ effects with antacids, caffeine, tobacco; ↓ effects of anticonvulsants, guanethidine, levodopa, sympathomimetics **Labs:** False + urine preg test; ↑ serum cholesterol, glucose, LFTs, ↓ uric acid **NIPE:** Photosensitivity – use sunscreen, urine may turn pink or red in color, ↑ risk of heatstroke in hot weather

Flurazepam (Dalmane) [C-IV]   Uses: Insomnia **Action:** Benzodiazepine **Dose:** Adults & Peds >15 y. 15–30 mg PO hs PRN; ↓ in elderly **Caution/Contra:** [X, ?/–] Respiratory depression, narrow-angle glaucoma **Supplied:** Caps 15, 30 mg **Notes/SE:** Hangover due to accumulation of metabolites, apnea **Interactions:** ↑ effects with amprenavir, anticonvulsants, azole antifungals, BBs, CNS depressants, cimetidine, ciprofloxin, clozapine, digoxin, disulfiram, diltizem, isoniazid, levodopa, macrolides, oral contraceptives, rifampin, ritonavir, SSRIs,

valporic acid, verapamil, alcohol, grapefruit juice, kava kava, valerian; ↓ effects with aminophylline, carbamazepine, rifampin, rifabutin, theophylline; ? ↓ effects of levodopa **Labs:** ↑ LFTs, false neg urine glucose **NIPE:** ⊘ PRG, breast-feeding

Flurbiprofen (Ansaid) **Uses:** Arthritis **Action:** NSAID **Dose:** 50–100 mg bid–qid to a max of 300 mg/d **Caution/Contra:** [B (D in 3rd trimester), +] **Supplied:** Tabs 50, 100 mg **Notes/SE:** Dizziness, GI upset, peptic ulcer disease **Interactions:** ↑ effects with aminoglycosides, phenytoin, sulfonylureas, sulfonamides, feverfew, garlic, ginger, gingko biloba; ↑ effects of lithium, anticoagulants, methotrexate, phenytoin, sulfonylureas, sulfonamides; ↓ effects with ASA; ↓ effects of antihypertensives, diuretics **Labs:** ↑ LFTs, cortisol; ↓ HMG, HCT, leukocytes, platelets **NIPE:** Take with food

Flutamide (Eulexin) **WARNING:** Liver failure and death have been reported. Measure LFT before, monthly, and periodically after; DC immediately if ALT 2× uln or jaundice develops **Uses:** Advanced prostate CA (in combination with GnRH agonists, eg, leuprolide or goserelin) with radiation and GnRH for localized prostate CA **Action:** Nonsteroidal antiandrogen **Dose:** 250 mg PO tid (750 mg total) **Caution/Contra:** [D, ?] Severe hepatic impairment **Supplied:** Caps 125 mg **Notes/SE:** Hot flashes, loss of libido, impotence, diarrhea, N/V, gynecomastia; follow LFTs **Interactions:** ↑ effects with anticoagulants **Labs:** ↑ LFTs, BUN **NIPE:** Urine amber/yellow-green in color

Fluticasone, Nasal (Flonase) **Uses:** Seasonal allergic rhinitis **Action:** Topical steroid **Dose:** *Adults & Adolescents.* Nasal: 1–2 sprays/nostril/d. *Peds 4–11 y.* Nasal: 1–2 sprays/nostril/d **Caution/Contra:** [C, M] **Supplied:** Nasal spray 50 μg/actuation **Notes/SE:** HA, dysphonia, oral candidiasis **Interactions:** ↑ effects with ketoconazole **Labs:** ↑ cholesterol **NIPE:** Clear nares of exudate before use

Fluticasone, Oral (Flovent, Flovent Rotadisk) **Uses:** Chronic Rx of asthma **Action:** Topical steroid **Dose:** *Adults & Adolescents.* 2–4 puffs bid. *Peds 4–11 y.* 50 μg bid **Caution/Contra:** [C, M] **Supplied:** Multidose inhaler 44, 110, 220 μg/activation; Rotadisk dry powder 50, 100, 250 μg/activation; risk of thrush **Notes/SE:** Counsel patients carefully on use of device; HA, dysphonia, oral candidiasis **Interactions:** ↑ effects with ketoconazole **Labs:** ↑ cholesterol **NIPE:** Rinse mouth after use, avoid & report exposure to measles & chickenpox

Fluticasone Propionate and Salmeterol Xinafoate (Advair Diskus) **Uses:** Maint therapy for asthma **Action:** Corticosteroid and long-acting bronchodilator **Dose:** *Adults & Peds >12 y.* Inhal BID CQ 12h **Caution/Contra:** [C, M] Not for acute attack or in conversion from oral steroids **Supplied:** Met-dose inhal powder (fluticasone in μg/salmeterol in μg) 100/50, 250/50, 500/50 **Notes/SE:** Not for acute asthma attack, combination of Flovent and Serevent; URI, pharyngitis, HA **Interactions:** ↑ bronchospasm with BBs; ↑ hypokalemia with loop and thiazide diuretics; ↑ effects with ketoconazole, MAOIs, TCAs **Labs:** ↑ cholesterol **NIPE:** Avoid & report exposure to measles & chickenpox, rinse mouth after use

Fluvastatin (Lescol)   **Uses:** Adjunct to diet in the treatment of ↑ total cholesterol **Action:** HMG-CoA reductase inhibitor **Dose:** 20–40 mg PO hs, may be ↑ to 80 mg/d; ↓ dose with hepatic impairment **Caution/Contra:** [X, –] Myopathy **Supplied:** Caps 20, 40 mg **Notes/SE:** Avoid concurrent use with gemfibrozil, niacin **Interactions:** ↑ effects with azole antifungals, cimetidine, danazol, glyburide, macrolides, phenytoin, ritonavir, alcohol, grapefruit juice; ↑ effects of diclofenac, glyburide, phenytoin, warfarin; ↓ effects with cholestyramine, colestipol, isradipine, rifampin **Labs:** ↑ LFTs, CPK, thyroid function **NIPE:** Take at bedtime, ↑ photosensitivity

Fluvoxamine (Luvox)   **Uses:** OCD **Action:** SSRI **Dose:** Initial 50 mg as single hs dose, may be ↑ to 300 mg/d in ÷ doses **Caution/Contra:** [C, ?/–] Numerous drug interactions (MAOIs) **Supplied:** Tabs 25, 50, 100 mg **Notes/SE:** ÷ Doses of >100 mg; HA, GI upset, somnolence, insomnia **Interactions:** ↑ effects with melatonin, MAOIs; ↑ effects of BBs, benzodiazepines, methadone, carbamazepine, haloperidol, lithium, phenytoin, TCAs, theophylline, warfarin, St. John's Wort; ↑ risks of serotonin syndrome with buspirone, dexfenfluramine, fenfluramine, tramadol, nefazodone, sibutramine, tryptophan; ↓ effects with buspirone, cyproheptadine, tobacco; ↓ effects of buspirone, HMG-CoA reductase inhibitors **NIPE:** ⊘ MAOIs for 14 d <start of drug; ⊘ alcohol

Folic Acid   **Uses:** Megaloblastic anemia; recommended for all women of childbearing age **Action:** Dietary supplementation **Dose:** *Adults. Supplement:* 0.4 mg/d PO. *PRG:* 0.8 mg/d PO. *Folate deficiency:* 1.0 mg PO qd–tid. *Peds. Supplement:* 0.04–0.4 mg/24 h PO, IM, IV, or SC. *Folate deficiency:* 0.5–1.0 mg/24 h PO, IM, IV, or SC **Caution/Contra:** [A, +] **Supplied:** Tabs 0.1, 0.4, 0.8, 1.0 mg; inj 5 mg/mL **Notes/SE:** ↓ Incidence of fetal neural tube defects by 50%; no effect on normocytic anemias; well tolerated **Interactions:** ↓ effects with anticonvulsants, sulfasalazine, aminosalicyclic acid, chloramphenicol, methotrexate, oral contraceptives, pyrimethamine, triamterene, trimethoprim; ↓ effects of phenobarbital, phenytoin

Fondaparinux (Arixtra)   **WARNING:** When epidural/spinal anesthesia or spinal puncture is used, patients anticoagulated or scheduled to be anticoagulated with LMW heparins, heparinoids, or fondaparinux for prevention of thromboembolic complications are at risk for epidural or spinal hematoma, which can result in long-term or permanent paralysis **Uses:** Prevents DVT in hip fracture or replacement or knee replacement surgery **Action:** Synthetic and specific inhibitor of activated factor X; an LMW heparin **Dose:** 2.5 mg/d SC, up to 5–9 d; start at least 6 h postop **Caution/Contra:** [B, ?] Contra in weight <50 kg and CrCl <30 mL/min, active major bleeding, bacterial endocarditis, thrombocytopenia associated with antiplatelet antibody **Supplied:** Prefilled syringes 2.5 mg **Notes/SE:** Thrombocytopenia, DC if platelets <100,000 mm³; anemia, fever, nausea, constipation, reversible ↑ LFTs **Interactions:** ↑ effects with anticoagulants, cephalosporins, NSAIDs, penicillins, salicylates **Labs:** ↑ LFTs

Formoterol (Foradil Aerolizer) **Uses:** Long term in the maint treatment of asthma and prevention of bronchospasm with reversible obstructive airways disease **Action:** Long-acting β_2-adrenergic receptor agonist, bronchodilator **Dose:** *Adults & Peds >5 y.* Inhal of one 12-μg capsule q12h using the aerosolizer inhaler, 24 μg/d max; patient must not exhale into device; prevent exercise-induced bronchospasm. *Adults & Peds >12 y.* One inhal 12-μg cap 15 min before exercise **Caution/Contra:** [C, ?] Do not start with significantly worsening or acutely deteriorating asthma, which may be life-threatening **Supplied:** 12-μg blister pack for use in aerosolizer **Notes/SE:** Paradoxical bronchospasm, can be life-threatening; URI, pharyngitis, back pain **Interactions:** ↑ effects with adrenergics; ↑ effects of BBs; ↑ risk of hypokalemia with corticosteroids, diuretics, xanthines; ↑ risk of arrhythmias with MAOIs, TCAs

Foscarnet (Foscavir) **Uses:** CMV; acyclovir-resistant herpes infections **Action:** Inhibits viral DNA polymerase and reverse transcriptase **Dose:** *Induction:* 60 mg/kg IV q8h for 14–21 d. *Maint:* 90–120 mg/kg/d IV (Mon–Fri) **Caution/Contra:** [C, –] Significant renal impairment **Supplied:** Inj 24 mg/mL **Notes/SE:** Adjust in ↓ renal function; nephrotoxic; monitor ionized Ca closely (causes electrolyte abnormalities); administer through central line **Interactions:** ↑ risks of seizure with quinolines; ↑ risks of nephrotoxicity with aminoglycosides, amphotericin B, didanosine, pentamidine, vancomycine **Labs:** ↑ LFTs, CPK, BUN, serum creatinine; ↓ HMG, HCT, calcium, magnesium, K⁺, phosphorus **NIPE:** ↑ fluids; perioral tingling, extremity numbness & paresthesia indicates electrolyte imbalance

Fosfomycin (Monurol) **Uses:** Uncomplicated UTI **Action:** Inhibits bacterial cell wall synthesis **Dose:** 3 g PO dissolved in 90–120 mL of water as single dose; ↓ in renal impairment **Caution/Contra:** [B, ?] **Supplied:** Granule packets 3 g **Notes/SE:** May take 2–3 d for symptoms to improve; HA, GI upset **Interactions:** ↓ effects with antacids, metoclopramide **Labs:** ↑ LFTs; ↓ HMG, HCT **NIPE:** May take w/o regard to food

Fosinopril (Monopril) **Uses:** HTN, CHF, DN **Action:** ACE inhibitor **Dose:** Initially 10 mg/d PO; may be ↑ to a max of 80 mg/d PO ÷ qd–bid; ↓ dose in elderly **Caution/Contra:** [D, +] Renal impairment **Supplied:** Tabs 10, 20, 40 mg **Notes/SE:** Nonproductive cough, dizziness, angioedema, hyperkalemia **Interactions:** ↑ effects with antihypertensives, diuretics; ↑ effects of lithium; ↑ risk of hyperkalemia with K⁺-sparing diuretics, salt substitutes; ↑ cough with capsaicin; ↓ effects with antacids, ASA, NSAIDs **Labs:** ↓ HMG, HCT **NIPE:** ⊘ PRG, breast-feeding

Fosphenytoin (Cerebyx) **Uses:** Status epilepticus **Action:** Inhibits seizure spread in motor cortex **Dose:** Dosed as phenytoin equivalents (PEs), loading 15–20 mg PE/kg, maint 4–6 mg PE/kg/d; dosage adjustment/plasma monitoring necessary in hepatic impairment **Caution/Contra:** [D, +] Rash development during treatment **Supplied:** Inj **Notes/SE:** Requires 15 min to convert fosphenytoin to phenytoin; administer at <150 mg PE/min to prevent hypotension; administer with BP monitoring; hypotension, dizziness, ataxia, pruritus, nystagmus **Interactions:** ↑ effects with amiodarone, chloramphenicol, cimetidine, diazepam, disulfiram, estrogens, isoniazid, omeprazole, phenothiazines, salicylates, sulfonamides, tolbutamide; ↓ effects with TCAs, antituberculosis drugs, carbamazepine, alcohol, nutritional supplements, ginkgo biloba; ↓ effects of anticoagulants, corticosteroids, digitoxin, doxycycline, oral contraceptives, folic acid, calcium, vitamin D, rifampin, quinidine, theophylline **Labs:** ↑ serum glucose, alkaline phosphatase; ↓ serum thyroxine, calcium **NIPE:** Breast-feeding, for short-term use

Frovatriptan (Frova) See Table 11, page 259

Fulvestrant (Faslodex) **Uses:** Hormone receptor-positive metastatic breast CA in postmenopausal women with disease progression following antiestrogen therapy **Action:** Estrogen receptor antagonist **Dose:** 250 mg monthly, either a single 5-mL inj or two concurrent 2.5-mL IM injs into buttocks **Caution/Contra:** [X, ?/–] **Supplied:** Prefilled syringes 50 mg/mL; single 5 mL, dual 2.5 mL **Notes/SE:** N/V/D, constipation, abdominal pain, HA, back pain, hot flushes, pharyngitis, inj site reactions **Interactions:** ↑ risk of bleeding with anticoagulants **NIPE:** ⊘ PRG, breast-feeding; use barrier contraception

Furosemide (Lasix) **Uses:** CHF, HTN, edema, ascites **Action:** Loop diuretic; inhibits Na and Cl reabsorption in ascending loop of Henle and distal tubule **Dose:** *Adults.* 20–80 mg PO or IV qd–bid. *Peds.* 1 mg/kg/dose IV q6–12h; 2 mg/kg/dose PO q12–24h; **Caution/Contra:** [C, +] Caution in hepatic disease, anuria **Supplied:** Tabs 20, 40, 80 mg; soln 10 mg/mL, 40 mg/5 mL; inj 10 mg/mL **Notes/SE:** Monitor for hypokalemia; high doses of the IV form may cause ototoxicity; hypotension, hyperglycemia **Interactions:** ↑ nephrotoxic effects with cephalosporins; ↑ ototoxicity with aminoglycosides, cisplatin; ↑ risk of hypokalemia with antihypertensives, carbenoxolone, corticosteroids, digitalis glycosides, terbutaline; ↓ effects with barbiturates, cholestyramine, colestipol, NSAIDs, phenytoin, dandelion, ginseng; ↓ effects of hypoglycemics **Labs:** ↑ BUN, serum amylase, cholesterol, glucose, triglycerides, uric acid, ↓ serum K⁺, sodium, calcium, magnesium **NIPE:** Risk of photosensitivity

Gabapentin (Neurontin) **Uses:** Adjunctive therapy in the treatment of partial seizures; chronic pain syndromes **Action:** Anticonvulsant **Dose:** 900–1800 mg/d PO in 3 ÷ doses; dosage adjustment in renal impairment **Caution/Contra:** [C, ?] **Supplied:** Caps 100, 300, 400 mg **Notes/SE:** Not necessary to monitor serum gabapentin levels; somnolence, dizziness, ataxia, fatigue **Interactions:** ↑ effects with cimetidine, CNS depressants; ↑ effects of phenytoin; ↓ effects with antacids, ginkgo biloba **Labs:** False + urinary protein **NIPE:** Take w/o regard to food

Galantamine (Reminyl) **Uses:** Alzheimer's disease **Action:** Acetylcholinesterase inhibitor **Dose:** 4 mg PO bid, ↑ to 8 mg bid after at least 4 wk; may ↑ to 12 mg in 4 wk **Caution/Contra:** [B, ?] Do not use in severe renal or hepatic impairment; caution with urinary outflow obstruction, Parkinson's disease, severe asthma or COPD, severe heart disease or hypotension **Supplied:** Tabs 4, 8, 12 mg **Notes/SE:** GI disturbances, weight loss, sleep disturbances, dizziness, HA **Interactions:** ↑ effects with amitriptyline, cimetidine, erythromycin, fluoxetine, fluvoxamine, ketoconazole, paroxetine, quinidine **Labs:** ↑ alkaline phosphatase **NIPE:** ↑ dosage q4wk, if d/c several days then restart at lowest dose; take with food and maintain adequate fluid intake

Gallium Nitrate (Ganite)   Uses: Hypercalcemia of malignancy; bladder
CA **Action:** Inhibits resorption of Ca^{2+} from the bones **Dose:** *CA:* 350 mg/m^2 cont inf for 5 d to 700 mg/m^2 rapid IV inf q2wk in antineoplastic settings **Caution/Contra:** [C, ?] **Supplied:** Inj 25 mg/mL **Notes/SE:** Can cause renal insufficiency; hypocalcemia, hypophosphatemia, and decreased bicarbonate; <1% of patients developed acute optic neuritis; for bladder CA, use in combination with vinblastine and ifosfamide **Interactions:** ↑ risks of nephrotoxicity with amphotericin B, aminoglycosides, vancomycin **NIPE:** Monitor serum creatinine, adequate fluids

Ganciclovir (Cytovene, Vitrasert)   Uses: Rx and prevention of CMV
retinitis and prevention of CMV disease in transplant recipients **Action:** Inhibits viral DNA synthesis **Dose:** *Adults & Peds.* *IV:* 5 mg/kg IV q12h for 14–21 d, then maint of 5 mg/kg/d IV for 7 d/wk or 6 mg/kg/d IV for 5 d/wk. *Ocular implant:* One implant q5–8mon *Adults.* *PO:* Following induction, 1000 mg PO tid. *Prevention:* 1000 mg PO tid; take caps with food; ↓ dose in renal impairment **Caution/Contra:** [C, –] Neutropenia, thrombocytopenia **Supplied:** Caps 250, 500 mg; inj 500 mg; ocular implant 4.5 mg **Notes/SE:** Not a cure for CMV; inj should be handled with cytotoxic cautions; implant confers no systemic benefit; granulocytopenia/ thrombocytopenia are major toxicities; fever, rash, GI upset **Interactions:** ↑ effects with cytotoxic drugs, immunosuppressive drugs, probenecid; ↑ risks of nephrotoxicity with amphotericin B, cyclosporine; ↑ effects with didanosine **Labs:** ↑ LFTs; ↓ blood glucose **NIPE:** Take with food, ⊘ PRG, breast-feeding, alcohol, NSAIDS; photosensitivity - use sunscreen

Gatifloxacin (Tequin)   Uses: Acute exacerbation of chronic bronchitis,
sinusitis, community-acquired pneumonia, UTI **Action:** Quinolone antibiotic, inhibits DNA-gyrase **Dose:** 400 mg/d PO or IV; avoid use with antacids; ↓ dose in renal impairment **Caution/Contra:** [C, M] Do not use in children <18 y or in pregnant or lactating women **Supplied:** Tabs 200, 400 mg; inj **Notes/SE:** Reliable activity against *S. pneumoniae;* prolonged QT interval, HA, nausea, diarrhea; tendon rupture, photosensitivity **Interactions:** ↑ effects with antiarrhythmics, antipsychotics, cimetidine, erythromycin, loop diuretics, probenecid, TCAs; ↑ CNS effects and seizures with NSAIDs; ↓ effects of digoxin, warfarin; ↓ effects with antacids, didanosine, H_2 antagonists, proton pump inhibitors, iron

Gefitinib (Iressa)   Uses: Locally advanced/metastatic non-small-cell lung
cancer after failure of both platinum-based and docetaxel chemotherapies **Action:** Inhibits intracellular phosphorylation of numerous tyrosine kinases **Dose:** 250 mg

PO daily **Caution:** [D,–] **Contra:** N/A **Supplied:** Tabs 250 mg **SE:** Rash, acne, dry skin, N/V/D, interstitial lung disease, increased liver transaminases **Notes:** Periodically check LFTs **Interactions:** ↑ effects with ketoconazole, itraconazole and other CYP3A4 inhibitors; ↑ risk of bleeding with warfarin; ↓ effects with cimetidine, ranitidine and other H₂ receptor antagonists; ↓ effects with phenytoin, rifampicin and other CYP3A4 inducers **Labs:** ↑ ALT, AST, PT **NIPE:** ⊘ PRG or breast feeding; take w/o regard to food; ↑ risk of corneal erosion/ulcer

Gemcitabine (Gemzar) **Uses:** Pancreatic CA, gastric CA, and lung CA **Action:** Antimetabolite; inhibits ribonucleotide reductase; produces false nucleotide base-inhibiting DNA synthesis **Dose:** 1000 mg/m² as a 1-h IV inf/wk for 3–4 wk or 6–8 wk; dose modifications based on hematologic function **Caution/Contra:** [D, ?/–] **Supplied:** Inj 20 mg/mL **Notes/SE:** Myelosuppression, N/V/D, drug fever, and skin rash **Interactions:** ↑ bone marrow depression with radiation therapy, antineoplastic drugs; ↓ live virus vaccines **Labs:** ↑ LFTs, BUN, serum creatinine **NIPE:** ⊘ alcohol, NSAIDs, immunizations, PRG?

Gemfibrozil (Lopid) **Uses:** Hypertriglyceridemia and reduction of CHD risk **Action:** Lipid-regulating agent **Dose:** 1200 mg/d PO in 2 ÷ doses 30 min ac AM and PM **Caution/Contra:** [C, ?] Avoid concurrent use with the HMG-CoA reductase inhibitors; renal/hepatic impairment, gallbladder disease **Supplied:** Tabs 600 mg; caps 300 mg **Notes/SE:** Monitor LFTs and serum lipids; cholelithiasis may occur secondary to treatment; may enhance the effect of warfarin; GI upset **Interactions:** ↑ effects of anticoagulants, sulfonylureas; ↓ effects with rifampin; ↓ effects of cyclosporine **Labs:** ↑ LFTs, + ANA, ↓ HMG, HCT, WBCs

Gentamicin (Garamycin, G-Myticin, others) **Uses:** Serious infections caused by *Pseudomonas, Proteus, E. coli, Klebsiella, Enterobacter,* and *Serratia* and initial treatment of gram– sepsis **Action:** Bactericidal; inhibits protein synthesis **Dose:** *Adults.* 3–5 mg/kg/24 h IV ÷ q8–24h. *Peds. Infants <7 d <1200 g:* 2.5 mg/kg/dose q18–24h. *Infants >1200 g:* 2.5 mg/kg/dose q12–18h. *Infants >7 d:* 2.5 mg/kg/dose IV q8–12h. *Children:* 2.5 mg/kg/dose IV q8h; ↓ dose with renal insufficiency **Caution/Contra:** [C, +/–] Monitor CrCl and serum conc for dosage adjustments (Table 2, page 242). **Supplied:** Inj 10, 40 mg/mL, IT preservative-free 2 mg/mL **Notes/SE:** Nephrotoxic and ototoxic, ataxia; daily dosing becoming popular; follow Cr **Interactions:** ↑ ototoxicity, neurotoxicity, nephrotoxicity with aminoglycosides, amphotericin B, cephalosporins, loop diuretics, penicillins; ↑ effects with NSAIDs; ↓ effects with carbenicillin **Labs:** False ↑ AST, urine protein; ↑ urine amino acids **NIPE:** Photosensitivity - use sunscreen

Gentamicin, Ophthalmic (Garamycin, Genoptic, Gentacidin, Gentak, others) **Uses:** Conjunctival infections **Action:** Bactericidal; inhibits protein synthesis **Dose:** Oint apply bid or tid; soln: 1–2 gtt q2–4h, up to 2 gtt/h for severe infections **Caution/Contra:** [C, ?] **Supplied:** Soln and oint 0.3% **Notes/SE:** Local irritation see **Gentamicin**. **NIPE:** ⊘ other eye gtts for 10 min >drug

Gentamicin, Topical (Garamycin, G-Myticin) Uses: Skin infections caused by susceptible organisms **Action:** Bactericidal; inhibits protein synthesis **Dose:** *Adults & Peds >1 y.* Apply tid–qid **Caution/Contra:** [C, ?] **Supplied:** Cream; oint; soln 0.3% **Notes/SE:** Irritation; see Gentamicin. **NIPE:** ⊘ apply to large denuded areas

Gentamicin and Prednisolone, Ophthalmic (Pred-G Ophthalmic) Uses: Steroid-responsive ocular and conjunctival infections sensitive to gentamicin (eg, *Staphylococcus, E. coli, H. influenzae, Klebsiella, Neisseria, Pseudomonas, Proteus,* and *Serratia* spp) **Action:** Bactericidal; inhibits protein synthesis plus antiinflammatory **Dose:** Oint apply bid or tid; Soln: 1–2 gtt q2–4h, up to 2 gtt/h for severe infections **Caution/Contra:** [C, ?] **Supplied:** *Oint, ophth:* Prednisolone acetate 0.6% and gentamicin sulfate 0.3% (3.5 g). *Susp, ophth:* Prednisolone acetate 1% and gentamicin sulfate 0.3% (2 mL, 5 mL, 10 mL). *Soln and oint:* 0.3% **Notes/SE:** Local irritation; see Gentamicin. **Additional NIPE:** systemic effects with long-term use

Glimepiride (Amaryl) Uses: Type 2 DM **Action:** Sulfonylurea; stimulates pancreatic insulin release; ↑ peripheral insulin sensitivity; ↓ hepatic glucose output and production **Dose:** 1–4 mg/d, up to max of 8 mg **Caution/Contra:** [C, –] **Supplied:** Tabs 1, 2, 4 mg **Notes/SE:** HA, hypoglycemia **Interactions:** ↑ effects with ACEIs, adrenergic antagonists, BBs, chloramphenicol, MAOIs, NSAIDs, probenecid, salicylates, sulfonamides, warfarin, ginseng, garlic; ↓ effects with corticosteroids, estrogens, isoniazid, oral contraceptives, nicotinic acid, phenytoin, sympathomimetics, thiazide diuretics, thyroid hormones **NIPE:** Antabuse-like effect with alcohol

Glipizide (Glucotrol XL) Uses: Type 2 DM **Action:** Sulfonylurea; stimulates pancreatic insulin release; ↑ peripheral insulin sensitivity; ↓ hepatic glucose output and production; ↓ intestinal absorption of glucose **Dose:** 5–15 mg qd–bid **Caution/Contra:** [C, ?/–] Contra in type 1 DM, sensitivity to sulfonamides; caution in severe liver disease **Supplied:** Tabs 5, 10 mg; ER tabs 5, 10 mg **Notes/SE:** Counsel patient about diabetes management; wait several days before adjusting dose; monitor glucose; HA, anorexia, N/V/D, constipation, fullness, rash, urticaria, photosensitivity **Interactions:** ↑ effects with azole antifungals, anabolic steroids, chloramphenicol, cimetidine, clofibrate, MAOIs, NSAIDs, probenecid, salicylates, sulfonamides, TCAs, warfarin, celery, coriander, dandelion root, fenugreek, ginseng, garlic, juniper berries; ↓ effects with amphetamines, corticosteroids, epinephrine, estrogens, glucocorticoids, oral contraceptives, phenytoin, rifampin, sympathomimetics, thiazide diuretics, thyroid hormones, tobacco **NIPE:** Antabuse-like effect with alcohol

Glucagon Uses: Severe hypoglycemic reactions in DM with sufficient liver glycogen stores or β-blocker and Ca channel blocker overdose **Action:** Accelerates liver gluconeogenesis **Dose:** *Adults.* 0.5–1.0 mg SC, IM, or IV; repeat after 20 min PRN. *β-Blocker overdose:* 3–10 mg IV; repeat in 10 min PRN; may be given as cont inf. **Peds.** *Neonates:* 0.3 mg/kg/dose SC, IM, or IV q4h PRN. *Children:* 0.025–0.1 mg/kg/dose SC, IM, or IV; repeat after 20 min PRN **Caution/Contra:** [B, M] **Supplied:** Inj 1 mg **Notes/SE:** Administration of glucose IV necessary; ineffective in states of starvation, adrenal insufficiency, or chronic hypoglycemia; hypotension **Interactions:** ↑ effect with epinephrine, phenytoin; ↑ effects of anticoagulants **Labs:** ↓ serum K⁺; **NIPE:** Response w/n 20 min >inj

Glyburide (DiaBeta, Micronase, Glynase)
Uses: Type 2 DM **Action:** Sulfonylurea; stimulates pancreatic insulin release; ↑ peripheral insulin sensitivity; ↓ hepatic glucose output and production; ↓ intestinal absorption of glucose **Dose:** *Nonmicronized:* 1.25–10 mg qd-bid. *Micronized:* 1.5–6 mg qd-bid **Caution/Contra:** [C, ?] Not recommended in renal impairment **Supplied:** Tabs 1.25, 2.5, 5 mg; micronized tabs 1.5, 3, 4.5, 6 mg **Notes/SE:** HA, hypoglycemia **Interactions:** ↑ effects with anticoagulants, anabolic steroids, BBs, chloramphenicol, cimetidine, clofibrate, MAOIs, NSAIDs, probenecid, salicylates, sulfonamides, TCAs, alcohol, celery, coriander, dandelion root, fenugreek, ginseng, garlic, juniper berries; ↓ effects with amphetamines, corticosteroids, baclofen, epinephrine, glucocorticoids, oral contraceptives, phenytoin, rifampin, sympathomimetics, thiazide diuretics, thyroid hormones, tobacco **Labs:** False ↑ urine protein **NIPE:** Antabuse-like effect with alcohol

Glyburide/Metformin (Glucovance)
Uses: Type 2 DM **Action:** Sulfonylurea; stimulates pancreatic insulin release; ↑ peripheral insulin sensitivity; ↓ hepatic glucose output and production; ↓ intestinal absorption of glucose **Dose:** 1st line (naive patients), 1.25/250 mg PO qd-bid; 2nd line, 2.5/500 mg or 5/500 mg bid, take with meals, ↑ dose gradually **Caution/Contra:** [C, –] Do not use if SCr >1.3 in females or >1.4 in males; contra in hypoxemic conditions (CHF, sepsis); avoid alcohol; hold dose prior to and 48 h after ionic contrast media **Supplied:** Tabs 1.25/250 mg, 2.5/500 mg, 5/500 mg **Notes/SE:** HA, hypoglycemia, lactic acidosis, anorexia, N/V, rash; **see Glyburide. Additional Interactions:** ↑ effects with amiloride, ciprofloxacin cimetidine, digoxin, miconazole, morphine, nifedipine, procainamide, quinidine, quinine, ranitidine, triamterene, trimethoprim, vancomycin; ↓ effects with CCBs, isoniazid, phenothiazines

Glycerin Suppository
Uses: Constipation **Action:** Hyperosmolar laxative **Dose:** *Adults.* 1 adult supp PR PRN. **Peds.** 1 infant supp PR qd–bid PRN **Caution/Contra:** [C, ?] **Supplied:** Supp (adult, infant); liq 4 mL/applicatorful **Notes/SE:** Can cause diarrhea **Interactions:** ↑ effects with diuretics **Labs:** ↑ serum triglycerides, phosphatidylglycerol in amniotic fluid; ↓ serum calcium **NIPE:** Insert and retain for 15 min

Gonadorelin (Lutrepulse)
Uses: Primary hypothalamic amenorrhea **Action:** Stimulates the pituitary to release the gonadotropins LH and FSH **Dose:** 5–20 μg IV q90min for 21 d using a reservoir and pump **Caution/Contra:** [B, M] **Supplied:** Inj 0.8 mg, 3.2 mg **Notes/SE:** Risk of multiple PRG; inj site pain **Interactions:** ↑ effects with androgens, estrogens, glucocorticoids, levodopa, pro-

gestins, spironolactone; ↓ effects with digoxin, dopamine antagonists, oral contraceptives, phenothiazines

Goserelin (Zoladex) **Uses:** Advanced prostate CA and with radiation for localized prostate CA; endometriosis **Action:** LHRH agonist, inhibits LH, resulting in ↓ testosterone **Dose:** 3.6 mg SC (implant) q28d or 10.8 mg SC q3mo; usually into lower abdominal wall **Caution/Contra:** [X, –] **Supplied:** Subcutaneous implant 3.6, 10.8 mg **Notes/SE:** Hot flashes, ↓ libido, gynecomastia, and transient exacerbation of CA-related bone pain ("flare reaction" 7–10 d after 1st dose) **Interactions:** none noted **Labs:** ↑ alkaline phosphatase, estradiol, HDL, LDL, triglycerides; initial ↑ then ↓ >1–2 wk FSH, LH, testosterone

Granisetron (Kytril) **Uses:** Prevention of N/V **Action:** Serotonin receptor antagonist **Dose:** *Adults & Peds.* 10 mg/kg IV 30 min prior to initiation of chemotherapy; 0.1–1 mg before end of operative case. *Adults.* 1 mg PO 1 h prior to chemotherapy, 1 mg 1 h later **Caution/Contra:** [B, +/–] **Supplied:** Tabs 1 mg; inj 1 mg/mL **Notes/SE:** HA **Interactions:** ↑ serotonergic effects with horehound; ↑ extrapyramidal reactions with drugs causing these effects **Labs:** ↑ ALT, AST **NIPE:** May cause anaphylactic reaction

Guaifenesin (Robitussin, others) **Uses:** Symptomatic relief of dry, nonproductive cough **Action:** Expectorant **Dose:** *Adults.* 200–400 mg (10–20 mL) PO q4h. *Peds.* <2 y: 12 mg/kg/d in 6 ÷ doses. 2–5 y: 50–100 mg (2.5–5 mL) PO q4h. 6–11 y: 100–200 mg (5–10 mL) PO q4h **Caution/Contra:** [C, ?] **Supplied:** Tabs 100, 200, 1200 mg; SR tabs 600 mg; caps 200 mg; SR caps 300 mg; liq 100, 200 mg/5 mL **Notes/SE:** GI upset **Interactions:** ↑ bleeding with heparin **Labs:** False results of urine 5-HIAA, VMA; **NIPE:** ↑ fluid intake

Guaifenesin and Codeine (Robitussin AC, Brontex, others) [C-V] **Uses:** Symptomatic relief of dry, nonproductive cough **Action:** Antitussive with expectorant **Dose:** *Adults.* 10 mL or 1 tab PO q6–8h. *Peds.* 2–6 y: 1–1.5 mg/kg codeine/d ÷ dose q4–6h; 6–12 y: 5 mL q4h; >12 y: 10 mL q4h, max 60 mL/24 h **Caution/Contra:** [C, +] **Supplied:** Brontex tab contains 10 mg codeine; Brontex liq 2.5 mg codeine/5 mL; others 10 mg codeine/5 mL **Notes/SE:** Somnolence; **see Guaifenesin. Additional Interactions:** ↑ CNS depression with barbiturates, antihistamines, glutethimide, methocarbamol, cimetidine, alcohol; ↓ effects with quinidine **Labs:** ↑ urine morphine; Take with food ↑ amylase, lipase **NIPE:** Take with food

Guaifenesin and Dextromethorphan (many OTC brands) **Uses:** Cough due to upper respiratory tract irritation **Action:** Antitussive with expectorant **Dose:** *Adults & Peds >12 y.* 10 mL PO q6h. *Peds.* 2–6 y: 2.5 mg q6–8h, 10 mL/d max. 6–12 y: 5 mL q6–8h, 20 mL max/d **Caution/Contra:** [C, +] **Supplied:** Many OTC formulations **Notes/SE:** Somnolence; **see Guaifenesin. Additional Interactions:** ↑ effects with quinidine, terbinafine; ↑ effects of isocarboxazid, MAOIs, phenelzine; ↑ risk of serotonin syndrome with sibutramine

Haemophilus B Conjugate Vaccine (ActHIB, HibTITER, PedvaxHIB, Prohibit, others) **Uses:** Routine immunization of children against *H. influenzae* type B diseases **Action:** Active immunization against *Haemophilus* B **Dose:** *Peds.* 0.5 mL (25 mg) IM in deltoid or vastus lateralis **Caution/Contra:** [C, +] Febrile illness, immunosuppression **Supplied:** Inj 7.5, 10, 15, 25 µg/0.5 mL **Notes/SE:** Booster not required; observe for anaphylaxis **Interactions:** ↓ effects with immunosuppressives, steroids

Haloperidol (Haldol) **Uses:** Psychotic disorders, agitation, Tourette's disorders, and hyperactivity in children **Action:** Antipsychotic, neuroleptic **Dose:** *Adults.* *Moderate symptoms:* 0.5–2.0 mg PO bid–tid. *Severe symptoms/agitation:* 3–5 mg PO bid–tid or 1–5 mg IM q4h PRN (max 100 mg/d). *Peds.* *3–6 y:* 0.01–0.03 mg/kg/24 h PO qd. *6–12 y:* Initially, 0.5–1.5 mg/24 h PO; ↑ by 0.5 mg/24 h to maint of 2–4 mg/24 h (0.05–0.1 mg/kg/24 h) or 1–3 mg/dose IM q4–8h to a max of 0.1 mg/kg/24 h; Tourette's may require up to 15 mg/24 h PO; ↓ dose in elderly **Caution/Contra:** [C, ?] Narrow-angle glaucoma **Supplied:** Tabs 0.5, 1, 2, 5, 10, 20 mg; conc liq 2 mg/mL; inj 5 mg/mL; decanoate inj 50, 100 mg/mL **Notes/SE:** Extrapyramidal symptoms, hypotension, anxiety, dystonias **Interactions:** ↑ effects with CNS depressants, quinidine, alcohol; ↑ hypotension with antihypertensives, nitrates; ↑ anticholinergic effects with antihistamines, antidepressants, atropine, phenothiazines, quinidine, disopyramide; ↓ effects with antacids, carbamazepine, lithium, nutmeg, tobacco; ↓ effects of anticoagulants, levodopa, guanethidine **Labs:** False + PRG test, ↓ serum cholesterol **NIPE:** ↑ risk of photosensitivity - use sunscreen

Haloprogin (Halotex) **Uses:** Topical Rx of tinea pedis, tinea cruris, tinea corporis, tinea manus **Action:** Topical antifungal **Dose:** *Adults.* Apply bid for up to 2 wk; intertriginous may require up to 4 wk **Caution/Contra:** [B, ?] **Supplied:** 1% cream; soln **Notes/SE:** Local irritation

Heparin **Uses:** Rx and prevention of DVT and PE, unstable angina, AF with emboli formation, and acute arterial occlusion **Action:** Acts with antithrombin to inactivate thrombin and inhibit thromboplastin formation **Dose:** *Adults.* *Prophylaxis:* 3000–5000 U SC q8–12h. *Thrombosis Rx:* Loading dose of 50–75 U/kg IV, then 10–20 U/kg IV qh (adjust based on PTT). *Peds.* *Infants:* Loading dose 50 U/kg IV bolus, then 20 U/kg/h IV by cont inf. *Children:* Loading dose 50 U/kg IV, then 15–25 U/kg cont inf or 100 U/kg/dose q4h IV intermittent bolus **Caution/Contra:** [B, +] Uncontrolled bleeding **Supplied:** Inj 10, 100, 1000, 2000, 2500, 5000, 7500, 10,000, 20,000, 40,000 U/mL **Notes/SE:** Follow PTT, thrombin time, or activated clotting time to assess effectiveness; little effect on the PT; therapeutic PTT is 2–3 for most conditions; thrombocytopenia (HIT); follow platelet counts **Interactions:** ↑ effects with anticoagulants, antihistamines, ASA, clopidogrel, cardiac glycosides, cephalosporins, pyridamole, NSAIDs, quinine, tetracycline, ticlopidine, feverfew, ginkgo biloba, ginger, valerian; ↓ effects with nitroglycerine, ginseng, goldenseal, ↓ effects of insulin **Labs:** ↑ LFTs, thyroid function tests

Hepatitis A Vaccine (Havrix, Vaqta) **Uses:** Prevents hepatitis A in high-risk individuals (eg, travelers, certain professions, or high-risk behaviors) **Ac-**

tion: Provides active immunity **Dose:** (Expressed as ELISA units [EL.U.]) *Havrix: Adults.* 1440 EL.U. single IM dose. *Peds >2 y.* 720 EL.U. single IM dose. *Vaqta: Adults.* 50 U single IM dose. *Peds.* 25 U single IM dose **Caution/Contra:** [C, +] **Supplied:** Inj 720 EL.U./0.5 after, 1440 EL.U./1 mL.; 50 U/mL **Notes/SE:** Booster recommended 6–12 mon after primary vaccination. Fever, fatigue, pain in inj site, HA **Interactions:** None noted **NIPE:** ○ if pt febrile

Hepatitis A (inactivated) and Hepatitis B Recombinant Vaccine (Twinrix) **Uses:** Active immunization against hepatitis A/B **Action:** Provides active immunity **Dose:** 1 mL IM at 0, 1, and 6 mon **Caution/Contra:** [C, +] **Supplied:** Single-dose vials, syringes **Notes/SE:** Booster recommended 6–12 mon after primary vaccination; fever, fatigue, pain in inj site, HA **Interactions:** ↓ immune response with corticosteroids, immunosuppressants **NIPE:** ↑ response if inj in deltoid vs gluteus

Hepatitis B Immune Globulin (HyperHep, H-BIG) **Uses:** Exposure to HBsAg-positive materials, eg, blood, plasma, or serum (accidental needle-stick, mucous membrane contact, or oral ingestion) **Action:** Passive immunization **Dose:** *Adults & Peds.* 0.06 mL/kg IM to a max of 5 mL; w/n 24 h of needle-stick or percutaneous exposure; w/n 14 d of sexual contact; repeat 1 and 6 mon after exposure **Caution/Contra:** [C, ?] Thimerosal allergy **Supplied:** Inj **Notes/SE:** Administered in gluteal or deltoid muscle; if exposure continues, patient should also receive the hepatitis B vaccine; pain at inj site, dizziness **Interactions:** ↓ immune response if given with live virus vaccines

Hepatitis B Vaccine (Engerix-B, Recombivax HB) **Uses:** Prevention of hepatitis B **Action:** Active immunization **Dose:** *Adults.* 3 IM doses of 1 mL each, the 1st 2 doses given 1 mon apart, the 3rd 6 mon after the 1st. *Peds.* 0.5 mL IM given on the same schedule as for adults **Caution/Contra:** [C, +] Yeast hypersensitivity **Supplied:** *Engerix-B:* Inj 20 µg/mL; peds inj 10 µg/0.5 mL. *Recombivax HB:* Inj 10 and 40 µg/mL; peds inj 5 µg/0.5 mL **Notes/SE:** Administer IM injs for adults and older peds in the deltoid; in other peds, administer in the anterolateral thigh; may cause fever, inj site soreness; derived from recombinant DNA technology **Interactions:** ↓ immune response with corticosteroids, immunosuppressants **NIPE:** ↑ response inj in deltoid vs gluteus

Hetastarch (Hespan) **Uses:** Plasma volume expansion as an adjunct in the treatment of shock and leukapheresis **Action:** Synthetic colloid with actions similar to those of albumin **Dose:** 500–1000 mL (do not exceed 1500 mL/d) IV at a rate not to exceed 20 mL/kg/h. *Leukapheresis:* 250–700 mL; ↓ dose in renal failure **Caution/Contra:** [C, +] Severe bleeding disorders, severe CHF, or renal failure with oliguria or anuria **Supplied:** Inj 6 g/100 mL **Notes/SE:** Not a substitute for blood or plasma; bleeding side effect (prolongs PT, PTT, bleed time, etc) **NIPE:** Monitor CBC, PT, PTT; observe for anaphylactic reactions

Hydralazine (Apresoline, others) **Uses:** Moderate–severe HTN; CHF (with Isordil) **Action:** Peripheral vasodilator **Dose:** *Adults.* Begin at 10 mg

PO qid, then ↑ to 25 mg qid to max of 300 mg/d. *Peds.* 0.75–3 mg/kg/24 h PO ÷ q12–6h; ↓ in renal impairment; check CBC and ANA before starting **Caution/Contra:** [C, +] Caution with impaired hepatic function and CAD **Supplied:** Tabs 10, 25, 50, 100 mg; inj 20 mg/mL **Notes/SE:** Compensatory sinus tachycardia eliminated with use of a β-blocker; chronically high doses cause SLE-like syndrome; SVT following IM administration, peripheral neuropathy **Interactions:** ↑ effects with antihypertensives, diazoxide, diuretics, MAOIs, nitrates, alcohol; ↓ pressor response with epinephrine; ↓ effects with NSAIDs; **NIPE:** Take with food

Hydrochlorothiazide (HydroDIURIL, Esidrix, others)
Uses: Edema, HTN **Action:** Thiazide diuretic; inhibits Na⁺ reabsorption in the distal tubule **Dose:** *Adults.* 25–100 mg/d PO in single or ÷ doses. *Peds. <6 mon:* 2–3 mg/kg/d in 2 ÷ doses. *>6 mon:* 2 mg/kg/d in 2 ÷ doses **Caution/Contra:** [D, +] Contra in anuria; sulfonamide allergy **Supplied:** Tabs 25, 50, 100 mg; caps 12.5 mg; oral soln 50 mg/5 mL **Notes/SE:** Hypokalemia frequent; hyperglycemia, hyperuricemia, hyponatremia **Interactions:** ↑ hypotension with ACEIs, antihypertensives, carbenoxolone, ↑ hypokalemia with carbenoxolone, corticosteroids; ↑ hyperglycemia with BBs, diazoxide, hypoglycemic drugs; ↑ effects of lithium, methotrexate; ↓ effects with amphetamines, cholestyramine, colestipol, NSAIDs, quinidine, dandelion **Labs:** False ↓ urine estriol **NIPE:** Monitor uric acid, take with food, ↑ risk of photosensitivity – use sunscreen

Hydrochlorothiazide and Amiloride (Moduretic)
Uses: HTN **Action:** Combined effects of a thiazide diuretic and a K⁺-sparing diuretic **Dose:** 1–2 tabs/d PO **Caution/Contra:** [D, ?] Do not give to diabetics or patients with renal failure, sulfonamide allergy. **Supplied:** Tabs (amiloride/hydrochlorothiazide) 5 mg/50 mg **Notes/SE:** Hypotension, photosensitivity, hyper-/hypokalemia

Hydrochlorothiazide and Spironolactone (Aldactazide)
Uses: Edema, HTN **Action:** Combined effects of a thiazide diuretic and a K⁺-sparing diuretic **Caution/Contra:** [D, +] Sulfonamide allergy **Dose:** 25–200 mg each component/d in ÷ doses **Supplied:** Tabs (hydrochlorothiazide/spironolactone) 25 mg/25 mg, 50 mg/50 mg **Notes/SE:** Photosensitivity, hypotension, hyper-/hypokalemia; **see Hydrochlorothiazide. Additional Interactions:** ↑ risk of hyperkalemia with ACEIs, K⁺-sparing diuretics, K⁺ supplements, salt substitutes; ↓ effects of digoxin **NIPE:** d/c drug 3 d <glucose tolerance test

Hydrochlorothiazide and Triamterene (Dyazide, Maxzide)
Uses: Edema and HTN **Action:** Combined effects of a thiazide diuretic and a K⁺-sparing diuretic **Dose:** *Dyazide:* 1–2 caps PO qd–bid. *Maxzide:* 1 tab/d PO **Caution/Contra:** [D, +/–] Sulfonamide allergy **Supplied:** (triamterene/HCTZ) 37.5 mg/25 mg, 50 mg/25 mg, 75 mg/50 mg **Notes/SE:** HCTZ component in Maxzide more bioavailable than in Dyazide; can cause hyperkalemia as well as hypokalemia; follow serum K⁺ levels; hypotension, photosensitivity; **see Hydrochlorothiazide. Additional Interactions:** ↑ risk of hyperkalemia with ACEIs,

K⁺-sparing diuretics, K⁺ supplements, salt substitutes; ↑ effects with cimetidine, licorice root, ↓ effects of digoxin **Labs:** ↑ serum glucose, BUN, creatinine K⁺, magnesium, uric acid, urinary calcium; interference with assay of quinidine & lactic dehydrogenase **NIPE:** Urine may turn blue

Hydrocodone and Acetaminophen (Lorcet, Vicodin, others) [C-III]

Uses: Moderate–severe pain; hydrocodone has antitussive properties **Action:** Narcotic analgesic with nonnarcotic analgesic **Dose:** 1–2 caps or tabs PO q4–6h PRN **Caution/Contra:** [C, M] **Supplied:** Many different combinations; specify hydrocodone/APAP dose. Caps 5/500; tabs 2.5/500, 5/400, 5/500, 7.5/400, 10/400, 7.5/500, 7.5/650, 7.5/750, 10/325, 10/400, 10/500, 10/650; elixir and soln (fruit punch flavor) 2.5 mg hydrocodone/167 mg APAP/5 mL **Notes/SE:** GI upset, sedation, fatigue **Interactions:** ↑ effects with antihistamines, cimetidine, CNS depressants, dextroamphetamines, glutethimide, MAOIs, protease inhibitors, TCAs, alcohol, St. John's Wort; ↑ effects of warfarin; ↓ effects with phenothiazines **Labs:** False ↑ amylase, lipase **NIPE:** Take with food, ↑ fluid intake

Hydrocodone and Aspirin (Lortab ASA, others) [C-III]

Uses: Moderate–severe pain **Action:** Narcotic analgesic with NSAID **Dose:** 1–2 PO q4–6h PRN **Caution/Contra:** [C, M] **Supplied:** 5 mg hydrocodone/500 mg ASA/tab **Notes/SE:** GI upset, sedation, fatigue; see Hydrocodone and Acetaminophen

Hydrocodone and Guaifenesin (Hycotuss Expectorant, others) [C-III]

Uses: Nonproductive cough associated with respiratory infection **Action:** Expectorant plus cough suppressant **Dose:** *Adults & Peds >12 y.* 5 mL q4h, pc and hs. *Peds.* *<2 y.* 0.3 mg/kg/d ÷ qid. *2–12 y.* 2.5 mL q4h pc and hs **Caution/Contra:** [C, M] **Supplied:** Hydrocodone 5 mg/guaifenesin 100 mg/5 mL **Notes/SE:** GI upset, sedation, fatigue; see Hydrocodone and Acetaminophen. **Additional Interactions:** ↑ bleeding with heparin **Labs:** False results of urine 5-HIAA, VMA

Hydrocodone and Homatropine (Hycodan, others) [C-III]

Uses: Relief of cough **Action:** Combination antitussive **Dose:** Dose based on hydrocodone. *Adults.* 5–10 mg q4–6h. *Peds.* 0.6 mg/kg/d ÷ tid–qid **Caution/Contra:** [C, M] Narrow-angle glaucoma **Supplied:** Syrup 5 mg hydrocodone/5 mL; tabs 5 mg hydrocodone **Notes/SE:** Sedation, fatigue, GI upset; see Hydrocodone and Acetaminophen. **Additional Labs:** ↑ ALT, AST

Hydrocodone and Ibuprofen (Vicoprofen) [C-III]

Uses: Moderate–severe pain (<10 d) **Action:** Narcotic with NSAID **Dose:** 1–2 tabs q4–6h PRN **Caution/Contra:** [C, M] Caution in renal insufficiency **Supplied:** Tabs 7.5 mg hydrocodone/200 mg ibuprofen **Notes/SE:** Sedation, fatigue, GI upset; see Hydrocodone and Acetaminophen. **Additional Interactions:** ↓ effects of ACEIs, diuretics

Hydrocodone and Pseudoephedrine (Entuss-D, Histussin-D, others) [C-III]

Uses: Cough and nasal congestion **Action:** Narcotic cough suppressant with decongestant **Dose:** 5 mL qid, PRN **Caution/Contra:** [C, M] MAOIs **Supplied:** *Entuss-D:* 5 mg hydrocodone/30 mg pseudoephedrine/5 mL. *Histussin-D:* 5 mg hydrocodone/60 mg pseudoephedrine/5 mL **Notes/SE:** ↑ blood pressure, GI upset, sedation, fatigue; **see Hydrocodone and Acetaminophen. Additional Interactions:** ↑ effects with sympathomimetics

Hydrocodone, Chlorpheniramine, Phenylephrine, Acetaminophen, and Caffeine (Hycomine Compound) [C-III]

Uses: Cough and symptoms of URI **Action:** Narcotic cough suppressant with decongestants and analgesic **Dose:** 1 tab PO q4h PRN **Caution/Contra:** [C, M] Narrow-angle glaucoma **Supplied:** Hydrocodone 5 mg/chlorpheniramine 2 mg/phenylephrine 10 mg/APAP 250 mg/caffeine 30 mg/tab **Notes/SE:** ↑ BP, GI upset, sedation, fatigue; **see Hydrocodone and Acetaminophen**

Hydrocortisone, Rectal (Anusol-HC Suppository, Cortifoam Rectal, Proctocort, others)

Uses: Painful anorectal conditions; radiation proctitis, management of ulcerative colitis **Action:** Antiinflammatory steroid **Dose:** *Adults. Ulcerative colitis:* 10–100 mg rectally qd–bid 2–3 wk, 1–2×/d for 2–3 wk **Caution/Contra:** [B, ?/–] **Supplied:** *Hydrocortisone acetate:* Rectal aerosol 90 mg/applicator; supp 25 mg. *Hydrocortisone base:* Rectal 1%; rectal susp 100 mg/60 mL **Notes/SE:** Minimal systemic effect **NIPE:** Administer >BM, insert supp blunt end first, admin enema with pt lying on side and retain for 1 h

Hydrocortisone, Topical and Systemic (Cortef, Solu-Cortef)

See Steroids, pages 209 and 210, and Tables 4 and 5, pages 248 and 249 **Caution/Contra:** [B, –] **Notes/SE:** Systemic **forms:** ↑ appetite, insomnia, hyperglycemia, bruising **Interactions:** ↑ effects with cyclosporine, estrogens; ↑ effects of cardiac glycosides, cyclosporine; ↑ risk of GI bleed with NSAIDs; ↓ effects with aminoglutethamide, antacids, barbiturates, cholestyramine, colestipol, ephedrine, phenobarbital, phenytoin, rifampin; ↓ effects of anticoagulants, hypoglycemics, insulin, isoniazid, salicylates **Labs:** False neg in skin allergy tests **NIPE:** ⊘ Alcohol, live virus vaccines, abrupt d/c of drug; take with food; may mask s/s infection

Hydromorphone (Dilaudid) [C–II]

Uses: Moderate–severe pain **Action:** Narcotic analgesic **Dose:** 1–4 mg PO, IM, IV, or PR q4–6h PRN; 3 mg PR q6–8h PRN; ↓ with hepatic failure **Caution/Contra:** [B (D if prolonged use or high doses near term), ?] **Supplied:** Tabs 1, 2, 3, 4, 8 mg; liq 5 mg/mL; inj 1, 2, 4, 10 mg/mL; supp 3 mg **Notes/SE:** 1.5 mg IM = 10 mg of morphine IM; sedation, dizziness, GI upset **Interactions:** ↑ effects with CNS depressants, phenothiazines, TCAs, alcohol, St. John's Wort; ↓ effects with nalbuphine, pentazocine **Labs:** ↑ serum amylase, lipase **NIPE:** Take with food, ↑ fluids & fiber to avoid constipation

Hydroxyurea (Hydrea, Droxia)

Uses: CML, head and neck, ovarian and colon CA, melanoma, acute leukemia, sickle cell anemia, polycythemia vera,

HIV Action: Probable inhibitor of the ribonucleotide reductase system **Dose:** 50–75 mg/kg for WBC counts of >100,000 cells/mL; 20–30 mg/kg in refractory CML. *HIV:* 1000–1500 mg/d in single or ÷ doses; ↓ in renal insufficiency **Caution/Contra:** [D, –] Severe anemia **Supplied:** Caps 200, 300, 400, 500 mg **Notes/SE:** Myelosuppression (primarily leukopenia), N/V, rashes, facial erythema, radiation recall reactions, and renal dysfunction **Interactions:** ↑ risk of pancreatitis with didanosine, indinavir, stavudine; ↑ bone marrow depression with antineoplastic drugs or radiation therapy **Labs:** ↑ serum uric acid, BUN, creatinine **NIPE:** ↑ fluids 10–12 glasses/d, use barrier contraception, ↑ risk of infertility

Hydroxyzine (Atarax, Vistaril)
Uses: Anxiety, tension, sedation, itching **Action:** Antihistamine, anxiety **Dose:** *Adults. Anxiety or sedation:* 50–100 mg PO or IM qid or PRN (max 600 mg/d). *Itching:* 25–50 mg PO or IM tid–qid. *Peds.* 0.5–1.0 mg/kg/24 h PO or IM q6h; ↓ in hepatic failure **Caution/Contra:** [C, +/–] **Supplied:** Tabs 10, 25, 50, 100 mg; caps 25, 50, 100 mg; syrup 10 mg/5 mL; susp 25 mg/5 mL; inj 25, 50 mg/mL **Notes/SE:** Useful in potentiating effects of narcotics; not for IV use; drowsiness, anticholinergic effects **Interactions:** ↑ effects with antihistamines, anticholinergics, CNS depressants, alcohol **Labs:** False neg skin allergy tests; false ↑ in urinary 17-hydroxycorticosteroid levels

Hyoscyamine (Anaspaz, Cystospaz, Levsin, others)
Uses: Spasm associated with GI and bladder disorders **Action:** Anticholinergic **Dose:** *Adults.* 0.125–0.25 mg (1–2 tabs) SL 3–4×/d, pc and hs; 1 SR caps q12h **Caution/Contra:** [C, +] Contra in obstructive uropathy, GI obstruction; narrow-angle glaucoma **Supplied:** *Cystospaz-M, Levsinex:* Cap timed release 0.375 mg; elixir (alcohol), soln 0.125 mg/5 mL; inj 0.5 mg/mL; Tab 0.125 mg. *Cystospaz:* Tab 0.15 mg. *Levbid:* ER tab 0.375 mg. *Levsin SL:* SL 0.125 mg **Notes/SE:** Dry skin, xerostomia, constipation, anticholinergic SE **Interactions:** ↑ effects with amantadine, antimuscarinics, haloperidol, phenothiazines, quinidine, TCAs, MAOIs; ↓ effects with antacids, antidiarrheals; ↓ effects of levodopa **NIPE:** ↑ risk of heat intolerance, photophobia

Hyoscyamine, Atropine, Scopolamine, and Phenobarbital (Donnatal, Barbidonna, others)
Uses: Irritable bowel, spastic colitis, peptic ulcer, spastic bladder **Dose:** 0.125–0.25 mg (1–2 tabs) 3–4×/d, 1 cap q12h (SR), 5–10 mL elixir 3–4×/d or q8h **Caution/Contra:** [D, M] Narrow-angle glaucoma **Supplied:** Many combinations/manufacturers available. *Caps* (Donnatal, others): Hyoscyamine 0.1037 mg/atropine 0.0194 mg/scopolamine 0.0065 mg/phenobarbital 16.2 mg. *Tabs* (Donnatal, others): Hyoscyamine 0.1037 mg/atropine 0.0194 mg/scopolamine 0.0065 mg/phenobarbital 16.2 mg. *Long-acting* (Donnatal): Hyoscyamine 0.311 mg/atropine 0.0582 mg/scopolamine 0.0195 mg/phenobarbital 48.6 mg. *Elixirs* (Donnatal, others): Hyoscyamine 0.1037 mg/atropine 0.0194 mg/scopolamine 0.0065 mg/phenobarbital 16.2 mg/5 mL **Notes/SE:** Sedation, xerostomia, constipation **Interactions:** ↑ effects with anticoagulants, amantadine, antihistamines, antidiarrheals, anticonvulsants, CNS depres-

sants, corticosteroids, digitalis, griseofulvin, MAOIs, phenothiazines, tetracyclines, TCAs **NIPE:** ↑ risk of photophobia, constipation, urinary hesitancy

Ibuprofen (Motrin, Rufen, Advil, others)
Uses: Arthritis and pain **Action:** NSAID **Dose:** *Adults*. 200–800 mg PO bid–qid. *Peds*. 30–40 mg/kg/d in 3–4 ÷ doses; best taken with food, caution when combined with other NSAIDs **Caution/Contra:** [B, +] Avoid in severe hepatic impairment; hypersensitivity to NSAIDs, UGI bleed, or ulcers **Supplied:** Tabs 100, 200, 400, 600, 800 mg; chew tabs 50, 100 mg; caps 200 mg; susp 100 mg/2.5 mL, 100 mg/5 mL, 40 mg/mL (200 mg is OTC preparation) **Notes/SE:** Dizziness, peptic ulcer, platelet inhibition, worsening of renal insufficiency; increases in lithium levels **Interactions:** ↑ effects with ASA, corticosteroids, probenecid, alcohol; ↑ effects of aminoglycosides, anticoagulants, digoxin, hypoglycemics, lithium, methotrexate; ↑ risks of bleeding with abciximab, cefotetan, valproic acid, thrombolytic drugs, warfarin, ticlopidine, garlic, ginger, ginkgo biloba; ↓ effects with feverfew; ↓ effects of antihypertensives **Labs:** ↑ BUN, creatinine; ↓ HMG, HCT, BS, platelets **NIPE:** Take with food

Ibutilide (Corvert)
Uses: Rapid conversion of AF or flutter **Action:** Class III antiarrhythmic agent **Dose:** 0.01 mg/kg (max 1 mg) IVinf over 1 min; may be repeated once **Caution/Contra:** [C, –] Do not administer class I or III antiarrhythmics concurrently or w/n 4 h of ibutilide inf. **Supplied:** Inj 0.1 mg/mL **Notes/SE:** Arrhythmias, HA **Interactions:** ↑ refractory effects with amiodarone, disopyramide, procainamide, quinidine, sotalol; ↑ QT interval with antihistamines, antidepressants, erythromycin, phenothiazines, TCAs

Idarubicin (Idamycin)
Uses: AML (in combination with cytarabine), CML in blast crisis, and ALL **Action:** DNA intercalating agent; inhibits DNA topoisomerases I and II **Dose:** 10–12 mg/m²/d for 3–4 d; ↓ in renal/hepatic dysfunction **Caution/Contra:** [D, –] **Supplied:** Inj 1 mg/mL (5-, 10-, 20-mg vials) **Notes/SE:** Myelosuppression, cardiotoxicity, N/V, mucositis, alopecia, and irritation at sites of IV administration; rare changes in renal/hepatic function **Interactions:** ↑ myelosuppression with antineoplastic drugs and radiation therapy; ↓ effects of live virus vaccines **NIPE:** ↑ fluids to 2–3 L/d

Ifosfamide (Ifex, Holoxan)
Uses: Lung and testicular CA, soft-tissue sarcoma, NHL **Action:** Alkylating agent **Dose:** 1.2 g/m²/d for 5 d by bolus or cont inf; 2.4 g/m²/d for 3 d; with mesna uroprotection; ↓ in renal, hepatic impairment (consider) **Caution/Contra:** [D, M] **Supplied:** Inj 1, 3 g **Notes/SE:** Hemorrhagic cystitis, nephrotoxicity, N/V, mild–moderate leukopenia, lethargy and confusion, alopecia, and hepatic enzyme elevations; dosage adjustment in renal impairment **Interactions:** ↑ effects with allopurinol, chloral hydrate, phenobarbital, phenytoin, grapefruit juice; ↑ myelosuppression with antineoplastic drugs and radiation therapy; ↓ effects of live virus vaccines **NIPE:** ↑ fluids to 2–3 L/d

Imatinib (Gleevec)
Uses: Treatment of CML, gastrointestinal stromal tumors (GIST) **Action:** Inhibits Bcl-Abl tyrosine kinase (signal transduction) **Dose:**

Chronic phase CML: 400–600 mg/d PO. *Accelerated/blast crisis:* 600–800 mg/d PO. *GIST:* 400–600/d mg **Caution/Contra:** [D, ?/–] Metabolized by CYP3A4 **Supplied:** Caps 100 mg **Notes/SE:** GI upset, fluid retention, muscle cramps, musculoskeletal pain, arthralgia, rash, HA; neutropenia and thrombocytopenia, follow CBCs; LFTs at baseline and monthly; caution with warfarin, cyclosporine, azole antifungals, erythromycin, phenytoin, rifampin, carbamazepine **Additional Interactions:** ↓ effects with St. John's Wort **NIPE:** Take with food, ↑ fluids, use barrier contraception

Imipenem-Cilastatin (Primaxin) **Uses:** Serious infections caused by a wide variety of susceptible bacteria; inactive against *S. aureus*, group A and B streptococci, etc **Action:** Bactericidal; interferes with cell wall synthesis **Dose: Adults.** 250–500 mg (imipenem) IV q6h. **Peds.** 60–100 mg/kg/24 h IV ÷ q6h; ↓ in renal disease if calculated CrCl is <70 mL/min **Caution/Contra:** [C, +/–] **Supplied:** Inj (imipenem/cilastatin) 250 mg/250 mg, 500 mg/500 mg **Notes/SE:** Seizures may occur if drug accumulates; GI upset, thrombocytopenia **Interactions:** ↑ risks of seizures with ganciclovir, theophylline; ↓ effects with aztreonam, cephalosporins, chloramphenicol, penicillins, probenicid **Labs:** ↑ LFTs, BUN, creatinine; ↓ HMG, HCT **NIPE:** Eval for superinfection

Imipramine (Tofranil) **Uses:** Depression, enuresis, panic attack, and chronic pain **Action:** TCA; ↑ synaptic conc of serotonin or norepinephrine in the CNS **Dose: Adults.** *Hospitalized:* Start at 100 mg/24 h PO in ÷ doses; can ↑ over several wk to 250–300 mg/24 h. *Outpatient:* Maint of 50–150 mg/24 h PO hs, not to exceed 200 mg/24 h. **Peds.** *Antidepressant:* 1.5–5.0 mg/kg/24 h ÷ 1–4×/d. *Enuresis:* >6 y: 10–25 mg PO hs; ↑ by 10–25 mg at 1–2 wk intervals; treat for 2–3 mon, then taper **Caution/Contra:** [D, ?/–] Do not use with MAOIs, narrow-angle glaucoma **Supplied:** Tabs 10, 25, 50 mg; caps 75, 100, 125, 150 mg **Notes/SE:** Less sedation than with amitriptyline; cardiovascular symptoms, dizziness, xerostomia, discolored urine **Interactions:** ↑ effects with amiodarone, anticholinergics, BBs, cimetidine, diltiazem, lithium, oral contraceptives, quinidine, phenothiazines, ritonavir, verapamil, alcohol, evening primrose oil; ↑ effects of CNS depressants, hypoglycemics, warfarin; ↑ risk of serotonin syndrome with MAOIs; ↓ effects with carbamazepine, phenobarbital, rifampin, tobacco; ↓ effects of clonidine, guanethidine, methyldopa, reserpine **Labs:** ↑ serum glucose, bilirubin, alkaline phosphatase **NIPE:** d/c 48 h <surgery, d/c MAOIs 2 wk <admin this drug, 4–6 wk for full effects, take with food

Imiquimod Cream, 5% (Aldara) **Uses:** External genital warts **Action:** Unknown; may induce cytokines **Dose:** Applied 3×/wk; leave on skin for 6–10 h, continue therapy for a max of 16 wk **Caution/Contra:** [B, ?] **Supplied:** Single-dose packets (250 mg of the cream) **Notes/SE:** Local skin reactions common **NIPE:** Condoms & diaphragms may be weakened – avoid contact

Immune Globulin, Intravenous (Gamimune N, Sandoglobulin, Gammar IV) **Uses:** IgG antibody deficiency disease states (eg, congenital agammaglobulinemia, CVH, and BMT), also ITP **Action:** IgG supplementation **Dose:** ***Adults & Peds.*** *Immunodeficiency:* 100–200 mg/kg/mon IV at a rate of 0.01–0.04 mL/kg/min to a max of 400 mg/kg/dose. *ITP:* 400 mg/kg/dose IV qd for ↓5 d. *BMT:* 500 mg/kg/wk; ↓ renal insufficiency **Caution/Contra:** [C, ?] **Supplied:** Inj **Notes/SE:** Adverse effects associated mostly with rate of inf; GI upset **Interactions:** ↓ effects of live virus vaccines **NIPE:** Give live virus vaccines 3 mon >this drug; rapid infusion can cause anaphylactoid reaction

Indapamide (Lozol) **Uses:** HTN and CHF **Action:** Thiazide diuretic; enhances Na+, Cl−, and water excretion in the proximal segment of the distal tubule **Dose:** 1.25–5 mg/d PO **Caution/Contra:** [D, ?] Thiazide/sulfonamide allergy **Supplied:** Tabs 1.25, 2.5 mg **Notes/SE:** Doses >5 mg do not have additional effects on lowering BP; hypotension, dizziness, photosensitivity **Interactions:** ↑ effects with antihypertensives, diazoxide, nitrates, alcohol; ↑ effects of ACEIs, lithium; ↑ risk of gout with cyclosporine, thiazides; ↑ risk of hypokalemia with amphotericin B, corticosteroids, mezlocillin, piperacillin, ticarcillin; ↓ effects with cholestyramine, colestipol, NSAIDs; ↓ effects of hypoglycemics **Labs:** ↑ serum glucose, uric acid, ↓ K+, sodium, choloride **NIPE:** ↑ risk photosensitivity, take with food

Indinavir (Crixivan) **Uses:** HIV infection **Action:** Protease inhibitor; inhibits maturation of immature noninfectious virions to mature infectious virus **Dose:** 800 mg PO q8h; use in combination with other antiretroviral agents; take on an empty stomach; ↓ in hepatic impairment **Caution/Contra:** [C, ?] Numerous drug interactions **Supplied:** Caps 200, 400 mg **Notes/SE:** Nephrolithiasis; drink six 8-oz glasses of water/d; dyslipidemia, lipodystrophy, GI effects **Interactions:** ↑ effects with aldesleukin, azole antifungals, clarithromycin, delavirdine, interleukins, quinidine, zidovudine; ↑ effects of amiodarone, cisapride, clarithromycin, ergot alkaloids, fentanyl, HMG-CoA reductase inhibitors, isoniazid, oral contraceptives, phenytoin, rifabutin, ritonavir, sildenafil, stavudine, zidovudine; ↓ effects with efavirenz, fluconazole, phenytoin, rifampin, St. John's Wort, high-fat/protein foods, grapefruit juice; ↓ effects of midazolam, triazolam **Labs:** ↑ serum glucose, LFTs, ↑ HMG, platelets, neutrophils **NIPE:** ↑ fluids 1–2 L/d, capsules moisture sensitive – keep dessicant in container

Indomethacin (Indocin) **Uses:** Arthritis; closure of the ductus arteriosus; tocolysis **Action:** Inhibits prostaglandin synthesis **Dose:** ***Adults.*** 25–50 mg PO bid–tid, to a max of 200 mg/d. *Tocolysis:* 50–100 10 PR, then 25 mg PO/PR q4–6h ×48 h. *Infants.* 0.2–0.25 mg/kg/dose IV; may be repeated in 12–24 h for up to 3 doses; take with food **Caution/Contra:** [B, +] ASA/NSAID sensitivity; peptic ulcer disease **Supplied:** Inj 1 mg/vial; caps 25, 50 mg; SR caps 75 mg; supp 50 mg; susp 25 mg/5 mL **Notes/SE:** Monitor renal function; GI bleeding or upset, dizziness, edema **Interactions:** ↑ effects with acetaminophen, antiinflammatories, gold compounds, diflunisal, probenicid; ↑ effects of aminoglycosides, anticoagulants, digoxin, hypoglycemics, lithium, methotrexate, nifedipine, phenytoin, penicillamine, verapamil; ↓ effects with ASA; ↓ effects of antihypertensives **Labs:** ↑ serum K⁺, BUN, creatinine, AST, ALT, urine glucose, protein, PT; ↓ HMG, HCT, leukocytes, platelets **NIPE:** Take with food

Infliximab (Remicade)   **Uses:** Moderate to severe Crohn's disease; RA (in combination with methotrexate) **Action:** IgG1κ; neutralizes biologic activity of TNFα **Dose:** *Crohn's disease:* 5 mg/kg IV inf, may follow with subsequent doses given at 2 and 6 wk after initial inf. *RA:* 3 mg/kg IV inf at 0, 2, 6 wk, followed by q8wk **Caution/Contra:** [C, ?/–] Murine hypersensitivity, active infection **Supplied:** Inj **Notes/SE:** May cause hypersensitivity reaction, made up of human constant and murine variable regions; patients are predisposed to infection (especially TB); HA, fatigue, GI upset, inf reactions **Interactions:** May ↓ effects of live virus vaccines; **Labs:** May ↑ + ANA **NIPE:** ↑ susceptibility to infection

Influenza Vaccine (Fluzone, FluShield, Fluvirin)   **Uses:** Prevents influenza; all adults >65 y, children 6–23 mon, pregnant women who will be in their 2nd or 3rd trimester during flu season, residents of nursing homes, patients with chronic diseases, health care workers and household contacts of high-risk patients, children < 9 y receiving vaccine for the first time **Actions:** Active immunization **Dose:** *Adults.* 0.5 mL/dose IM 0.5-mL IM *Peds.* = *3 y:* 0.5-mL dose. *6–35 mon:* 0.25 mL IM. *6– < 9 y who receive for the 1st time:* 2 doses at least 4 wk apart, the 2nd dose before December if possible. **Caution, Contra:** [C, +] Egg or thimerosal allergy, active infection at site, egg protein sensitivity **Supplied:** Based on specific manufacturer, 0.25 and 0.5 mL prefilled syringes **Notes:** Optimal dosing in the U.S. is Oct–Nov, protection begins 1–2 wk after and lasts up to 6 mon; Each y, specific vaccines manufactured based on predictions of the strains to be active in flu season (Dec–Spring in U.S.). Whole or split virus usually given to adults; give children <13 y split virus or purified surface antigen form to ↓ febrile reactions; soreness at the inj site, adverse fever, myalgia malaise, Guillain-Barré syndrome (controversial) **Interactions:** ↑ effects of theophylline, warfarin; ↓ effects with corticosteroids, immunosuppressants; ↓ effects of aminopyrine, phenytoin

Influenza Virus Vaccine Live, Intranasal (FluMist)   **Uses:** Prevention of influenza **Action:** Live-attenuated vaccine **Dose:** *Adults.* Age 9–49 y: 1 dose (0.5 mL) intranasal per season *Peds.* 5–8 y: not previously vaccinated with FluMist: 2 doses 0.25 mL in each nostril; 60 days apart + 14 days for initial season; previously vaccinated with FluMist: 1 dose (0.5 mL) per season. **Caution:** [C,?/–] **Contra:** Egg allergy, PRG, children/adolescents on aspirin, Hx Guillain-Barré syndrome, known/suspected immune deficiency, asthma or reactive airway disease **Supplied:** Prefilled, single-use, intranasal sprayer **SE:** Runny nose, nasal congestion, HA, sore throat, cough, myalgia, low-grade fever **Notes:** Do not administer concurrently with other vaccines **NIPE:** ⊘ Take with antivirals, ASA, NSAIDS, immunosuppressants, corticosteroids, radiation therapy

Insulin   **Uses:** Type 1 or type 2 DM refractory to diet change or oral hypoglycemic agents; management of acute life-threatening hyperkalemia **Action:** Insulin supplementation **Dose:** Based on serum glucose levels; usually SC but can be given IV (only regular)/IM; typical start dose for type 1 0.5–1 U/kg/d; type 2 0.3–0.4 U/kg/d; renal failure may ↓ insulin needs **Caution/Contra:** [B, +] **Supplied:** Table 6 (page 252) **Notes/SE:** Highly purified insulins ↑ free insulin; monitor patients closely for several wk when changing doses/agents **Interactions:** ↑ hypoglycemic effects with α-blockers, anabolic steroids, BBs, clofibrate, fenfluramine, guanethidine, MAOIs, NSAIDs, pentamidine, phenylbutazone, salicylates, sulfinpyrazone, tetracyclines, alcohol, celery, coriander, dandelion root, fenugreek, ginseng, garlic, juniper berries; ↓ hypoglycemic effects with corticosteroids, dextrothyroxine, diltiazem, dobutamine, epinephrine, niacin, oral contraceptives, protease inhibitor antiretrovirals, rifampin, thiazide diuretics, thyroid preps, marijuana, tobacco **NIPE:** If mixing insulins – draw up short-acting preps first in syringe

Interferon Alfa (Roferon-A, Intron A)
Uses: Hairy cell leukemia, Kaposi's sarcoma, multiple myeloma, CML, renal cell carcinoma, bladder CA, melanoma, and chronic hepatitis C **Action:** Direct antiproliferative action against tumor cells; modulation of the host immune response **Dose:** Dictated by treatment protocol. *Alfa-2a (Roferon-A):* 3 million IU/d for 16–24 wk SC or IM. *Alfa-2b (Intron A):* 2 million IU/m^2 IM or SC 3×/wk for 2–6 mon; intravesical 50–100 million IU in 50 mL/wk NS ×6 **Caution/Contra:** [C, +/–] Benzyl alcohol sensitivity **Supplied:** Injectable forms **Notes/SE:** May cause flu-like symptoms; fatigue common; anorexia occurs in 20–30% of patients; neurotoxicity may occur at high doses; neutralizing antibodies in up to 40% of patients receiving prolonged systemic therapy **Interactions:** ↑ effects of antineoplastics, CNS depressants, doxorubicin, theophylline; ↓ effects of live virus vaccine **Labs:** ↑ LFTs, BUN, serum creatinine, glucose, phosphorus, ↓ HMG, HCT, calcium **NIPE:** ASA & alcohol use may cause GI bleed, ↑ fluids to 2–3 L/d

Interferon Alfa-2b and Ribavirin Combination (Rebetron)
Uses: Chronic hepatitis C in patients with compensated liver disease who have relapsed following alfa-interferon therapy **Action:** Combination antiviral agents **Dose:** 3 MU Intron A SC 3×/wk with 1000–1200 mg of Rebetron PO ÷ bid dose for 24 wk. *Patients <75 kg:* 1000 mg of Rebetron/d **Caution/Contra:** [X, ?] **Supplied:** *Patients <75 kg:* Combination packs: 6 vials Intron A (3 MU/0.5 mL) with 6 syringes and alcohol swabs, 70 Rebetron caps; one 18 million-IU multidose vial of Intron A inj (22.8 MU/3.8 mL; 3 MU/0.5 mL) and 6 syringes and swabs, 70 Rebetron caps; one 18 million-IU Intron A inj multidose pen (22.5 million IU/1.5 mL; 3 million IU/0.2 mL) and 6 disposable needles and swabs, 70 Rebetron caps. *Patients >75 kg:* Identical except 84 Rebetron caps/pack **Notes/SE:** Instruct patients in self-administration of SC Intron A; flu-like syndrome, HA, anemia; see **Interferon Alfa. Additional Labs:** ↑ uric acid

Interferon Alfacon-1 (Infergen)
Uses: Management of chronic hepatitis C **Action:** Biologic response modifier **Dose:** 9 μg SC 3×/wk **Caution/Con-**

ra: [C, M] **Supplied:** Inj 9, 15 μg **Notes/SE:** Allow at least 48 h between inj; flu-like syndrome, depression, blood dyscrasias **Interactions:** ↑ effects of theophylline **Labs:** ↑ triglycerides, TSH; ↓ HMG, HCT **NIPE:** Refrigerate, ⊘ shake, use barrier contraception

Interferon Beta-1b (Betaseron)
Uses: Management of MS **Action:** Biologic response modifier **Dose:** 0.25 mg SC qod **Caution/Contra:** [C, ?] **Supplied:** Powder for inj 0.3 mg **Notes/SE:** Flu-like syndrome, depression, blood dyscrasias **Interactions:** ↑ effects of theophylline, zidovudine **Labs:** ↑ LFTs, BUN, urine protein **NIPE:** ↑ risk of photosensitivity, abortion; ↑ fluid intake, use barrier contraception

Interferon Gamma-1b (Actimmune)
Uses: ↓ Incidence of serious infections in chronic granulomatous disease (CGD), osteopetrosis **Action:** Biologic response modifier **Dose:** CGD: 50 μg/m² SC (1.5 MU/m²) BSA >0.5 m²; if BSA <0.5 m², give 1.5 μg/kg/dose; given 3×/wk **Caution/Contra:** [C, ?] **Supplied:** Inj 100 μg (3 MU) **Notes/SE:** Flu-like syndrome, depression, blood dyscrasias

Ipecac Syrup
Uses: Drug overdose and certain cases of poisoning **Action:** Irritation of the GI mucosa; stimulation of the chemoreceptor trigger zone **Dose:** *Adults.* 15–30 mL PO, followed by 200–300 mL of water; if no emesis in 20 min, may repeat. *Peds. 6–12 mon:* 5–10 mL PO, followed by 10–20 mL/kg of water; if no emesis in 20 min, repeat. *1–12 y:* 15 mL PO followed by 10–20 mL/kg of water; if no emesis in 20 min, repeat **Caution/Contra:** [C, ?] Do not use for petroleum distillates or strong acid, base, or other caustic agents; not for use in comatose or unconscious patients **Supplied:** Syrup 15, 30 mL **Notes/SE:** Caution in CNS depressant overdose; lethargy, cardiotoxicity, protracted vomiting. 2003 NIH panel may recommend removal from market due to lack of documented efficacy **Interactions:** ↑ effects of myelosuppressives, theophylline, zidovudine **NIPE:** ↑ fluids to 2–3 L/d, ⊘ alcohol, CNS depressants

Ipratropium (Atrovent)
Uses: Bronchospasm with COPD, bronchitis, emphysema, and rhinorrhea **Action:** Synthetic anticholinergic agent similar to atropine **Dose:** *Adults & Peds >12 y.* 2–4 puffs qid. *Nasal:* 2 sprays/nostril bid–tid **Caution/Contra:** [B, +] **Supplied:** Met-dose inhaler 18 μg/dose; soln for inhal 0.02%; nasal spray 0.03%, 0.06% **Notes/SE:** Not for acute bronchospasm; nervousness, dizziness, HA, cough **Interactions:** ↑ effects with albuterol; ↑ effects of anticholinergics, antimuscarinics; ↓ effects with jaborandi tree, pill-bearing spurge **NIPE:** Adequate fluids, separate inhalation of other drugs by 5 min

Irbesartan (Avapro)
Uses: HTN, DN, CHF **Action:** Angiotensin II receptor antagonist **Dose:** 150 mg/d PO, may be ↑ to 300 mg/d **Caution/Contra:** [C (in 1st trimester; D in 2nd and 3rd), ?/–] **Supplied:** Tabs 75, 150, 300 mg **Notes/SE:** Fatigue, hypotension **Interactions:** ↑ risk of hyperkalemia with K⁺-sparing diuretics, trimethoprim, K⁺ supplements; ↑ effects of lithium **Labs:** ↑ BUN, serum creatinine; ↓ HMG **NIPE:** ⊘ PRG, breast-feeding

Irinotecan (Camptosar)   **Uses:** Colorectal and lung CA **Action:** Topoisomerase I inhibitor; interferes with DNA synthesis **Dose:** 125–250 mg/m² weekly to qowk; ↓ hepatic dysfunction, as tolerated per toxicities **Caution/Contra:** [D, –] **Supplied:** Inj 20 mg/mL **Notes/SE:** Myelosuppression, N/V/D, abdominal cramping, alopecia. Diarrhea dose limiting in many studies; Rx acute diarrhea with atropine; Rx subacute diarrhea with loperamide. Diarrhea correlated to levels of metabolite SN-38 **Interactions:** ↑ effects of antineoplastics; ↑ risk of akathisia with prochlorperazine **Labs:** ↑ LFTs **NIPE:** Use barrier contraception, ⊘ exposure to infection

Iron Dextran (Dexferrum, INFeD)   **Uses:** Iron deficiency when oral supplementation not possible **Action:** Parenteral iron supplementation **Dose:** Estimate iron deficiency, given IM/IV. A 0.5-mL test dose (0.25 mL in infants) prior to starting iron dextran. Total replacement dose (mL) = 0.0476 × weight (kg) × [desired hemoglobin (g/dL) – measured hemoglobin (g/dL)] + 1 mL/5 kg weight (max 14 mL). *Adults >50 kg. Max daily dose:* 100 mg Fe. *Peds. Max daily dose: <5 kg:* 25 mg Fe. *5–10 kg:* 50 mg Fe. *10–50 kg:* 100 mg Fe **Caution/Contra:** [C, M] **Supplied:** Inj 50 mg Fe/mL **Notes/SE:** Use test dose because anaphylaxis possible; give deep IM using "Z-track" technique, IV route preferred; anaphylaxis, flushing, dizziness, inj site and inf reactions, metallic taste **Interactions:** ↓ effects with chloramphenicol, ↓ absorption of oral iron **Labs:** False ↓ serum calcium; false + guaiac test **NIPE:** ⊘ Take oral iron

Isoetharine (generic)   **Uses:** Bronchial asthma and reversible bronchospasm **Action:** Sympathomimetic bronchodilator **Dose:** *Adults.* 0.25–1 mL diluted 1:3 with NS q4–6h. *Peds.* 0.01 mL/kg; min dose 0.1 mL; max dose 0.5 mL; dilute with NS q4–6h **Caution/Contra:** [C, ?] **Supplied:** Soln for inhal; aerosol **Notes/SE:** Tachycardia, HTN, dizziness, trembling **Interactions:** ↑ effects with bronchodilators, MAOIs, sympathomimetics, TCAs; ↑ hypokalemia with furosemide; ↑ arrhythmias with halothane; ↓ effects with BBs **Labs:** ↓ serum K⁺ **NIPE:** ↑ fluid intake

Isoniazid (INH)   **Uses:** Rx and prophylaxis of *Mycobacterium* spp infections **Action:** Bactericidal; interferes with mycolic acid synthesis (disrupts cell wall) **Dose:** *Adults. Active TB:* 5 mg/kg/24 h PO or IM (usually 300 mg/d). *Prophylaxis:* 300 mg/d PO for 6–12 mon *Peds. Active TB:* 10–20 mg/kg/24 h PO or IM to a max of 300 mg/d. *Prophylaxis:* 10 mg/kg/24 h PO; ↓ in hepatic impairment **Caution/Contra:** [C, +] Acute liver disease, dialysis **Supplied:** Tabs 50, 100, 300 mg; syrup 50 mg/5 mL; inj 100 mg/mL **Notes/SE:** Given with 2–3 other drugs for active TB, based on INH resistance patterns where TB acquired; IM route rarely used. To prevent peripheral neuropathy, give pyridoxine 50–100 mg/d. Can cause severe hepatitis, peripheral neuropathy, GI upset, anorexia, dizziness **Interactions:** ↑ effects of acetaminophen, anticoagulants, carbamazepine, cycloserine, diazepam, meperidine, hydantoins, theophylline, valproic acid, alcohol; ↑ effects with rifampin; ↓ effects with aluminum salts; ↓ effects of anticoagulants, ketoconazole **Labs:** False + urine glucose, false ↑ AST, uric acid, false ↓ serum glucose **NIPE:** Only take with food if GI upset

Isoproterenol (Isuprel) **Uses:** Shock, cardiac arrest, and AV nodal block; antiasthmatic **Action:** β_1- and β_2-receptor stimulant **Dose:** *Adults. Shock:* 1–4 mg/min IV inf; titrate to effect. *AV nodal block:* 20–60 mg IV push; may repeat q3–5min; maint 1–5 mg/min IV inf. *Inhalation:* 1–2 inhal 4–6×/d. *Peds. Inhal:* 1–2 inhal 4–6×/d **Caution/Contra:** [C, ?] Tachycardia; pulse >130 may induce ventricular arrhythmias. **Supplied:** Met-inhaler; soln for neb 0.5%, 1%; inj 0.02, 0.2 mg/mL **Notes/SE:** Insomnia, arrhythmias, GI upset, trembling, dizziness **Interactions:** ↑ effects with albuterol, guanethidine, oxytocic drugs, sympathomimetics, TCAs; ↑ risk of arrhythmias with amitriptyline, bretylium, cardiac glycosides, K^+-depleting drugs, theophylline; ↓ effects with BBs **Labs:** false ↑ serum AST, bilirubin, glucose **NIPE:** Saliva may turn pink in color, ↑ fluids to 2–3 L/d

Isosorbide Dinitrate (Isordil, Sorbitrate) **Uses:** Rx and prevention of angina, CHF (with hydralazine) **Action:** Relaxation of vascular smooth muscle **Dose:** *Acute angina:* 5–10 mg PO (chew tabs) q2–3h or 2.5–10 mg SL PRN q5–10min; >3 doses should not be given in a 15–30-min period. *Angina prophylaxis:* 5–60 mg PO tid; do not give nitrates on a chronic q6h or qid basis >7–10 d because tolerance may develop **Caution/Contra:** [C, ?] Contra severe anemia, closed-angle glaucoma, orthostatic hypotension, cerebral hemorrhage, head trauma (can ↑ ICP) **Supplied:** Tabs 5, 10, 20, 30, 40 mg; SR tabs 40 mg; SL tabs 2.5, 5, 10 mg; chew tabs 5, 10 mg; SR caps 40 mg **Notes/SE:** HAs, ↓ BP, flushing, tachycardia, dizziness; higher oral dose usually needed to achieve same results as SL forms **Interactions:** ↑ hypotension with antihypertensives, ASA, CCBs, phenothiazides, sildenafil, alcohol **Labs:** False ↓ serum cholesterol **NIPE:** ⊘ nitrates for a 8–12 h period/d to avoid tolerance

Isosorbide Mononitrate (ISMO, Imdur) **Uses:** Prevention of angina pectoris **Action:** Relaxes vascular smooth muscle **Dose:** 20 mg PO bid, the 2 doses 7 h apart or ER (Imdur) 30–120 mg/d PO **Caution/Contra:** [C, ?] Contra in head trauma or cerebral hemorrhage (can ↑ ICP) **Supplied:** Tabs 10, 20 mg; ER 30, 60, 120 mg **Notes/SE:** HAs, dizziness, hypotension **Interactions:** ↑ hypotension with ASA, CCB, nitrates, sildenafil, alcohol **Labs:** False ↓ serum cholesterol

Isotretinoin [13-*cis*-Retinoic Acid] (Accutane) **WARNING:** Must not be used by pregnant females; patient must be capable of complying with mandatory contraceptive measures; Accutane must be prescribed under SMART (system to manage Accutane-related teratogenicity) **Uses:** Refractory severe acne **Action:** Retinoic acid derivative **Dose:** 0.5–2 mg/kg/d PO ÷ bid; ↓ in hepatic disease **Caution/Contra:** [X, –] Retinoid sensitivity **Supplied:** Caps 10, 20, 40 mg **Notes/SE:** Isolated reports of depression, psychosis, suicidal thoughts; dermatologic sensitivity, xerostomia, photosensitivity; SMART risk management programs require 2 negative PRG tests before therapy and use 2 forms of contraception 1 mon before, during, and 1 mon after therapy; informed consent recommended **In-**

teractions: ↑ effects with corticosteroids, phenytoin, vitamin A ; ↑ risk of pseudotumor cerebri with tetracyclines; ↑ triglyceride levels with alcohol; ↓ effects of carbamazepine **NIPE:** ↑ risk of photosensitivity, take with food, ⊘ PRG

Isradipine (DynaCirc) **Uses:** HTN w/wo diuretics **Action:** Ca^{2+} channel blocker **Dose:** 2.5–10 mg PO bid **Caution/Contra:** [C, ?] Heart block, CHF **Supplied:** Caps 2.5, 5 mg; tabs CR 5, 10 mg **Notes/SE:** HA, edema, flushing, fatigue, dizziness, palpitations **Interactions:** ↑effects with azole antifungals, BBs, cimetidine; ↑ effects of carbamazepine, cyclosporine, digitalis glycosides, prazosin, quinidine; ↓ effects with calcium, rifampi; ↓ effects of lovastatin **Labs:** ↑ LFTs **NIPE:** ⊘ d/c abruptly

Itraconazole (Sporanox) **WARNING:** Potential for negative inotropic effects on the heart; if signs or symptoms of CHF occur during administration, continued use should be assessed **Uses:** Systemic fungal infections (aspergillosis, blastomycosis, histoplasmosis, candidiasis) **Action:** Inhibits synthesis of ergosterol **Dose:** 200 mg PO or IV qd–bid with meals or cola/grapefruit juice **Caution/Contra:** [C, ?] Contra if CrCl <30 mL/min, Hx of CHF or ventricular dysfunction, or concurrently with H_2-antagonist, omeprazole, antacids; numerous other interactions **Supplied:** Caps 100 mg; soln 10 mg/mL; inj 10 mg/mL **Notes/SE:** Often used in patients who cannot take amphotericin B; nausea, rash, hepatitis **Interactions:** ↑ effects with clarithromycin, erythromycin; ↑ effects of alprazolam, anticoagulants, atevirdine, atorvastatin, buspirone, cerivastatin, chlordiazepoxide, cyclosporine, diazepam, digoxin, felodipine, fluvastatin, indinavir, lovastatin, methadone, methylprednisolone, midazolam, nelfinavir, pravastatin, ritonavir, saquinavir, simvastatin, tacrolimus, tolbutamide, triazolam, warfarin; ↑ QT prolongation with astemizole, cisapride, pimozide, quinidine, terfenadine; ↓ effects with antacids, calcium, cimetidine, didanosine, famotidine, lansoprazole, magnesium, nizatidine, omeprazole, phenytoin, rifampin, sucralfate, grapefruit juice **Labs:** ↑ LFTs, BUN, serum creatinine **NIPE:** Take capsule with food & soln w/o food, ⊘ PRG or breast-feeding, ↑ risk of disulfiram-like response with alcohol

Kaolin-Pectin (Kaodene, Kao-Spen, Kapectolin, Parepectolin) **Uses:** Diarrhea **Action:** Absorbent demulcent **Dose:** *Adults.* 60–120 mL PO after each loose stool or q3–4h PRN. *Peds. 3–6 y:* 15–30 mL/dose PO PRN. *6–12 y:* 30–60 mL/dose PO PRN **Caution/Contra:** [C, +] **Supplied:** Multiple OTC forms; also available with opium (Parepectolin) **Notes/SE:** Constipation, dehydration **Interaction:** ↓ effects of ciprofloxacin, clindamycin, digoxin, lincomycin, lovastatin, penicillamine, quinidine, tetracycline **NIPE:** Take other meds 2–3 h < or > this drug

Ketoconazole (Nizoral, Nizoral AD Shampoo [OTC]) **Uses:** Systemic fungal infections; topical cream for localized fungal infections due to dermatophytes and yeast; shampoo for dandruff, short term in prostate CA when rapid reduction of testosterone needed (ie, cord compression) **Action:** Inhibits fungal cell wall synthesis **Dose:** *Adults. Oral:* 200 mg PO qd; ↑ to 400 mg/d PO for serious infections; prostate CA 400 mg PO tid (short term). *Topical:* Apply to the affected area qd (cream or shampoo). **Peds >2 y.** 5–10 mg/kg/24 h PO ÷ q12–24h; drug interaction with any agent increasing gastric pH will prevent absorption of ketoconazole; ↓ in hepatic disease **Caution/Contra:** [C, +/–] Contra in CNS fungal infections (poor CNS penetration); may enhance oral anticoagulants; may react with alcohol to produce a disulfiram-like reaction; numerous other drug interactions **Supplied:** Tabs 200 mg; topical cream 2%; shampoo 2% **Notes/SE:** Monitor LFTs with systemic use; can cause nausea; oral form multiple drug interactions **Interactions:** ↑ effects of alprazolam, anticoagulants, atevirdine, atorvastatin, buspirone, chlordiazepoxide, cyclosporine, diazepam, felodipine, fluvastatin, indinavir, lovastatin, methadone, methylprednisolone, midazolam, nelfinavir, pravastatin, ritonavir, saquinavir, simvastatin, tacrolimus, tolbutamide, triazolam, warfarin; ↑ QT prolongation with astemizole, cisapride, quinidine, terfenadine; ↓ effects with antacids, calcium, cimetidine, didanosine, famotidine, lansoprazole, magnesium, nizatidine, omeprazole, phenytoin, rifampin, sucralfate **Labs:** ↑ LFTs **NIPE:** Take tabs with citrus juice, take with food; shampoo wet hair 1 min, rinse, repeat for 3 min; ⊘ PRG or breast-feeding

Ketoprofen (Orudis, Oruvail)   Uses: Arthritis and pain **Action:** NSAID; inhibits prostaglandin synthesis **Dose:** 25–75 mg PO tid–qid to a max of 300 mg/d; take with food **Caution/Contra:** [B (D 3rd trimester), ?] NSAID/ASA sensitivity **Supplied:** Tabs 12.5 mg; caps 25, 50, 75 mg; caps, SR 100, 150, 200 mg **Notes/SE:** GI upset, peptic ulcers, dizziness, edema, rash **Interactions:** ↑ effects with ASA, corticosteroids, NSAIDs, probenicid, alcohol; ↑ effects of antineoplastics, hypoglycemics, insulin, lithium, methotrexate; ↑ risk of nephrotoxicity with aminoglycosides, cyclosporines; ↑ risk of bleeding with anticoagulants, defamandole, cefotetan, cefoperazone, clopidogrel, eptifibatide, plicamycine, thrombolytics, tirofiban, valproic acid, dong quai, feverfew, garlic, ginkgo biloba, ginger, horse chestnut, red clover; ↓ effects of antihypertensives, diuretics **Labs:** ↑ LFTs, BUN, serum sodium, creatinine, chloride, K⁺, PT; ↑ or ↓ glucose; ↓ HMG, HCT, platelets, leukocytes **NIPE:** ↑ risk of photosensitivity, take with food

Ketorolac (Toradol)   **WARNING:** Indicated for short term (up to 5 d) of moderately severe acute pain that requires analgesia at opioid level **Uses:** Pain **Action:** NSAID; inhibits prostaglandin synthesis **Dose:** 15–30 mg IV/IM q6h or 10 mg IV/IM q6h; max IV/IM 120 mg/d, max PO 40 mg/d; do not use for longer than 5 days; ↓ for age and renal dysfunction **Caution/Contra:** [B (D 3rd trimester), –] Contra peptic ulcer disease, NSAID sensitivity, advanced renal disease, CNS bleeding, anticipated major surgery, labor and delivery, nursing mothers **Supplied:** Tabs 10 mg; inj 15 mg/mL, 30 mg/mL **Notes/SE:** Bleeding, peptic ulcer disease, renal failure, edema, dizziness, hypersensitivity; PO used only as continuation of IM/IV therapy **Interactions:** ↑ effects with ASA, corticosteroids, NSAIDs, probenicid, alcohol; ↑ effects of antineoplastics, hypoglycemics, insulin, lithium, methotrexate; ↑ risk of nephrotoxicity with aminoglycosides, cyclosporines; ↑ risk of bleeding with anticoagulants, defamandole, cefotetan, cefoperazone, clopidogrel, eptifibatide, plicamycine, thrombolytics, tirofiban, valproic acid, dong quai, feverfew, garlic, ginkgo biloba, ginger, horse chestnut, red clover; ↓ effects of antihypertensives, diuretics **Labs:** ↑ LFTs, PT, BUN, serum creatinine, sodium, chloride, K⁺ **NIPE:** 30-mg dose equals comparative analgesia of meperidine 100 mg or morphine 12 mg

Ketorolac Ophthalmic (Acular)   **Uses:** Relief of ocular itching caused by seasonal allergic conjunctivitis **Action:** NSAID **Dose:** 1 gt qid **Caution/Contra:** [C, +] **Supplied:** Soln 0.5% **Notes/SE:** Local irritation; see Ketorolac **NIPE:** ⊘ soft contact lenses

Ketotifen (Zaditor)   **Uses:** Allergic conjunctivitis **Action:** H₁-receptor antagonist and mast cell stabilizer **Dose:** *Adults & Peds.* 1 gt in affected eye(s) q8–12h **Caution/Contra:** [C, ?/–] **Supplied:** Solution 0.025%/5 mL **Notes/SE:** Local irritation, HA, rhinitis **NIPE:** Insert soft contact lenses 10 min >drug use

Labetalol (Trandate, Normodyne)   **Uses:** HTN and hypertensive emergencies **Action:** α- and β-adrenergic blocking agent **Dose:** *Adults.* *HTN:* Initially, 100 mg PO bid, then 200–400 mg PO bid. *Hypertensive emergency:* 20–80 mg IV bolus, then 2 mg/min IV inf, titrated to effect. *Peds.* *Oral:* 3–20 mg/kg/d in ÷ doses. *Hypertensive emergency:* 0.4–1.5 mg/kg/h IV cont inf **Caution/Contra:** [C (D in 2nd or 3rd trimester), +] Cardiogenic shock, uncompensated CHF, heart block **Supplied:** Tabs 100, 200, 300 mg; inj 5 mg/mL **Notes/SE:** Dizziness, nausea, ↓ BP, fatigue, cardiovascular effects **Interactions:** ↑ effects with cimetidine, diltiazem, nitroglycerine, quinidine, paroxetine, propalenone, verapamil; ↑ tremors with TCAs; ↓ effects with glutethimide, NSAIDs, salicylates; ↓ effects of antihypertensives, β-adrenergic bronchodilators, sulfonylureas **Labs:** False ÷ urine catecholamines **NIPE:** May have transient tingling of scalp

Lactic Acid and Ammonium Hydroxide [Ammonium Lactate] (Lac-Hydrin)   **Uses:** Severe xerosis and ichthyosis **Action:** Emollient moisturizer **Dose:** Apply bid **Caution/Contra:** [C, ?] **Supplied:** Lactic acid 12% with ammonium hydroxide **Notes/SE:** Local irritation

Lactobacillus (Lactinex Granules)   **Uses:** Control of diarrhea, especially after antibiotic therapy **Action:** Replaces normal intestinal flora **Dose:** *Adults & Peds >3 y.* 1 packet, 2 caps, or 4 tabs with meals or liq tid–qid **Caution/Contra:** [A, +] Contra in milk/lactose allergy **Supplied:** Tabs; caps; EC caps; powder in packets **Notes/SE:** Flatulence

Lactulose (Chronulac, Cephulac)   **Uses:** Hepatic encephalopathy; laxative **Action:** Acidifies the colon, allowing ammonia to diffuse into the colon **Dose:** *Adults.* *Acute hepatic encephalopathy:* 30–45 mL PO q1h until soft stools, then tid–qid. *Chronic laxative therapy:* 30–45 mL PO tid–qid; adjust q1–2d to produce 2–3 soft stools/d. *Rectally:* 200 g in 700 mL of water PR. *Peds.* *Infants:* 2.5–10 mL/24 h ÷ tid–qid. *Children:* 40–90 mL/24 h ÷ tid–qid **Caution/Contra:** [B, ?] Galactosemia **Supplied:** Syrup 10 g/15 mL **Notes/SE:** Severe diarrhea, flatulence **Interactions:** ↓ effects with antacids, neomycin **Labs:** ↓ serum ammonia **NIPE:** May take 24–48 h for results

Lamivudine (Epivir, Epivir-HBV)
WARNING: Lactic acidosis and severe hepatomegaly with steatosis reported with nucleoside analogs **Uses:** HIV infection and chronic hepatitis B **Action:** Inhibits HIV reverse transcriptase, resulting in viral DNA chain termination **Dose:** *HIV: Adults & Peds >12 y.* 150 mg PO bid. *Peds <12 y.* 4 mg/kg bid. *HBV:* 100 mg/d. *Peds 2–17 y.* 3 mg/kg/d PO, 100 mg max; ↓ in renal impairment **Caution/Contra:** [C, ?] **Supplied:** Tabs 100, 150 mg (HBV); soln 5 mg/mL, 10 mg/mL **Notes/SE:** HA, pancreatitis, anemia, GI upset **Interactions:** ↑ effects with co-trimoxazole, trimethoprim/sulfamethoxazole; ↑ risk of lactic acidosis with antiretrovirals, reverse transcriptase inhibitors **Labs:** ↑ LFTs

Lamotrigine (Lamictal)
WARNING: Serious rashes requiring hospitalization and DC of treatment reported with Lamictal use; this rash occurs more frequently in children than adults **Uses:** Partial seizures **Action:** Phenyltriazine antiepileptic **Dose:** *Adults.* Initial 50 mg/d PO, then 50 mg PO bid for 2 wk, then maint 300–500 mg/d in 1–2 doses. *Peds.* 0.15 mg/kg in 1–2 doses for wk 1 and 2, then 0.3 mg/kg for wk 3 and 4, then maint 1 mg/kg/d in 1–2 doses **Caution/Contra:** [C, –] **Supplied:** Tabs 25, 100, 150, 200 mg; chew tabs 5, 25 mg **Notes/SE:** May cause rash and photosensitivity; value of therapeutic monitoring not established; interacts with other antiepileptics; HA, GI upset, dizziness, ataxia, rash (potentially life-threatening in children >adults) **Interactions:** ↑ effects valproic acid; ↑ effects of carbamazepine; ↓ effects with phenobarbital, phenytoin, primidone; **NIPE:** ↑ risk of photosensitivity

Lansoprazole (Prevacid)
Uses: Duodenal ulcers, prevent and Rx NSAID gastric ulcers, *H. pylori* infection, erosive esophagitis, and hypersecretory conditions **Action:** Proton pump inhibitor **Dose:** 15–30 mg/d PO; NSAID ulcer prevention 15 mg/d PO up to 12 wk, NSAID ulcers 30 mg/d PO, ×8 wk; ↓ in severe hepatic impairment **Caution/Contra:** [B, ?/–] **Supplied:** Caps 15, 30 mg **Notes/SE:** HA, fatigue **Interactions:** ↑ effects of hypoglycemics, nifedipine; ↓ effects with sucralfate; ↓ effects of ampicillin, cefpodoxime, cefuroxime, digoxin, enoxacin, ketoconazole, theophylline **Labs:** ↑ LFTs, serum creatinine, LDH, gastrin, lipids **NIPE:** Take <meals

Latanoprost (Xalatan)
Uses: Refractory glaucoma **Action:** Prostaglandin **Dose:** 1 gt eye(s) hs **Caution/Contra:** [C, ?] **Supplied:** 0.005% soln **Notes/SE:** May darken light irises; blurred vision, ocular stinging, and itching **Interactions:** ↑ risk of precipitation if mixed with eye gtts with thimerosal

Leflunomide (Arava)
WARNING: PRG must be excluded prior to start of treatment **Uses:** Active RA **Action:** Inhibits pyrimidine synthesis **Dose:** Initial 100 mg/d for 3 d, then 10–20 mg/d **Caution/Contra:** [X, –] **Supplied:** Tabs 10, 20, 100 mg **Notes/SE:** Monitor LFTs during initial therapy; diarrhea, infection, HTN, alopecia, rash, nausea, joint pain, hepatitis **Interactions:** ↑ effects with ri-

fampin; ↑ risk of hepatotoxicity with hepatotoxic drugs, methotrexate; ↑ effects of NSAIDs; ↓ effects with activated charcoal, cholestyramine **Labs:** ↑ LFTs **NIPE:** ⊘ PRG, breast-feeding, live virus vaccines

Lepirudin (Refludan) **Uses:** Heparin-induced thrombocytopenia **Action:** Direct inhibitor of thrombin **Dose:** Bolus 0.4 mg/kg IV, then 0.15 mg/kg inf; ↓ dose and inf rate if CrCl <60 mL/min **Caution/Contra:** [B, ?/–] Caution in patients who have suffered hemorrhagic event **Supplied:** Inj 50 mg **Notes/SE:** Adjust dose based on aPTT ratio, maintain aPTT ratio of 1.5–2.0; bleeding, anemia, hematoma **Interactions:** ↑ risk of bleeding with antiplatelet drugs, cephalosporins, NSAIDs, thrombolytics, salicylates, feverfew, ginkgo biloba, ginger, valerian

Letrozole (Femara) **Uses:** Advanced breast CA **Action:** Nonsteroidal inhibitor of the aromatase enzyme system **Dose:** 2.5 mg/d **Caution/Contra:** [D, ?] **Supplied:** Tabs 2.5 mg **Notes/SE:** Requires periodic CBC, thyroid function, electrolyte, LFT, and renal monitoring; anemia, nausea, hot flashes, arthralgia **Interactions:** ↑ risk of interference with action of drug with estrogens and oral contraceptives **Labs:** ↑ LFTs, cholesterol, calcium, ↓ lymphocytes

Leucovorin (Wellcovorin) **Uses:** Overdose of folic acid antagonist; augmentation of 5-FU **Action:** Reduced folate source; circumvents action of folate reductase inhibitors (ie, MTX) **Dose:** *Adults & Peds. MTX rescue:* 10 mg/m²/dose IV or PO q6h for 72 h until MTX level <10⁻⁸. *5-FU:* 200 mg/m²/d IV 1–5 d during daily 5-FU treatment or 500 mg/m²/wk with weekly 5-FU therapy. *Adjunct to antimicrobials:* 5–15 mg/d PO **Caution/Contra:** [C, ?/–] Pernicious anemia; should not be administered intrathecally/intraventricularly **Supplied:** Tabs 5, 15, 25 mg; inj **Notes/SE:** Many dosing schedules for leucovorin rescue following MTX therapy; allergic reaction **Interactions:** ↑ effects of fluorouracil; ↓ effects of methotrexate, phenobarbital, phenyotin, primidone, trimethoprim/sulfamethoxazole **NIPE:** ↑ fluids 3 L/d

Leuprolide (Lupron, Lupron Depot, Lupron Depot-Ped, Viadur, Eligard) **Uses:** Advanced prostate CA (CAP), endometriosis, uterine fibroids, and CPP **Action:** LHRH agonist; paradoxically inhibits release of gonadotropin, resulting in decreased pituitary gonadotropins (ie, ↓ LH); in men ↓ testosterone **Dose:** *Adults. CAP:* 7.5 mg IM q28d or 22.5 mg IM q3mon or 30 mg IM q4mon of depot; Viadur implant (CAP only), insert in inner upper arm using local anesthesia, replace q12mon. *Endometriosis (depot only):* 3.75 mg IM qmon ×6. *Fibroids:* 3.75 mg IM qmon ×3. *Peds. CPP:* 50 µg/kg/d as a daily SC inj; ↑ by 10 µg/kg/d until total down-regulation achieved. *Depot: <25 kg:* 7.5 mg IM q4wk. *>25–37.5 kg:* 11.25 mg IM q4wk. *>37.5 kg:* 15 mg IM q4wk **Caution/Contra:** [X, ?] Contra in undiagnosed vaginal bleeding **Supplied:** Inj 5 mg/mL; Lupron depot 3.75 mg (1 mon for fibroids, endometriosis), Lupron depot for CAP 7.5 (1 mon), 22.5 (3 mon), 30 mg (4 mon); Eligard depot for CAP 7.5 mg (1 mon); Viadur 12-mon SC implant; Lupron-PED 7.5, 11.25, 15 mg **Notes/SE:** Hot flashes, gynecomastia, N/V, constipation, anorexia, dizziness, HA, insomnia, paresthesias, peripheral edema, and bone pain (transient "flare reaction" at 7–14 d after the 1st dose due to LH and testosterone surge before suppression) **Interactions:** ↓ effects with androgens, estrogens **Labs:** ↓ LFTs, BUN, serum calcium, uric acid, glucose, lipids, WBC, PT; ↓ serum K+, platelets

Levalbuterol (Xopenex) Uses: Rx and prevention of bronchospasm **Action:** Sympathomimetic bronchodilator **Dose:** 0.63 mg neb q6–8h **Caution/Contra:** [C, +] **Supplied:** Soln for inhal 0.63, 1.25 mg/3 mL **Notes/SE:** Therapeutically active *R*-isomer of albuterol; tachycardia, nervousness, trembling **Interactions:** ↑ effects with MAOIs, TCAs; ↑ risk of hypokalemia with loop & thiazide diuretics; ↓ effects with BBs; ↓ effects of digoxin **Labs:** ↑ serum glucose, ↓ serum K+ **NIPE:** Use other inhalants 5 min >this drug

Levamisole (Ergamisol) Uses: Adjuvant therapy of Dukes' C colon CA (in combination with 5-FU) **Action:** Poorly understood immunostimulatory effects **Dose:** 50 mg PO q8h for 3 d q14d during 5-FU therapy; ↓ in hepatic dysfunction **Caution/Contra:** [C, ?/–] **Supplied:** Tabs 50 mg **Notes/SE:** N/V/D, abdominal pain, taste disturbance, anorexia, hyperbilirubinemia, disulfiram-like reaction on alcohol ingestion, minimal bone marrow depression, fatigue, fever, conjunctivitis **Interactions:** ↑ effects of phenytoin, warfarin **NIPE:** Avoid exposure to infection

Levetiracetam (Keppra) Uses: Partial onset seizures **Action:** Unknown **Dose:** 500 mg PO bid, may ↑ to max 3000 mg/d; ↓ in renal insufficiency **Caution/Contra:** [C, ?/–] **Supplied:** Tabs 250, 500, 750 mg **Notes/SE:** May cause dizziness and somnolence; may impair coordination **Interactions:** ↑ effects with antihistamines, TCAs, benzodiazepines, narcotics, alcohol **NIPE:** May take with food

Levobunolol (A-K Beta, Betagan) Uses: Glaucoma **Action:** β-Adrenergic blocker **Dose:** 1–2 gtt/d 0.5% or 1–2 gtt 0.25% bid **Caution/Contra:** [C, ?] **Supplied:** Soln 0.25, 0.5% **Notes/SE:** Ocular stinging or burning; possible systemic effects if absorbed **Interactions:** ↑ effects with BBs; ↑ risk of hypotension & bradycardia with quinidine, verapamil; ↓ intraocular pressure with carbonic anhydrase inhibitors, epinephrine, pilocarpine **NIPE:** Night vision and acuity may be decreased

Levocabastine (Livostin) Uses: Allergic seasonal conjunctivitis **Action:** Antihistamine **Dose:** 1 gt in eye(s) qid up to 4 wk **Caution/Contra:** [C, +/–] **Supplied:** 0.05% gtt **Notes/SE:** Ocular discomfort **NIPE:** ⊘ insert soft contact lenses

Levofloxacin (Levaquin, Quixin Ophthalmic) Uses: Lower respiratory tract infections, sinusitis, UTI; topical for bacterial conjunctivitis **Action:** Quinolone antibiotic, inhibits DNA gyrase **Dose:** 250–500 mg/d PO or IV; ophth 1–2 gtt in eye(s) q2h while awake for 2 d, then q4h while awake for 5 d; ↓ in renal insufficiency **Caution/Contra:** [C, –] **Supplied:** Tabs 250, 500 mg; premixed bags 250, 500 mg; ophth 0.5% soln **Notes/SE:** Reliable activity against *S. pneumoniae*; interactions with cation-containing products; dizziness, rash, GI upset, photosensitivity **Interactions:** ↑ effects of cyclosporine, digoxin, theophylline, warfarin, caffeine; ↑ risk of seizures with foscarnet, NSAIDs; ↑ risk of hyper- or hypoglycemia with hypoglycemic drugs; ↓ effects with antacids, antineoplastics, calcium, cimetidine, didanosine, famotidine, iron, lansoprazole, magnesium, nizatidine, omeprazole, phenytoin, ranitidine, sodium bicarbonate, sucralfate, zinc **NIPE:** Risk of tendon rupture & tendonitis – d/c if pain or inflammation; ↑ fluids, use sunscreen, antacids 2 h < or > this drug

Levonorgestrel (Plan B) **Uses:** Emergency contraceptive ("morning-after pill"); can prevent PRG if taken <72 h after unprotected sex (contraceptive fails or if no contraception used) **Action:** Progestin **Dose:** 1 pill q12h × 2 **Supplied:** tablets, 0.75 mg, 2 blister pack **Contra/Caution:**[X, M] Contra known suspected PRG, abnormal uterine bleeding **Notes:** Will not induce abortion; may increase risk of ectopic PRG; N/V, abdominal pain, fatigue HA, menstrual changes **Interactions:** ↓ effects with barbiturates, carbamazepine, modafinil, phenobarbital, phenytoin, pioglitazone, rifabutin, rifampin, ritonavir, topiramate

Levonorgestrel Implant (Norplant) **Uses:** Contraceptive **Action:** Progestational agent **Dose:** Implant 6 caps in the midforearm **Caution/Contra:** [X, +/–] Hepatic disease, thromboembolism, breast CA **Supplied:** Kits containing 6 implantable caps, each containing 36 mg **Notes/SE:** Prevents PRG for up to 5 y; may be removed if PRG desired; uterine bleeding, HA, acne, nausea **Interactions:** ↓ effects with barbiturates, carbamazepine, modafinil, phenobarbital, phenytoin, pioglitazone, rifabutin, rifampin, ritonavir, topiramate **Labs:** ↑ uptake of T3, ↓ T4 sex hormone binding globulin levels **NIPE:** Menstrual irregularities first y >implant, use barrier contraception if taking anticonvulsants, may cause vision changes or contact lens tolerability

Levorphanol (Levo-Dromoran) [C-II] **Uses:** Moderate–severe pain **Action:** Narcotic analgesic **Dose:** 2 mg PO or SC PRN q6–8h; ↓ in hepatic failure **Caution/Contra:** [B, ?] **Supplied:** Tabs 2 mg; inj 2 mg/mL **Notes/SE:** Tachycardia, hypotension, drowsiness, GI upset, constipation, respiratory depression **Interactions:** ↑ CNS effects with antihistamines, cimetidine, CNS depressants, glutethimide, methocarbamol, alcohol, St. John's Wort **Labs:** False ↑ amylase, lipase **NIPE:** ↑ fluids & fiber, take with food

Levothyroxine (Synthroid, others) **Uses:** Hypothyroidism **Action:** Supplementation of L-thyroxine **Dose:** *Adults.* Initially, 25–50 μg/d PO or IV; ↑ by 25–50 μg/d every mon; usual dose 100–200 μg/d. *Peds. 0–1 y:* 8–10 μg/kg/24 h PO or IV. *1–5 y:* 4–6 μg/kg/24 h PO or IV. *>5 y:* 3–4 μg/kg/24 h PO or IV; titrate dosage based on clinical response and thyroid function tests; dosage can ↑ more rapidly in young to middle-aged patients. **Caution/Contra:** [A, +] Contra recent MI, uncorrected renal insufficiency **Supplied:** Tabs 25, 50, 75, 88, 100, 112, 125, 150, 175, 200, 300 μg; inj 200, 500 μg **Notes/SE:** Insomnia, weight loss, alopecia, arrhythmia **Interactions:** ↑ effects of anticoagulants, sympathomimetics, TCAs, warfarin; ↓ effects with antacids, BBs, carbamazepine, cholestyramine, estrogens, iron salts, phenytoin, phenobarbital, rifampin, simethicone, sucralfate, ↓ effects of forms; ↓ with liver disease or CHF;

sociated with amprenavir, parecin... BBs; cimetidine; ↑ cardiac depression with... with tubocurarine, parecin... **Labs:** False ↑ serum creatinine; ↑ sides; tubocurarine/choline may impair swallowing **Action:** Topical anesthetic **Uses:** Topical anesthetic; adjunct to phlebotomy effects of succinylcholine **Supplied:** Inj local: 0.5, 1, 1.5, 2, 4, 10, 20%; liq 2.5%; soln 2–4%; viscous 2% 0.4%; Inj admixture 4, 10, 20%. IV inj: 0.2%; 0.4%; Inj 2.5, 5%; in emergency cardiac care; for local or nose anesthesia to ↑ effect and ↓ bleeding; for drug levels **Interactions:** ↑ effects associated with amprenavir, procainamide, tocainide; ↓ neuromuscular blockade with procainamide, tocainide; ↓ dizziness; paresthesias, ↑ CPK for 48 h >IM inj **Action/Contra:** [C, +] Do not use in ears, or nose because vasoconstriction **Caution/Contra:** dilute ET dose 1–2 mL with **Notes/SE:** ↑ NIPE: Oral spray/solution

Lidocaine (ELA-Max) **Uses:** Topical anesthetic: adjunct to phlebotomy or dermal procedures **Action:** Topical anesthetic **Dose:** Apply a 1⁄4-in. thick layer to intact skin at least 30 min before **Caution/Contra:** [C, +] Not for ophth use; methemoglobinemia **Supplied:** Cream 4% **Notes/SE:** Longer contact time gives greater effect; invasive dermal procedures **Caution/Contra:** see **Lidocaine.** NIPE: ☉ apply to broken skin areas

Lidocaine/Prilocaine (EMLA) **Uses:** Topical anesthetic; adjunct to phlebotomy or dermal procedures **Action:** Topical anesthetic **Dose:** *Adults,* EMLA cream and anesthetic disc (1 g/10 cm²); Apply thick layer 2–2.5 g to intact skin and cover with an occlusive dressing (eg. Tegaderm) for at least 1 h. Anesthetic disc: 1 g/10 cm² for at least 1 h. *Peds.* Max dose: 3 mon or <5 kg: 1 g/10 cm² for 1 h, 3–12 mon and >5 kg: 2 g/20 cm² for 4 h, 1–6 y and >10 kg: 10 g/100 cm² for 4 h, 7–12 y and >20 kg: 20 g/200 cm² for 4 h **Caution/Contra:** [B, +] Contra on mucous membranes; broken skin. ophth use; methemoglobinemia **Supplied:** Cream 2.5% lidocaine/2.5% prilocaine; anesthetic disc (1 g) **Notes/SE:** Longer contact time gives greater effect; burning, stinging, methemoglobinemia, see **Lidocaine.** NIPE: Low risk of systemic adverse effects

see Table 3 (page 247) for local anesthesia

... total up ...: Antiarrhyth-/ dose of 5 mg/kg./ mg/kg/dose. Local inj anes-/ tion; [C, +] Do not use/ ... because vasoconstriction /e: drug NIPE: / nds

NS: epi... nical 0 μg IV. **Contra:** [A, +]; ↓
cream 2%... gel 1%... *thetic:* ... IV: 1% (10) epinephrine... 2% 2.5...
lidocaine ... may cause necrosis; heart block Sm... of anticoagulants; ↓
... then IV Inf 2–4 ... *loading dose:* ... Max 4.5 ... epinephrine on the digit... **Notes/SE:** [A, +]; ... phenytoin, rifampin; CHF, prevent DN and AMI
to 200–300 ... *rhythmic* **Dose:** *Addit:* ... qd-bid. *AMI:* 5 mg w/in 24 h of
mic: ET, ... 8 h, then 10 mg/d; ↓ in renal insuffi-
anesthetic: ... *Anti:* ... *Topical:* Apply max 4.5
Lidocaine (Anes... *Additi:* ... *Antiar:* ... page digit... (Table ... 245) Co...
Levothyroxine...

(Kwell) **Uses:** Head lice, crab lice...
ovicide **Dose:** *Adults & Peds.* Ca...
leave on for 8–12 h (6 ...
ply 30 mL ...

Liothyronine (C... Lindane
food-... avoiding tyramine-
containing foods; ... **Lisinopril (Prinivil, Zestril...**
Dose: *Adults.* Initial 25–75 μg/24...
response Initial dose of ... MI **Supplied:** 5–40 m...
tervals; recent arrhythmias, che...
Contra: alopecia, acid sequestrant...
TFT: with hypoglycemics, theoph...
↓ effects of hypo... **Lisinopril** ACE inhibitor **Dose:** 5–40 m...

Action: ... by 5 mg after 24 h. 10 m... **↓ Suppl.ed:** Tabs 2.5, 5, 10, 20, 30, 40 mg
MI followed **Contra:** HA, cough, hypotension, angioedema, hyperkalemia; ↑ effects with
ciency **SE:** Dizziness, ↑ risk of hyperkalemia with K+-sparing diuretics, trimetho-
Notes: start when urinary ↑ risk of cough with capsaicin; ↑ effects of insulin, lithium;
tem DN: diuretics ↑ risk ... indomethacin, NSAIDs **Labs:** ↑ serum K+, creatinine, BUN
α-blockers substitutes, ASA, indomethacin, ... take several wk
prints salt with ASA, maint effect may ...
NifeL: Carbonate ... **Uses:** Manic episodes of
Lithium Carbonate (Eskalith, others) **Uses:** Manic episodes of
effects in recurrent disease **Action:** Effects shift toward in-
bipolar illness, maint therapy in recurrent disease **Action:** Effects shift toward in-

traneuronal metabolism of catecholamines **Dose:** *Adults. Acute mania:* 600 mg PO tid or 900 mg SR bid. *Maint:* 300 mg PO tid–qid. *Peds 6–12 y.* 15–60 mg/kg/d in 3–4 ÷ doses; dosage must be titrated; follow serum levels; ↓ in renal insufficiency, elderly **Caution/Contra:** [D, –] Severe renal impairment or cardiovascular disease **Supplied:** Caps 150, 300, 600 mg; tabs 300 mg; SR tabs 300, 450 mg; syrup 300 mg/5 mL **Notes/SE:** Table 2 (page 245) for drug levels. Polyuria, polydipsia, nephrogenic DI, tremor; Na retention or diuretic use may potentiate toxicity, arrhythmias, dizziness **Interactions:** ↑ effects of TCA; ↑ effects with ACEIs, bumetanide, carbamazepine, ethacrynic acid, fluoxetine, furosemide, methyldopa, NSAIDs, phenytoin, phenothiazines, probenecid, tetracyclines, thiazide diuretics, dandelion, juniper; ↓ effects with acetazolamide, antacids, mannitol, theophyllines, urea, verapamil, caffeine **Labs:** False + urine glucose; ↑ serum glucose, creatinine kinase, TSH, Iodine 131 uptake; ↓ uric acid, T3, T4 **NIPE:** Several weeks before full effects of med, ↑ fluid intake to 2–3 L/d

Lodoxamide (Alomide)   **Uses:** Seasonal allergic conjunctivitis **Action:** Stabilizes mast cells **Dose:** *Adults & Peds >2 y.* 1–2 gtt in eye(s) qid up to 3 mon **Caution/Contra:** [B, ?] **Supplied:** Soln 0.1% **Notes/SE:** Ocular burning, stinging, HA

Lomefloxacin (Maxaquin)   **Uses:** UTI and lower respiratory tract infections caused by gram– bacteria; prophylaxis in transurethral procedures **Action:** Quinolone antibiotic; inhibits DNA gyrase **Dose:** 400 mg/d PO; ↓ in renal insufficiency **Caution/Contra:** [C, –] **Supplied:** Tabs 400 mg **Notes/SE:** Photosensitivity, seizures, HA, dizziness **Interactions:** ↑ effects with cimetidine, probenecid; ↑ effects of cyclosporine, warfarin, caffeine; ↓ effects with antacids **Labs:** ↑ LFTs, ↓ K⁺ **NIPE:** ↑ risk of photosensitivity – use sunscreen, ↑ fluids to 2 L/d

Loperamide (Imodium)   **Uses:** Diarrhea **Action:** Slows intestinal motility **Dose:** *Adults.* Initially 4 mg PO, then 2 mg after each loose stool, up to 16 mg/d. *Peds.* 0.4–0.8 mg/kg/24 h PO q6–12h until diarrhea resolves or for 7 d max **Caution/Contra:** [B, +] Do not use in acute diarrhea caused by *Salmonella*, *Shigella*, or *C. difficile.* **Supplied:** Caps 2 mg; tabs 2 mg; liq 1 mg/5 mL, 1 mg/mL **Notes/SE:** Constipation, sedation, dizziness **Interactions:** ↑ effects with antihistamines, CNS depressants, phenothiazines, TCAs, alcohol

Lopinavir/Ritonavir (Kaletra)   **Uses:** HIV infection **Action:** Protease inhibitor **Dose:** *Adults.* 3 caps or 5 mL PO bid with food. *Peds. 7–15 kg:* 12/3 mg/kg PO bid. *15–40 kg:* 10/2.5 mg/kg PO bid. *>40 kg:* Adult dose **Caution/Contra:** [C, ?/–] Numerous drug interactions **Supplied:** Caps 133.3 mg/33.3 mg (lopinavir/ritonavir), solution 400 mg/100 mg/5 mL **Notes/SE:** Soln contains alcohol, avoid disulfiram and metronidazole; GI upset, asthenia, ↑ cholesterol and triglycerides, pancreatitis; protease metabolic syndrome **Interactions:** ↑ effects with clarithromycin, erythromycin; ↑ effects of amiodarone, amprenavir, azole antifungals, bepredil, cisapride, cyclosporine, CCBs, ergot alkaloids, flecainide, flurazepam, HMG-CoA reductase inhibitors, indinavir, lidocaine, meperidine, midazolam, pimozide, propafenone, propoxyphene, quinidine, rifabutin, saquinavir, sildenafil, tacrolimus, terfenadine, triazolam, zolpidem; ↓ effects with barbiturates, carbamazepine, dexamethasone, didanosine, efavirenz, nevirapine, phenytoin, rifabutin, rifampin, St. John's Wort; ↓ effects of oral contraceptives, warfarin **NIPE:** Take with food, use barrier contraception

Loracarbef (Lorabid) Uses: Upper and lower respiratory tract, skin, bone, urinary tract, abdomen, and gynecologic system bacterial infections **Action:** 2nd-gen. cephalosporin; inhibits cell wall synthesis **Dose:** *Adults.* 200–400 mg PO bid. *Peds.* 7.5–15 mg/kg/d PO ÷ bid; take on empty stomach; ↓ in severe renal insufficiency **Caution/Contra:** [B, +] **Supplied:** Caps 200, 400 mg; susp 125, 250 mg/5 mL **Notes/SE:** More gram– activity than 1st-gen. cephalosporins; causes diarrhea **Interactions:** ↑ effects with probenecid; ↑ effects of warfarin; ↑ nephrotoxicity with aminoglycosides, furosemide **NIPE:** Take w/o food

Loratadine (Claritin) Uses: Allergic rhinitis, chronic idiopathic urticaria **Action:** Nonsedating antihistamine **Dose:** *Adults.* 10 mg PO qd. *Peds. 2–5 y:* 5 mg PO qd. *>6 y:* adult dose; should be taken on an empty stomach; ↓ in hepatic insufficiency **Caution/Contra:** [B, +/–] **Supplied:** Tabs 10 mg; rapid disintegration; Reditabs 10 mg; syrup 1 mg/mL **Notes/SE:** HA, somnolence, xerostomia **Interactions:** ↑ effects with CNS depressants, erythromycin, ketoconazole, MAOIs, protease inhibitors, procarbazine, alcohol **NIPE:** Take w/o food

Lorazepam (Ativan, others) [C-IV] Uses: Anxiety and anxiety with depression; preop sedation; control of status epilepticus; alcohol withdrawal; antiemetic **Action:** Benzodiazepine; antianxiety agent **Dose:** *Adults. Anxiety:* 1–10 mg/d PO in 2–3 ÷ doses. *Preop sedation:* 0.05 mg/kg to 4 mg max IM 2 h before surgery. *Insomnia:* 2–4 mg PO hs. *Status epilepticus:* 4 mg/dose IV PRN q10–15 min; usual total dose 8 mg. *Antiemetic:* 0.5–2 mg IV or PO q4–6h PRN. *Peds. Status epilepticus:* 0.05 mg/kg/dose IV repeated at 1–20-min intervals × 2 PRN. *Antiemetic, 2–15 y:* 0.05 mg/kg (to 2 mg/dose) prechemotherapy; ↓ in elderly; do not administer IV >2 mg/min or 0.05 mg/kg/min **Caution/Contra:** [D, ?/–] Contra in severe pain, severe hypotension, narrow-angle glaucoma **Supplied:** Tabs 0.5, 1, 2 mg; soln, oral conc 2 mg/mL; inj 2, 4 mg/mL **Notes/SE:** May take up to 10 min to see effect when given IV; sedation, ataxia, tachycardia, constipation, respiratory depression **Interactions:** ↑ effects with cimetidine, disulfiram, probenecid, calendula, catnip, hops, lady's slipper, passionflower, kava kava, valerian; ↑ effects of phenytoin; ↑ CNS depression with anticonvulsants, antihistamines, CNS depressants, MAOIs, scopolamine, alcohol; ↓ effects with caffeine, tobacco; ↓ effects of levodopa **Labs:** ↑ LFTs **NIPE:** ⊘ d/c abruptly

Losartan (Cozaar) Uses: HTN, CHF, DN **Action:** Angiotensin II antagonist **Dose:** 25–50 mg PO qd–bid; ↓ dose in elderly or hepatic impairment **Caution/Contra:** [C (1st trimester, D 2nd and 3rd trimesters), ?/–] **Supplied:** Tabs 25, 50, 100 mg **Notes/SE:** Symptomatic hypotension may occur in patients on diuretics; GI upset, angioedema **Interactions:** ↑ risk of hyperkalemia with K⁺-sparing diuretics, K$^+$ supplements, trimethoprim; ↑ effects of lithium; ↓ effects with diltiazem, fluconazole, phenobarbital, rifampin **NIPE:** ⊘ PRG, breast-feeding

Lovastatin (Mevacor, Altocor)
Uses: Hypercholesterolemia; slows progression of atherosclerosis **Action:** HMG-CoA reductase inhibitor **Dose:** 20 mg/d PO with PM meal; may ↑ at 4-wk intervals to a max of 80 mg/d taken with meals; avoid grapefruit juice **Caution/Contra:** [X, −] Avoid concurrent use with gemfibrozil if possible; active liver disease **Supplied:** Tabs 10, 20, 40 mg **Notes/SE:** Patient must maintain standard cholesterol-lowering diet throughout treatment; monitor LFT q12wk × 1 y, then q6mo; HA and GI intolerance common; patient should promptly report any unexplained muscle pain, tenderness, or weakness (myopathy) **Interactions:** ↑ effects with grapefruit juice; ↑ risk of severe myopathy with azole antifungals, cyclosporine, erythromycin, gemfibrozil, HMG-CoA inhibitors, niacin; ↑ effects of warfarin; ↓ effects with isradipine, pectin **Labs:** ↑ LFTs **NIPE:** ⊘ PRG, take drug in evening, periodic eye exams

Lymphocyte Immune Globulin [Antithymocyte Globulin, ATG] (Atgam)
Uses: Allograft rejection in transplant patients; aplastic anemia if not candidates for BMT **Action:** ↓ Number of circulating, thymus-dependent lymphocytes **Dose:** *Adults.* *Prevent rejection:* 15 mg/kg/day IV ×14 d, then qod ×7; initial w/n 24 h before/after transplant. *Treat rejection:* Same except use 10–15 mg/kg/day **Caution/Contra:** [C, ?] Acute viral illness, Hx reaction to other equine γ-globulin preparation **Supplied:** Inj 50 mg/mL **Notes/SE:** Test dose 0.1 mL of a 1:1000 dilution in NS; DC with severe thrombocytopenia or leukopenia; rash, fever, chills, HA, ↑ K$^+$ **Interactions:** ↑ immunosuppression with azathioprine, corticosteroids, immunosuppressants **Labs:** ↑ LFTs **NIPE:** Risk of febrile reaction

Magaldrate (Riopan, Lowsium)
Uses: Hyperacidity associated with peptic ulcer, gastritis, and hiatal hernia **Action:** Low-Na antacid **Dose:** 5–10 mL PO between meals and hs **Caution/Contra:** [B, ?] Do not use in renal insufficiency due to Mg content. **Supplied:** Susp **Notes/SE:** <0.3 mg Na/tab or tsp; GI upset **Interactions:** ↑ effects of levodopa, quinidine; ↓ effects of allopurinol, anticoagulants, cefpodoxime, ciprofloxacin, clindamycin, digoxin, indomethacin, isoniazid, ketoconazole, lincomycin, phenothiazines, quinolones, tetracyclines **NIPE:** ⊘ other meds w/n 1–2 h

Magnesium Citrate (generic OTC)
Uses: Vigorous bowel preparation; constipation **Action:** Cathartic laxative **Dose:** *Adults.* 120–240 mL PO PRN. *Peds.* 0.5 mL/kg/dose, to a max of 200 mL PO; take with a beverage **Caution/Contra:** [B, +] Renal insufficiency or intestinal obstruction **Supplied:** Effervescent soln **Notes/SE:** Abdominal cramps, gas **Interactions:** ↓ effects of anticoagulants, digoxin, fluoroquinolones, ketoconazole, nitrofurantoin, phenothiazines, tetracyclines **Labs:** ↑ magnesium, ↓ protein, calcium, K$^+$ **NIPE:** ⊘ Other meds w/n 1–2 hr

Magnesium Hydroxide (Milk of Magnesia)
Uses: Constipation **Action:** NS laxative **Dose:** *Adults.* 15–30 mL PO PRN. *Peds.* 0.5 mL/kg/dose PO

PRN **Caution/Contra:** [B, +] Renal insufficiency or intestinal obstruction **Supplied:** Tabs 311 mg, liq 400, 800 mg/5 mL **Notes/SE:** Diarrhea, abdominal cramps **Interactions:** ↓ effects of chlordiazepoxide, dicumarol, digoxin, indomethacin, isoniazid, quinolones, tetracyclines **Labs:** ↑ magnesium, ↓ protein, calcium, K⁺ **NIPE:** ⊘ other meds w/n 1–2 h

Magnesium Oxide (Mag-Ox 400, others) **Uses:** Replacement for low plasma levels **Action:** Mg supplementation **Dose:** 400–800 mg/d ÷ qd–qid with full glass of water **Caution/Contra:** [B, +] Renal insufficiency **Supplied:** Caps 140 mg; tabs 400 mg **Notes/SE:** Diarrhea, nausea **Interactions:** ↓ effects of chlordiazepoxide, dicumarol, digoxin, indomethacin, isoniazid, quinolones, tetracyclines **Labs:** ↑ magnesium, ↓ protein, calcium, K⁺ **NIPE:** ⊘ Other meds w/n 1–2 h

Magnesium Sulfate (generic) **Uses:** Replacement for low Mg levels; refractory hypokalemia and hypocalcemia; preeclampsia and premature labor **Action:** Mg supplement **Dose:** *Adults. Supplement:* 1–2 g IM or IV; repeat PRN. *Preeclampsia/premature labor:* 4 g load then 1–4 g/h IV inf. *Peds.* 25–50 mg/kg/dose IM or IV q4–6h for 3–4 doses; repeat if ↓ Mg persists; ↓ dose with low urine output or renal insufficiency **Caution/Contra:** [B, +] Heart block, renal failure **Supplied:** Inj 100, 125, 250, 500 mg/mL; oral soln 500 mg/mL; granules 40 mEq/5 g **Notes/SE:** CNS depression, diarrhea, flushing, heart block **Interactions:** ↑ CNS depression with antidepressants, antipsychotics, anxiolytics, barbiturates, hypnotics, narcotics; alcohol; ↑ neuromuscular blockade with aminoglycosides, atracurium, gallamine, pancuronium, tubocurarine, vecuronium **Labs:** ↑ magnesium; ↓ protein, calcium, K⁺ **NIPE:** Check for absent patellar reflexes

Mannitol (coheric) **Uses:** Cerebral edema, oliguria, anuria, myoglobinuria **Action:** Osmotic diuretic **Dose:** *Adults. Diuresis:* 0.2 g/kg/dose IV over 3–5 min; if no diuresis w/n 2 h, DC. *Peds. Diuresis:* 0.75 g/kg/dose IV over 3–5 min; if no diuresis w/n 2 h, DC. *Adults & Peds. Cerebral edema:* 0.25 g/kg/dose IV push, repeated at 5-min intervals PRN; ↑ incrementally to 1 g/kg/dose PRN for ↑ ICP; caution with CHF or volume overload **Caution/Contra:** [C, ?] Anuria, dehydration, PE **Supplied:** Inj 5, 10, 15, 20, 25% **Notes/SE:** Initial volume increase may exacerbate CHF; monitor for volume depletion **Interactions:** ↑ effects of cardiac glycosides; ↓ effects of barbiturates, imipramine, lithium, salicylates **Labs:** ↑ / ↓ serum phosphate

Maprotiline (Ludiomil) **Uses:** Depressive neurosis, bipolar illness, major depressive disorder, anxiety with depression **Action:** Tetracyclic antidepressant **Dose:** 75–150 mg/d hs to a max of 300 mg/d; patients >60 y, give only 50–75 mg/d **Caution/Contra:** [B, +/−] Contra with MAOIs or seizure Hx **Supplied:** Tabs 25, 50, 75 mg **Notes/SE:** Anticholinergic side effects, arrhythmias **Interactions:** ↑ effects with cimetidine, fluoxetine, fluvoxamine, methylphenidate, neuroleptics, propoxphene, quinidine, alcohol, grapefruit juice; ↑ effects of anticoagulants, MAOIs, tolazemide; ↑ HTN with levodopa, sympathomimetics; ↑ risk of seizures with benzodiazepines, phenothiazines, alcohol; ↑ cardiac effects with thyroid meds; ↓ effects with carbamazepine; ↓ effects of antihypertensives **NIPE:** Full effects may take 2–3 wk, risk of photosensitivity

Mechlorethamine (Mustargen) **WARNING:** Highly toxic agent, handle with care **Uses:** Hodgkin's and NHL, cutaneous T-cell lymphoma (mycosis fungoides), lung CA, CLL, CML, and malignant pleural effusions **Action:** Alkylating agent (bifunctional) **Dose:** 0.4 mg/kg single dose or 0.1 mg/kg/d for 4 d; 6 mg/m² 1–2 ×/mon; highly volatile; must be administered w/in 30–60 min of preparation **Caution/Contra:** [D, ?] **Supplied:** Inj 10 mg **Notes/SE:** *Toxicity symptoms:* Myelosuppression, thrombosis, or thrombophlebitis at inj site; tissue damage with extravasation (Na thiosulfate may be used topically to treat); N/V, skin rash, amenorrhea, and sterility. High rates of sterility (especially in men) and secondary leukemia in patients treated for Hodgkin's disease **Interactions:** ↑ risk of blood dyscrasias with amphotericin B; ↑ risk of bleeding with anticoagulants, NSAIDs, platelet inhibitors, salicylates; ↑ myelosuppression with antineoplastic drugs, radiation therapy; ↓ effects of live virus vaccines **Labs:** ↑ serum uric acid **NIPE:** ↑ fluids to 2–3 L/d; ⊘ PRG, breast-feeding, vaccines, exposure to infection; ↑ risk of tinnitus

Meclizine (Antivert) **Uses:** Motion sickness; vertigo associated with diseases of the vestibular system **Action:** Antiemetic, anticholinergic, and antihistaminic properties **Dose:** *Adults & Peds >12 y.* 25 mg PO tid–qid PRN **Caution/Contra:** [B, ?] **Supplied:** Tabs 12.5, 25, 50 mg; chew tabs 25 mg; caps 25, 30 mg **Notes/SE:** Drowsiness, xerostomia, and blurred vision common **Interactions:** ↑ sedation with antihistamines, CNS depressants, neuroleptics, alcohol; ↑ anticholinergic effects with anticholinergics, atropine, disopyramide, haloperidol, phenothiazines, quinidine **NIPE:** Use prophylactically

Medroxyprogesterone (Provera, Depo-Provera) **Uses:** Contraception; secondary amenorrhea, and AUB caused by hormonal imbalance; endometrial CA **Action:** Progestin supplement **Dose:** *Contraception:* 150 mg IM q3mon or 450 mg IM q6mon. *Secondary amenorrhea:* 5–10 mg/d PO for 5–10 d. *AUB:* 5–10 mg/d PO for 5–10 d beginning on the 16th or 21st d of menstrual cycle. *Endometrial CA:* 400–1000 mg/wk IM; ↓ in hepatic insufficiency **Caution/Contra:** [X, +] Contra with Hx past thromboembolic disorders or with hepatic disease **Supplied:** Tabs 2.5, 5, 10 mg; depot inj 100, 150, 400 mg/mL **Notes/SE:** Perform breast exam and Pap smear before therapy; breakthrough bleeding, spotting, altered menstrual flow, anorexia, edema, thromboembolic complications, depression, weight gain **Interactions:** ↓ effects with aminoglutethimide, phenytoin, carbamazepine, phenobarbital, rifampin, rifabutin **NIPE:** Sunlight exposure may cause melasma, if GI upset take with food

Megestrol Acetate (Megace) **Uses:** Breast and endometrial CAs; appetite stimulant in CA and HIV-related cachexia **Action:** Hormone; progesterone analogue **Dose:** *CA:* 40–320 mg/d PO in ÷ doses. *Appetite:* 800 mg/d PO **Cau-**

tion/Contra: [X, –] Thromboembolism **Supplied:** Tabs 20, 40 mg; soln 40 mg/mL **Notes/SE:** May induce DVT; do not DC therapy abruptly; edema, menstrual bleeding; photosensitivity, insomnia, rash, myelosuppression **Interactions:** ↑ effects of warfarin **Labs:** ↑ LDH **NIPE:** ↑ risk of photosensitivity - use sunscreen

Meloxicam (Mobic) **Uses:** Osteoarthritis **Action:** NSAID with ↑ COX-2 activity **Dose:** 7.5–15 mg/d PO; ↓ in renal insufficiency; take with food **Caution/Contra:** [C, ?/–] Peptic ulcer, NSAID, or ASA sensitivity **Supplied:** Tabs 7.5 mg **Notes/SE:** HA, dizziness, GI upset, GI bleeding, edema **Interactions:** ↑ effects of ASA, anticoagulants, corticosteroids, lithium, alcohol, tobacco; ↓ effects with cholestyramine; ↓ effects of antihypertensives **Labs:** False + guaiac test, ↑ LFTs **NIPE:** Take with food, may take several d for full effect

Melphalan [L-PAM] (Alkeran) **WARNING:** Severe bone marrow depression; leukemogenic and mutagenic **Uses:** Multiple myeloma, breast, testicular, and ovarian CAs, melanoma; allogenic and ABMT in high doses **Action:** Alkylating agent (bifunctional) **Dose:** (Per protocol) 9 mg/m² or 0.25 mg/kg/d for 4–7 d, repeated at 4–6-wk intervals, or 1-mg/kg single dose once q4–6wk; 0.15 mg/kg/d for 5 d q6wk. *High dose for high-risk multiple myeloma:* Single dose 140 mg/m². *ABMT:* 140–240 mg/m² IV; ↓ in renal insufficiency; take on empty stomach **Caution/Contra:** [D, ?] **Supplied:** Tabs 2 mg; inj 50 mg **Notes/SE:** Myelosuppression (leukopenia and thrombocytopenia), secondary leukemia, alopecia, dermatitis, stomatitis, and pulmonary fibrosis; very rare hypersensitivity reactions **Interactions:** ↑ risk of nephrotoxicity with cisplatin, cyclosporine; ↓ effects with cimetidine, interferon alfa **Labs:** ↑ uric acid, urine 5-HIAA **NIPE:** ↑ fluids, ⊘ PRG, breast-feeding

Meningococcal Polysaccharide Vaccine (Menomune) **Uses:** Immunizes against *N. meningitidis* (meningococcus); recommended in certain complement deficiencies, asplenia, lab workers with exposure; recommended for college students by some professional groups **Action:** Live bacterial vaccine, active immunization **Dose:** *Adults & Peds >2 y.* 0.5 mL SC; do not inject intradermally or IV; epinephrine (1:1000) must be available for anaphylactic/allergic reactions **Caution/Contra:** [C, ?/–] Contra in thimerosal sensitivity **Supplied:** Inj **Notes/SE:** Active against meningococcal serotypes groups A, C, Y, and W-135 but not group B; local inj site reactions, HA **Interactions:** ↓ effects with immunoglobulin if admin. w/n 1 mon **NIPE:** Pain & inflam at inj site

Meperidine (Demerol) [C-II] **Uses:** Moderate to severe pain **Action:** Narcotic analgesic **Dose:** *Adults.* 50–150 mg PO or IM q3–4h PRN. *Peds.* 1–1.5 mg/kg/dose PO or IM q3–4h PRN, up to 100 mg/dose; ↓ dose in elderly and renal impairment **Caution/Contra:** [B, +] Do not use in renal failure; MAOIs **Supplied:** Tabs 50, 100 mg; syrup 50 mg/mL; inj 10, 25, 50, 75, 100 mg/mL **Notes/SE:** 75 mg IM = 10 mg of morphine IM; respiratory depression, seizures, sedation, constipation, analgesic effects potentiated with use of Vistaril **Interactions:** ↑ effects with antihistamines, barbiturates, cimetidine, MAOIs, neuroleptics, selegiline,

TCAs, St. John's Wort, alcohol; ↑ effects of isoniazid; ↓ effects with phenytoin **Labs:** ↑ serum amylase, lipase

Meprobamate (Equanil, Miltown) [C-IV]
Uses: Short-term relief of anxiety **Action:** Mild tranquilizer; antianxiety **Dose:** *Adults.* 400 mg PO tid–qid up to 2400 mg/d; SR 400–800 mg PO bid. *Peds. 6–12 y.* 100–200 mg bid–tid; SR 200 mg bid; ↓ in renal insufficiency **Caution/Contra:** [D, +/–] Narrow-angle glaucoma, porphyria **Supplied:** Tabs 200, 400, 600 mg; SR caps 200, 400 mg **Notes/SE:** May cause drowsiness, syncope, tachycardia, edema **Interactions:** ↑ effects with antihistamines, barbiturates, CNS depressants, narcotics, alcohol

Mercaptopurine [6-MP] (Purinethol)
Uses: Acute leukemias, 2nd-line Rx of CML and NHL, maint therapy of ALL in children, and immunosuppressant therapy for autoimmune diseases (Crohn's disease) **Action:** Antimetabolite; mimics hypoxanthine **Dose:** 80–100 mg/m^2/d or 2.5–5 mg/kg/d; maint 1.5–2.5 mg/kg/d; concurrent allopurinol therapy requires a 67–75% dose reduction of 6-MP because of interference with metabolism by xanthine oxidase; ↓ in renal, hepatic insufficiency; empty stomach; adequate hydration **Caution/Contra:** [D, ?] Severe hepatic disease **Supplied:** Tabs 50 mg **Notes/SE:** Mild hematologic toxicity; uncommon GI toxicity, except mucositis, stomatitis, and diarrhea; rash, fever, eosinophilia, jaundice, and hepatitis **Interactions:** ↑ effects with allopurinol; ↑ risk of bone marrow suppression with trimethoprim-sulfamethoxazole; ↓ effects of warfarin **Labs:** False ↑ serum glucose, uric acid **NIPE:** ↑ fluid intake to 2–3 L/d, may take 4+ wk for improvement

Meropenem (Merrem)
Uses: Serious infections caused by a wide variety of bacteria; bacterial meningitis **Action:** Carbapenem; inhibits cell wall synthesis, a β-lactam **Dose:** *Adults.* 1 g IV q8h. *Peds.* 20–40 mg/kg IV q8h; ↓ in renal insufficiency; beware of possible anaphylaxis **Caution/Contra:** [B, ?] β-Lactam sensitivity **Supplied:** Inj **Notes/SE:** Less seizure potential than imipenem; diarrhea, thrombocytopenia **Interactions:** ↑ effects with probenecid **Labs:** ↑ LFTs, BUN, creatinine, eosinophils ↓ HMG, HCT, WBCs **NIPE:** Monitor for superinfection

Mesalamine (Rowasa, Asacol, Pentasa)
Uses: Mild–moderate distal ulcerative colitis, proctosigmoiditis, or proctitis **Action:** Unknown; may topically inhibit prostaglandins **Dose:** Retention enema qd hs or insert 1 supp bid. *Oral:* 800–1000 mg PO 3–4×/d **Caution/Contra:** [B, M] Sulfite or salicylate sensitivity **Supplied:** Tabs 400 mg; caps 250 mg; supp 500 mg; rectal susp 4 g/60 mL **Notes/SE:** HA, malaise, abdominal pain, flatulence, rash, pancreatitis, pericarditis **Interactions:** ↓ effect of digoxin **Labs:** ↑ LFTs, amylase, lipase

Mesna (Mesnex)
Uses: ↑ Incidence of ifosfamide- and cyclophosphamide-induced hemorrhagic cystitis **Antidote:** None **Dose:** 20% of the ifosfamide dose (+/–) or cyclophosphamide dose IV 15 min prior to and 4 and 8 h after chemotherapy **Caution/Contra:** [B, ?/–] Thiol sensitivity **Supplied:** Inj 100 mg/mL **Notes/SE:** Hypotension, allergic reactions, HA, GI upset, taste perversion **Interactions:** ↓ effects of warfarin **Labs:** False + urine ketones

152

Mesoridazine

Mesoridazine (Serentil) **WARNING:** Can prolong QT interval in a dose-related fashion; torsades de points reported **Uses:** Schizophrenia, acute and chronic alcoholism, chronic brain syndrome **Action:** Phenothiazine antipsychotic **Dose:** Initially, 25–50 mg PO or IV tid; ↑ to 300–400 mg/d max **Caution/Contra:** [C, ?/–] Phenothiazine sensitivity **Supplied:** Tabs 10, 25, 50, 100 mg; oral conc 25 mg/mL; inj 25 mg/mL **Notes/SE:** Low incidence of extrapyramidal side effects; hypotension, xerostomia, constipation, skin discoloration, tachycardia, lowered seizure threshold, blood dyscrasias, pigmentary retinopathy at high doses **Interactions:** ↑ effects with antimalarials, BBs, chloroquine, TCAs, alcohol; ↑ effects of antidepressants, nitrates, antihypertensives; ↑ QT interval with amiodarone, azole antifungals, disopyramide, fluoxetine, macrolides, paroxetine, procainamide, quinidine, quinolones, TCAs, verapamil; ↓ effects with attapulgite, barbiturates, caffeine, tobacco; ↓ effects of barbiturates, guanethidine, guanadrel, levodopa, lithium, sympathomimetics **Labs:** False + PRG test; ↑ serum glucose, cholesterol; ↓ uric acid **NIPE:** Photosensitivity – use sunscreen

Metaproterenol (Alupent, Metaprel) **Uses:** Asthma and reversible bronchospasm **Action:** Sympathomimetic bronchodilator **Dose:** *Adults.* Inhal: 1–3 inhal q3–4h, 12 inhal max/24 h; allow at least 2 min between inhal. *Oral:* 20 mg q6–8h. **Peds.** Inhal: 0.5 mg/kg/dose, 15 mg/dose max inhaled q4–6h by neb or 1–2 puffs q4–6h. *Oral:* 0.3–0.5 mg/kg/dose q6–8h **Caution/Contra:** [C, ?/–] Tachycardia or other arrhythmia **Supplied:** Aerosol 75, 150 mg; soln for inhal 0.4, 0.6, 5%; tabs 10, 20 mg; syrup 10 mg/5 mL **Notes/SE:** Fewer β₁ effects than isoproterenol and longer acting; nervousness, tremor, tachycardia, HTN **Interactions:** ↑ effects with sympathomimetic drugs, xanthines; ↑ risk of arrhythmias with cardiac glycosides, halothane, levodopa, theophylline, thyroid hormones; ↑ HTN with MAOIs; ↓ effects with BBs **Labs:** ↑ serum K⁺ **NIPE:** Separate additional aerosol use by 5 min

Metaraminol (Aramine) **Uses:** Prevention and Rx of hypotension due to spinal anesthesia **Action:** α-Adrenergic agent **Dose:** *Adults.* Prevention: 2–10 mg IM q10–15min PRN. *Rx:* 0.5–5 mg IV bolus followed by IV inf of 1–4 mg/kg/min titrated to effect. *Peds.* Prevention: 0.1 mg/kg/dose IM PRN. *Rx:* 0.01-mg/kg IV bolus followed by IV inf of 5 mg/kg/min titrated to effect **Caution/Contra:** [D, ?] **Supplied:** Injectable forms **Notes/SE:** Allow 10 min for max effect; use other shock management techniques, eg, fluid resuscitation, as needed; may cause cardiac arrhythmias, skin blanching, flushing **Interactions:** ↑ effects with cyclopropane, halothane, MAOIs, digoxin, oxytocin, reserpine; ↑ cardiac effects with cardiac glycosides, levodopa, sympathomimetics, thyroid hormones; ↑ pressor effects with doxapram, ergot alkaloids, MAOIs, trimethaphan; ↓ effects with TCAs; ↓ effects of antihypertensives, guanadrel, guamethidine

Metaxalone (Skelaxin) **Uses:** Relief of painful musculoskeletal conditions **Action:** Centrally acting skeletal muscle relaxant **Dose:** 800 mg PO 3–4×/d **Caution/Contra:** [X, ?/–] Do not use in hepatic/renal impairment; caution in anemia **Supplied:** Tabs 400 mg **Notes/SE:** N/V, HA, drowsiness, hepatitis **Interactions:** ↑ sedating effects with CNS depressants, alcohol **Labs:** False + urine glucose using Benedict's test

Metformin (Glucophage, Glucophage XR) WARNING: Associated with lactic acidosis
Uses: Type 2 DM **Action:** Decreases hepatic glucose production; ↓ intestinal absorption of glucose; improves insulin sensitivity **Dose:** Initial dose 500 mg PO bid; may ↑ 2500 mg/d max; administer with AM and PM meals; can convert total daily dose to qd dose of XR formulation **Caution/Contra:** [B, +/−] Do not use if SCr >1.4 in females or >1.5 in males; contra in hypoxemic conditions, including acute CHF/sepsis; avoid alcohol; hold dose before and 48 h after ionic contrast **Supplied:** Tabs 500, 850, 1000 mg; XR tabs 500 mg **Notes/SE:** Anorexia, N/V, rash **Interactions:** ↑ effects with amiloride, cimetidine, digoxin, furosemide, MAOIs, morphine, procainamide, quinidine, quinine, ranitidine, triamterene, trimethoprim, vancomycin; ↓ effects with corticosteroids, CCBs, diuretics, estrogens, isoniazid, oral contraceptives, phenothiazines, phenytoin, sympathomimetics, thyroid drugs, tobacco **NIPE:** Take with food; avoid dehydration, alcohol

Methadone (Dolophine) [C-II]
Uses: Severe pain; detoxification and maint of narcotic addiction **Action:** Narcotic analgesic **Dose:** *Adults.* 2.5–10 mg IM q3–8h or 5–15 mg PO q8h; titrate as needed. *Peds.* 0.7 mg/kg/24 h PO or IM ÷ q8h; ↑ slowly to avoid respiratory depression; ↓ in renal disease **Caution/Contra:** [B, + (with doses = 20 mg/24 h)] Severe liver disease **Supplied:** Tabs 5, 10, 40 mg; oral soln 5, 10 mg/5 mL; oral conc 10 mg/mL; inj 10 mg/mL **Notes/SE:** Equianalgesic with parenteral morphine; longer half-life; respiratory depression, sedation, constipation, urinary retention **Interactions:** ↑ effects with cimetidine, CNS depressants, alcohol; ↑ effects of anticoagulants, alcohol, antihistamines, barbiturates, glutethimide, methocarbamol; ↓ effects with carbamazepine, nelfinavir, phenobarbital, phenytoin, primidone, rifampin, ritonavir **Labs:** ↑ serum amylase, lipase

Methenamine (Hiprex, Urex, others)
Uses: Suppression or elimination of bacteriuria associated with chronic/recurrent UTI **Dose:** *Adults.* Hippurate: 1 g bid. Mandelate: 1 g qid pc and hs. *Peds. 6–12 y.* Hippurate: 25–50 mg/kg/d ÷ bid. Mandelate: 50–75 mg/kg/d ÷ qid; take with food and ascorbic acid; adequate hydration **Caution/Contra:** [C, +] Contra in patients with renal insufficiency, severe hepatic disease, and severe dehydration; allergy to sulfonamides **Supplied:** *Methenamine hippurate (Hiprex, Urex):* 1-g tabs. *Methenamine mandelate:* 500 mg/1 g EC tabs **Notes/SE:** Rash, GI upset, dysuria, ↑ LFTs **Interactions:** ↓ effects with acetazolamide, antacids; ↑ serum catecholamines, urine glucose, urobilinogen; ↓ urine estriol, estrogens **NIPE:** ↑ fluids to 2–3 L/d; take with food

Methimazole (Tapazole)
Uses: Hyperthyroidism and prep for thyroid surgery or radiation **Action:** Blocks the formation of T_3 and T_4 **Dose:** *Adults.* Ini-

tial: 15–60 mg/d PO ÷ tid. *Maint:* 5–15 mg PO qd. **Peds.** *Initial:* 0.4–0.7 mg/kg/24 h PO ÷ tid. *Maint:* 1/3–2/3 of the initial dose PO qd; take with food **Caution/Contra:** [NA, D] Avoid in nursing mothers **Supplied:** Tabs 5, 10 mg **Notes/SE:** Follow clinically and with TFT; GI upset, dizziness, blood dyscrasias **Interactions:** ↑ effects of digitalis glycosides, metroprolol, propranolol; ↑ effects of anticoagulants, theophylline; ↓ effects with amiodarone **Labs:** ↑ LFTs, PT **NIPE:** Take with food

Methocarbamol (Robaxin) Uses: Relief of discomfort associated with painful musculoskeletal conditions **Action:** Centrally acting skeletal muscle relaxant **Dose:** *Adults.* 1.5 g PO qid for 2–3 d, then 1-g PO qid maint therapy; IV form rarely indicated. **Peds.** 15 mg/kg/dose may repeat PRN (recommended for tetanus only) **Caution/Contra:** [C, +] Contra with myasthenia gravis, renal impairment; caution in seizure disorders **Supplied:** Tabs 500, 750 mg; inj 100 mg/mL **Notes/SE:** Can discolor urine; drowsiness, GI upset **Interactions:** ↑ effects with CNS depressant, alcohol **Labs:** ↑ urine 5-HIAA, urine vanillylmandelic acid **NIPE:** Monitor for blurred vision, nausea

Methotrexate (Folex, Rheumatrex) Uses: ALL and AML (including leukemic meningitis), trophoblastic tumors (choriepithelioma, choriocarcinoma, chorioadenoma destruens, hydatidiform mole), breast CA, Burkitt's lymphoma, mycosis fungoides, osteosarcoma, head and neck CA, Hodgkin's and NHL, lung CA; psoriasis; RA **Action:** Inhibits dihydrofolate reductase-mediated gen. of tetrahydrofolate **Dose:** *CA,* "conventional dose": 15–30 mg PO or IV 1–2×/wk q1–3 wk. "Intermediate dose": 50–240 mg or 0.5–1 g/m² IV once q4d to 3 wk. "High dose": 1–12 g/m² IV once q1–3wk; 12 mg/m² (max 15 mg) IT, weekly until the CSF cell count returns to normal. *RA:* 7.5 mg/wk PO as a single dose or 2.5 mg q12h PO for 3 doses/wk; "high dose" Rx requires leucovorin rescue to limit hematologic and mucosal toxicity; ↓ in renal/hepatic impairment **Caution/Contra:** [D, –] Severe renal/hepatic impairment **Supplied:** Tabs 2.5 mg; inj 2.5, 25 mg/mL; preservative-free inj 25 mg/mL **Notes/SE:** Myelosuppression, N/V/D, anorexia, mucositis, hepatotoxicity (transient and reversible; may progress to atrophy, necrosis, fibrosis, cirrhosis), rashes, dizziness, malaise, blurred vision, renal failure, pneumonitis, and, rarely, pulmonary fibrosis. Chemical arachnoiditis and HA with IT delivery; monitor blood counts and MTX levels **Interactions:** ↑ effects with chloramphenicol, cyclosporine, etretinate, NSAIDs, phenylbutazone, phenytoin, penicillin, probenecid, salicylates, sulfonamides, sulfonylureas, alcohol; ↑ effects of cyclosporine, tetracycline, theophylline; ↓ effects with antimalarials, aminoglycosides, binding resins, cholestyramine, folic acid; ↓ effects of digoxin **Labs:** ↑ AST, alkaline phosphatase, bilirubin, cholesterol **NIPE:** ↑ risk of photosensitivity - use sunscreen, ↑ fluids 2–3 L/d

Methoxamine (Vasoxyl) Uses: Support, restoration, or maint of BP during anesthesia; for termination of some episodes of PSVT **Action:** α-Adrenergic **Dose:** *Adults.* *Anesthesia:* 10–15 mg IM; if emergency, 3–5 mg slow IV push. *PSVT:* 10 mg by slow IV push. **Peds.** 0.25 mg/kg/dose IM or 0.08 mg/kg/dose slow

IV push **Caution/Contra:** [C, ?] **Supplied:** Injectable forms **Notes/SE:** IM dose requires 15 min to act; use 5–10 mg phentolamine locally in case of extravasation; MAOIs and TCAs potentiate methoxamine effect **Interactions:** ↑ effects with atropine, BBs, TCAs; ↑ risk of HTN crisis with ergot alkaloids, furazolidone, indomethacin, MAOIs, oxytocics, vasopressin **NIPE:** ⊘ admin for 2 wk >MAOI use

Methyldopa (Aldomet)
Uses: Essential HTN **Action:** Centrally acting antihypertensive **Dose:** *Adults.* 250–500 mg PO bid-tid (max 2–3 g/d) or 250 mg–1 g IV q6–8h. *Peds.* 10 mg/kg/24 h PO in 2–3 ÷ doses (max 40 mg/kg/24 h + q6–12h) or 5–10 mg/kg/dose IV q6–8h to total dose of 20–40 mg/kg/24 h; ↓ dose in renal insufficiency and in elderly **Caution/Contra:** [B (oral), C (IV), +] Contra in liver disease; MAOIs **Supplied:** Tabs 125, 250, 500 mg; oral susp 50 mg/mL; inj 50 mg/mL **Notes/SE:** Can discolor urine; initial transient sedation or drowsiness frequent; edema, hemolytic anemia; hepatic disorders **Interactions:** ↑ effects with anesthetics, diuretics, levodopa, lithium, methotrimeprazine, thioxanthenes, vasodilators, verapamil; ↑ effects of haloperidol, lithium, tolbutamide; ↓ effects with amphetamines, iron, phenothiazines, TCAs; ↓ effects of ephedrine **Labs:** Interference with serum creatinine, glucose, AST, catecholamines; urine catecholamines, uric acid; false ↓ serum cholesterol, triglycerides **NIPE:** >1–2 mon tolerance may develop

Methylergonovine (Methergine)
Uses: Prevention and Rx postpartum hemorrhage caused by uterine atony **Action:** Ergotamine derivative **Dose:** 0.2 mg IM after delivery of placenta, may repeat at 2–4-h intervals, or 0.2–0.4 mg PO q6–12h for 2–7 d **Caution/Contra:** [C, ?] **Supplied:** Injectable forms; tabs 0.2 mg **Notes/SE:** IV doses should be given over a period of >1 min with frequent BP monitoring; HTN, N/V **Interactions:** ↑ vasoconstriction with ergot alkaloids, sympathomimetics, tobacco **NIPE:** ⊘ smoking

Methylprednisolone (Solu-Medrol)
See **Steroids,** page 209, Table 4, page 248 **Interactions:** ↑ effects with cyclosporine, clarithromycin, erythromycin, estrogens, ketoconazole, oral contraceptives, troleandomycin, grapefruit juice; ↑ effects of cyclosporine; ↓ effects with aminoglutethimide, barbiturates, carbamazepine, cholestyramine, colestipol, isoniazid, phenytoin, phenobarbital, rifampin; ↓ effects of anticoagulants, hypoglycemics, isoniazid, salicylates, vaccines **Labs:** ↓ skin test reactions; false ↑ serum cortisol, digoxin, theophylline, & urine glucose **NIPE:** ⊘ d/c abruptly, ⊘ infections or vaccines

Metoclopramide (Reglan, Clopra, Octamide)
Uses: Relief of diabetic gastroparesis, symptomatic GERD; chemotherapy-induced N/V; stimulate gut in prolonged postop ileus **Action:** Stimulates motility of the upper GI tract; blocks dopamine in the chemoreceptor trigger zone **Dose:** *Adults. Diabetic gastroparesis:* 10 mg PO 30 min ac and hs for 2–8 wk PRN, or same dose given IV for 10 d, then switch to PO. *Reflux:* 10–15 mg PO 30 min ac and hs. *Antiemetic:* 1–3 mg/kg/dose IV 30 min before chemotherapy, then q2h for 2 doses, then q3h for 3

doses. **Peds.** *Reflux:* 0.1 mg/kg/dose PO qid. *Antiemetic:* 1–2 mg/kg/dose IV as for adults **Caution/Contra:** [B, –] Seizure disorders **Supplied:** Tabs 5, 10 mg; syrup 5 mg/5 mL; soln 10 mg/mL; inj 5 mg/mL **Notes/SE:** Dystonic reactions common with high doses, treat with IV diphenhydramine; used to facilitate small-bowel intubation and radiologic evaluation of the upper GI tract; restlessness, drowsiness, diarrhea **Interactions:** ↑ risk of serotonin syndrome with sertraline, venlafaxine; ↑ effects of acetaminophen, ASA, CNS depressants, cyclosporine, levodopa, lithium, succinylcholine, tetracyclines, alcohol; ↓ effects with anticholinergics, narcotics; ↓ effects of cimetidine, digoxin **Labs:** ↑ serum ALT, AST, amylase **NIPE:** Monitor for extrapyramidal effects

Metolazone (Mykrox, Zaroxolyn) Uses: Mild/moderate essential HTN and edema of renal disease or cardiac failure **Action:** Thiazide-like diuretic; inhibits Na reabsorption in the distal tubules **Dose:** *Adults. HTN:* 2.5–5 mg/d PO. *Edema:* 5–20 mg/d PO. **Peds.** 0.2–0.4 mg/kg/d PO ÷ q12h–qd **Caution/Contra:** [D, +] Thiazide or sulfonamide sensitivity **Supplied:** Tabs Mykrox (rapid acting) 0.5 mg, Zaroxolyn 2.5, 5, 10 mg **Notes/SE:** Monitor fluid and electrolyte status during treatment; dizziness, hypotension, tachycardia, chest pain, photosensitivity; Mykrox and Zaroxolyn not bioequivalent **Interactions:** ↑ effects with antihypertensives, barbiturates, narcotics, nitrates, alcohol, food; ↑ effects of digoxin, lithium; ↑ hyperglycemia with BBs, diazoxide; ↑ hypokalemia with amphotericin B, corticosteroids, mezlocillin, piperacillin, ticarcillin; ↓ effects with cholestyramine, colestipol, hypoglycemics, insulin, NSAIDs, salicylates; ↓ effects of methenamine **Labs:** ↑ serum and urine glucose, serum cholesterol, triglycerides, uric acid **NIPE:** ↑ risk of photosensitivity - use sunscreen; ↑ risk of gout; monitor electrolytes

Metoprolol (Lopressor, Toprol XL) WARNING: Do not acutely stop therapy as marked worsening of angina can result Uses: HTN, angina, AMI, and CHF **Action:** Competitively blocks β-adrenergic receptors, β$_1$. **Dose:** *Angina:* 50–100 mg PO bid. *HTN:* 100–450 mg/d PO. *AMI:* 5 mg IV ×3 doses, then 50 mg PO q6h ×48 h, then 100 mg PO bid; *CHF:* 12–25 mg/d PO ×2 wk, increase at 2-wk intervals to 200 mg/max, use low dose in patients with greatest severity; ↓ in hepatic failure **Caution/Contra:** [C, +] Uncompensated CHF, bradycardia, heart block **Supplied:** Tabs 50, 100 mg; ER tabs 50, 100, 200 mg; inj 1 mg/mL **Notes/SE:** Drowsiness, insomnia, erectile dysfunction, bradycardia, bronchospasm **Interactions:** ↑ effects with cimetidine, dihydropyridines, diltiazem, fluoxetine, hydralazine, methimazole, oral contraceptives, propylthiouracil, quinidine, quinolones; ↑ effects of hydralazine; ↑ bradycardia with digoxin, dipyridamole, verapamil; ↓ effects with barbiturates, NSAIDs, rifampin; ↓ effects of isoproterenol, theophylline **Labs:** ↑ BUN, serum creatinine, LFTs, uric acid **NIPE:** Take with food, ⊘ d/c abruptly—withdraw over 2 wk

Metronidazole (Flagyl, MetroGel) Uses: Amebiasis, trichomoniasis, *C. difficile, H. pylori,* anaerobic infections, and bacterial vaginosis **Action:** Inter-

feres with DNA synthesis **Dose:** *Adults. Anaerobic infections:* 500 mg IV q6–8h. *Amebic dysentery:* 750 mg/d PO for 5–10 d. *Trichomoniasis:* 250 mg PO tid for 7 d or 2 g PO ×1. *C. difficile infection:* 500 mg PO or IV q8h for 7–10 d (PO preferred; IV only if patient NPO). *Vaginosis:* 1 applicatorful intravaginally bid or 500 mg PO bid for 7 d. *Acne rosacea/skin:* Apply bid. **Peds.** *Anaerobic infections:* 15 mg/kg/24 h PO or IV ÷ q6h. *Amebic dysentery:* 35–50 mg/kg/24 h PO in 3 ÷ doses for 5–10 d; ↓ in hepatic failure **Caution/Contra:** [B, M] Avoid alcohol **Supplied:** Tabs 250, 500 mg; ER tabs 750 mg; caps 375 mg; topical lotion and gel 0.75%; gel, vaginal 0.75% (5 g/applicator 37.5 mg in 70-g tube) **Notes/SE:** For *Trichomonas* infections, Rx patient's partner; no aerobic bacteria activity; used in combination in serious mixed infections; may cause disulfiram-like reaction with alcohol; dizziness, HA, GI upset, anorexia, urine discoloration; **Interactions:** ↑ effects with cimetidine; ↑ effects of carbamazepine, fluorouracil, lithium, warfarin; ↓ effects with barbiturates, cholestyramine, colestipol, phenytoin **Labs:** May cause ↓/zero values for LFTs, triglycerides, glucose **NIPE:** Take with food, possible metallic taste

Metyrosine (Demser)
Uses: Pheochromocytoma; short-term preop and long term when surgery contraindicated **Action:** Tyrosine hydroxylase inhibitor **Dose:** *Adults & Peds >12 y.* 250 mg PO qid, ↑ by 250–500 mg/d up to 4 g/d. *Maint dose:* 2–3 g/d ÷ qid **Caution/Contra:** [C, ?] **Supplied:** 250-mg caps **Notes/SE:** Hydrate well to prevent crystallization; administer at least 5–7 d preop; drowsiness, extrapyramidal symptoms, diarrhea **Interactions:** ↑ sedative effects with CNS depressants, alcohol; ↑ extrapyramidal effects with droperidol, haloperidol, phenothiazines **Labs:** False ↑ urine catecholamines **NIPE:** ↑ fluids to 2–3 L/d

Mexiletine (Mexitil)
Uses: Suppression of symptomatic ventricular arrhythmias; diabetic neuropathy **Action:** Class IB antiarrhythmic **Dose:** Administer with food or antacids; 200–300 mg PO q8h; 1200 mg/d max; drug interactions with hepatic enzyme inducers and suppressors requiring dosage changes **Caution/Contra:** [C, +] Contra in cardiogenic shock or 2nd/3rd-degree AV block w/o pacemaker; may worsen severe arrhythmias **Supplied:** Caps 150, 200, 250 mg **Notes/SE:** Monitor LFTs; lightheadedness, dizziness, anxiety, incoordination, GI upset, ataxia, hepatic damage, blood dyscrasias **Interactions:** ↑ effects with fluvoxamine, quinidine, caffeine; ↑ effects of theophylline; ↓ effects with atropine, hydantoins, phenytoin, phenobarbital, rifampin, tobacco **Labs:** ↑ LFTs, + ANA

Mezlocillin (Mezlin)
Uses: Infections caused by susceptible gram– bacteria (including *Klebsiella, Proteus, E. coli, Enterobacter, P. aeruginosa,* and *Serratia*) involving the skin, bone, respiratory tract, urinary tract, abdomen, and septicemia **Action:** Bactericidal; inhibits cell wall synthesis **Dose:** *Adults.* 3 g IV q4–6h. *Peds.* 200–300 mg/kg/d ÷ q4–6h; ↓ in renal/hepatic insufficiency **Caution/Contra:** [B, M] Penicillin sensitivity **Supplied:** Inj **Notes/SE:** Often used in combination with aminoglycoside; GI upset, agranulocytosis, thrombocytopenia **Interactions:** ↑ effects with probenecid; ↑ effects of methotrexate **Labs:** ↑ LFTs, BUN, serum creatinine; ↓ serum K+

Miconazole (Monistat, others) **Uses:** Various tinea forms; cutaneous candidiasis; vulvovaginal candidiasis; tinea versicolor; occasionally used for severe systemic fungal infections **Action:** Fungicidal; alters permeability of the fungal cell membrane **Dose:** *Adults.* Apply to area bid for 2–4 wk. *Intravaginally:* 1 applicatorful or supp hs for 7 d; 200–1200 mg/d IV, ÷ tid **Caution/Contra:** [C, ?] Azole sensitivity **Supplied:** Topical cream 2%; lotion 2%; powder 2%; spray 2%; vaginal supp 100, 200 mg; vaginal cream 2%; inj **Notes/SE:** Antagonistic to amphotericin B in vivo; may potentiate warfarin **Interactions:** ↑ effects of anticoagulants, cisapride, loratadine, phenytoin, quinidine; ↓ effects with amphotericin B; ↓ effects of amphotericin B **Labs:** ↑ protein

Midazolam (Versed) [C-IV] **Uses:** Preoperative sedation, conscious sedation for short procedures, induction of general anesthesia **Action:** Short-acting benzodiazepine **Dose:** *Adults.* 1–5 mg IV or IM; titrate to effect. *Peds.* Preop: 0.25–1 mg/kg, 20 mg max PO. *Conscious sedation:* 0.08 mg/kg IM ×1. *General anesthesia:* 0.15 mg/kg IV, then 0.05 mg/kg/dose q2min for 1–3 doses PRN to induce anesthesia; ↓ in elderly, with use of narcotics or CNS depressants **Caution/Contra:** [D, +/–] Narrow-angle glaucoma; use of amprenavir, nelfinavir, ritonavir **Supplied:** Inj 1, 5 mg/mL; syrup 2 mg/mL **Notes/SE:** Monitor for respiratory depression; hypotension in conscious sedation, nausea **Interactions:** ↑ effects with azole antifungals, antihistamines, cimetidine, CCBs, CNS depressants, erythromycin, isoniazid, phenytoin, protease inhibitors, grapefruit juice, alcohol; ↓ effects with rifampin, tobacco; ↓ effects of levodopa

Mifepristone [RU 486] (Mifeprex) **WARNING:** Patient counseling and information required **Uses:** Termination of intrauterine pregnancies of <49 d **Action:** Antiprogestin; ↑ prostaglandins, resulting in uterine contraction **Dose:** Administered with 3 office visits: day 1, three 200-mg tabs PO; day 3 if no abortion, two 200-mg misoprostol PO; on or about day 14, verify termination of PRG **Caution/Contra:** [X, –] Must be administered under physician's supervision **Supplied:** Tabs 200 mg **Notes/SE:** Abdominal pain and 1–2 wk of uterine bleeding **Interactions:** ↑ effects with azole antifungals, erythromycin, grapefruit juice; ↓ effects with carbamazepine, dexamethasone, phenytoin, phenobarbital, rifampin, St. John's Wort

Miglitol (Glyset) **Uses:** Type 2 DM **Action:** α-Glucosidase inhibitor; delays digestion of ingested carbohydrates **Dose:** Initial 25 mg PO tid with 1st bite of each meal; maint 50–100 mg tid with meals **Caution/Contra:** [B, –] Obstructive or inflammatory GI disorders; avoid if SCr >2 **Supplied:** Tabs 25, 50, 100 mg **Notes/SE:** Used alone or in combination with sulfonylureas; flatulence, diarrhea, abdominal pain **Interactions:** ↑ effects with celery, coriander, juniper berries, ginseng, garlic; ↓ effects with isoniazid, niacin; ↓ effects of digoxin, propranolol, ranitidine

Milrinone (Primacor) **Uses:** CHF **Action:** Positive inotrope and vasodilator; little chronotropic activity **Dose:** 50 µg/kg, then 0.375–0.75 µg/kg/min inf; ↓ dose in renal impairment **Caution/Contra:** [C, ?] **Supplied:** Inj 1 μg/mL **Notes/SE:** Carefully monitor fluid and electrolyte status; arrhythmias, hypotension, HA **Interactions:** ↑ hypotension with disopyramide

Mineral Oil (generic)
Uses: Constipation **Action:** Emollient laxative **Dose:** *Adults.* 5–45 mL PO PRN. *Peds >6 y.* 5–20 mL PO bid **Caution/Contra:** [C, ?] N/V, difficulty swallowing, bedridden patients **Supplied:** Liq **Notes/SE:** Lipid pneumonia, anal incontinence, impaired vitamin absorption **Interactions:** ↑ effects with stool softeners; ↓ effects of cardiac glycosides, oral contraceptives, sulfonamides, warfarin

Minoxidil (Loniten, Rogaine)
Uses: Severe HTN; male and female pattern baldness **Action:** Peripheral vasodilator; stimulates vertex hair growth **Dose:** *Adults.* 2.5–10 mg PO bid–qid. *Topical:* Apply bid to affected area. *Peds.* 0.2–1 mg/kg/24 h ÷ PO q12–24h; ↓ oral dose in elderly **Caution/Contra:** [C, +] **Supplied:** Tabs 2.5, 10 mg; topical soln (Rogaine) 2% **Notes/SE:** Pericardial effusion and volume overload may occur with oral use; hypertrichosis after chronic use; edema, ECG changes, weight gain **Interactions:** ↑ hypotension with guanethidine **Labs:** ↑ alkaline phosphatase, BUN, creatinine; ↓ HMG, HCT

Mirtazapine (Remeron)
Uses: Depression **Action:** Tetracyclic antidepressant **Dose:** 15 mg PO hs, up to 45 mg/d hs **Caution/Contra:** [C, ?] Contra with MAOIs w/n 14 d **Supplied:** Tabs 15, 30, 45 mg **Notes/SE:** Do not ↓ dose at intervals of less than 1–2 wk; somnolence, ↑ constipation, xerostomia, weight gain, agranulocytosis **Interactions:** ↑ effects with CNS depressants, fluvoxamine; ↑ risk of HTN crisis with MAOIs **Labs:** ↑ ALT, cholesterol, triglycerides

Misoprostol (Cytotec)
Uses: Prevention of NSAID-induced gastric ulcers; induction of labor, incomplete and therapeutic abortion **Action:** Prostaglandin with both antisecretory and mucosal protective properties **Dose:** *Ulcer prevention:* 200 μg PO qid with meals. In females, start on 2nd or 3rd day of next normal menstrual period; 25–50 μg; induction of labor (Term): 400 μg; induction of labor (2nd trimester): 600 μg **Caution/Contra:** [X, –] **Supplied:** Tabs 100, 200 μg **Notes/SE:** Can cause miscarriage with potentially dangerous bleeding; HA, GI SE common (diarrhea, abdominal pain, constipation) **Interactions:** ↑ HA & GI symptoms with phenylbutazone

Mitomycin (Mutamycin)
Uses: Stomach, breast, pancreas, colon CAs; squamous cell carcinoma of the anus; non-small-cell lung, head, neck, cervical, and breast CAs; bladder CA (intravesically) **Action:** Alkylating agent; may also generate oxygen free radicals, induces DNA strand breaks **Dose:** 20 mg/m² q6–8wk or 10 mg/m² in combination with other myelosuppressive drugs; bladder CA 20–40 mg in 40 mL NS via a urethral catheter once/wk for 8 wk, followed by monthly treatments for 1 y; ↓ dose in renal/hepatic impairment **Caution/Contra:** [D, –] Thrombocytopenia, leukopenia, serum creatinine (> 0.7 mg/dL) **Supplied:** Inj **Notes/SE:** Myelosuppression (may persist up to 3–8 wk after dose and may be cumulative minimized by a lifetime dose <50–60 mg/m²), N/V, anorexia, stomati-

tis, and renal toxicity; microangiopathic hemolytic anemia (similar to hemolytic-uremic syndrome) with progressive renal failure; venooclusive disease of the liver, interstitial pneumonia, alopecia (rare); extravasation reactions can be severe **Interactions:** ↑ bronchospasm with vinca alkaloids; ↑ bone marrow suppression with antineoplastics

Mitotane (Lysodren) **Uses:** Palliative treatment of inoperable adrenocortical carcinoma **Action:** Unclear; induces mitochondrial injury in adrenocortical cells **Dose:** 8–10 g/d in 3–4 ÷ doses (begin at 2 g/d with glucocorticoid replacement); ↓ in hepatic insufficiency; adequate hydration necessary **Caution/Contra:** [C, ?] **Supplied:** Tabs 500 mg **Notes/SE:** Anorexia, N/V/D; acute adrenal insufficiency may be precipitated by physical stresses (shock, trauma, infection), Rx with steroids; allergic reactions (rare), visual disturbances, hemorrhagic cystitis, albuminuria, hematuria, HTN or hypotension, minor aches, fever **Interactions:** ↑ effects of CNS depressants, alcohol; ↓ effects of corticosteroids, phenytoin, phenobarbital, warfarin **Labs:** ↓ protein bound iodine **NIPE:** Full effects may take 2–3 mo

Mitoxantrone (Novantrone) **Uses:** AML (with cytarabine), ALL, CML, breast and prostate CA, NHL, MS **Action:** DNA-intercalating agent; inhibitor of DNA topoisomerase II **Dose:** 12 mg/m²/d for 3 d (ALL induction), 12–14 mg/m² q3wk (advanced solid tumors); cumulative dose should not exceed 160 mg/m² with prior mediastinal radiation therapy or 120 mg/m² with prior anthracycline therapy; MS 12 mg/m² over 5–15 min q3mon up to cumulative 140 mg/m²; ↓ dose in hepatic failure, leukopenia, thrombocytopenia; maintain hydration **Caution/Contra:** [D, –] **Supplied:** Inj 20, 25, 30 mg **Notes/SE:** Myelosuppression, N/V, stomatitis, alopecia (infrequent), cardiotoxicity **Interactions:** ↑ bone marrow suppression with antineoplastics; ↓ effects of live virus vaccines **Labs:** ↑ AST, ALT, uric acid **NIPE:** ↑ fluids to 2–3 L/d, ⊘ vaccines, infection

Mivacurium (Mivacron) **Uses:** Adjunct to general anesthesia or mechanical ventilation **Action:** Nondepolarizing neuromuscular blocker **Dose:** **Adults.** 0.15 mg/kg/dose IV; repeat PRN at 15-min intervals. **Peds.** 0.2 mg/kg/dose IV; repeat PRN at 10-min intervals; ↓ dose in renal/hepatic impairment **Caution/Contra:** [C, ?] **Supplied:** Inj 0.5, 2 mg/mL **Notes/SE:** Flushing, hypotension, bronchospasm **Interactions:** ↑ neuromuscular blockage with aminoglycosides, anesthetics, bacitracin, BBs, CCBs, clindamycin, colistin, furosemide, lincomycin, lithium, polymyxins, procainamide, quinidine, tetracyclines; ↓ effects with carbamazepine, phenytoin, theophylline, caffeine

Moexipril (Univasc) **Uses:** HTN, post-MI, DN **Action:** ACE inhibitor **Dose:** 7.5–30 mg in 1–2 ÷ doses 1 h ac **Caution/Contra:** [C (1st trimester, D 2nd and 3rd trimesters). ?] ACE inhibitor sensitivity **Supplied:** Tabs 7.5, 15 mg; ↓ dose in renal impairment **Notes/SE:** Hypotension, edema, angioedema, HA, dizziness, cough

Molindone (Moban) **Uses:** Psychotic disorders **Action:** Piperazine phenothiazine **Dose:** **Adults.** 50–75 mg/d, ↑ to 225 mg/d if necessary. **Peds. 3–5 y:**

1–2.5 mg/d in 4 ÷ doses. **5–12 y:** 0.5–1.0 mg/kg/d in 4 ÷ doses **Caution/Contra:** [C, ?] Narrow-angle glaucoma **Supplied:** Tabs 5, 10, 25, 50, 100 mg; conc 20 mg/mL **Notes/SE:** Hypotension, tachycardia, arrhythmias, extrapyramidal symptoms, seizures, constipation, xerostomia **Interactions:** ↑ effects with antihypertensives; ↑ hyperkalemia with K⁺-sparing diuretics, K⁺ supplements, salt substitutes, trimethoprim; ↑ effects of insulin, lithium; ↓ effects with ASA, NSAIDs **Labs:** ↑ serum K⁺, BUN, creatinine **NIPE:** Take w/o food, monitor for persistant cough

Montelukast (Singulair)
Uses: Prophylaxis and Rx of chronic asthma, seasonal allergic rhinitis **Action:** Leukotriene receptor antagonist **Dose:** *Asthma:* **Adults >15 y:** 10 mg/d PO taken in PM. **Peds. 2–5 y:** 4 mg/d PO taken in PM. **6–14 y:** 5 mg/d PO taken in PM; *Rhinitis:* **Adults:** 10 mg/d. **Peds. 2–5 y:** 4 mg/d. **6–14 y:** 5 mg/d **Caution/Contra:** [B, M] **Supplied:** Tabs 10 mg; chew tabs 4, 5 mg **Notes/SE:** Not for acute asthma attacks; HA, dizziness, fatigue, rash, GI upset, Churg-Strauss syndrome **Interactions:** ↑ ↓ effects with phenobarbital, rifampin **Labs:** ↑ AST, ALT

Moricizine (Ethmozine)
WARNING: Proarrhythmic effects **Uses:** Ventricular arrhythmias **Action:** Class I antiarrhythmic **Dose:** 200–300 mg PO tid; ↓ dose in renal/hepatic insufficiency **Caution/Contra:** [B, +/–] AV block w/o pacemaker; cardiogenic shock **Supplied:** Tabs 200, 250, 300 mg **Notes/SE:** Dizziness, arrhythmias, CHF, HA, fatigue, GI upset, BP changes **Interactions:** ↑ effects with cimetidine; ↑ effects of warfarin; ↑ PR interval with digoxin, propranolol; ↓ effects of theophylline **Labs:** ↑ LFTs

Morphine (Avinza ER, Duramorph, MS Contin, Kadian SR, Oramorph SR, Roxanol) [C-II]
Uses: Relief of severe pain **Action:** Narcotic analgesic **Dose:** *Adults. Oral:* 10–30 mg q4h PRN; SR tabs 30–60 mg q8–12h. *IV/IM:* 2.5–15 mg q2–6h. *Peds.* 0.1–0.2 mg/kg/dose IM/IV q2–4h PRN to a max of 15 mg/dose **Caution/Contra:** [B (D if prolonged use or high doses at term), +/–] Respiratory depression **Supplied:** Immediate release tabs 10, 14, 20 mg; MS Contin CR tabs 15, 30, 60, 100, 200 mg; Oramorph SR CR tabs 15, 30, 60, 100 mg; Kadian SR caps 20, 30 50, 60, 100 mg; Avinza ER caps 30, 60, 90, 120 mg; soln 10, 20, 100 mg; supp 5, 10, 20 mg; inj 2, 4, 5, 8, 10, 15 mg/mL; Duramorph preservative-free inj 0.5, 1 mg/mL **Notes/SE:** May require scheduled dosing to relieve severe chronic pain; MS Contin commonly used SR form (do not crush); narcotic SE (respiratory depression, sedation, constipation, N/V, pruritus) **Interactions:** ↑ effects with cimetidine, CNS depressants, dextroamphetamine, TCAs, alcohol, kava kava, valerian, St. John's Wort; ↑ effects of warfarin; ↑ risk of HTN crisis with MAOIs; ↓ effects with opioids, phenothiazines **Labs:** ↑ serum amylase, lipase

Moxifloxacin (Avelox)
Uses: Acute sinusitis, acute bronchitis, and community-acquired pneumonia **Action:** Quinolone; inhibits DNA gyrase **Dose:** 400 mg/d once **Caution/Contra:** [C, ?/–] Quinolone sensitivity; interactions with

Mg^{2+}-, Ca^{2+}-, Al^{2+}-, and Fe^{2+}-containing products and class IA and III antiarrhythmic agents **Supplied:** Tabs 400 mg **Notes/SE:** Active against gram– bacteria and *S. pneumoniae*; dizziness, nausea, QT prolongation, seizures, photosensitivity, tendon rupture: take 4 h before or 8 h after antacids **Interactions:** ↑ effects with probenecid; ↑ effects of diazepam, theophylline, caffeine, metoprolol, propranolol, phenytoin, warfarin; ↓ effects with antacids, didanosine, iron salts, magnesium, sucralfate, sodium bicarbonate, zinc **Labs:** ↑ LFTs, BUN, serum creatinine, amylase, PT, triglycerides, cholesterol; ↓ HMG, HCT **NIPE:** ⊘ give to children <18 y; ↑ fluids to 2–3 L/d

Mupirocin (Bactroban)
Uses: Impetigo; eradication of MRSA in nasal carriers **Action:** Inhibits bacterial protein synthesis **Dose:** *Topical:* Apply small amount to affected area. *Nasal:* Apply bid in nostrils **Caution/Contra:** [B, ?] Do not use concurrently with other nasal products **Supplied:** Oint 2%; cream 2% **Notes/SE:** Local irritation, rash **Interactions:** ↓ bacterial action with chloramphenicol **NIPE:** ⊘ use with other nasal drugs

Muromonab-CD3 (Orthoclone OKT3)
WARNING: Can cause anaphylaxis; monitor fluid status **Uses:** Acute rejection following organ transplantation **Action:** Blocks T-cell function **Dose:** *Adults.* 5 mg/d IV for 10–14 d. *Peds.* 0.1 mg/kg/d for 10–14 d **Caution/Contra:** [C, ?/–] Murine sensitivity, fluid overload **Supplied:** Inj 5 mg/5 mL **Notes/SE:** Murine antibody; fever and chills after the 1st dose; monitor for anaphylaxis or pulmonary edema **Interactions:** ↑ effects with immunosuppressives; ↑ effects of live virus vaccines; ↑ risk of CNS effects & encephalopathy with indomethacin **Labs:** ↑ AST, ALT **NIPE:** ⊘ immunizations, exposure to infection

Mycophenolate Mofetil (CellCept)
WARNING: ↑ risk of infections, possible development of lymphoma **Uses:** Prevents organ rejection after transplant **Action:** Inhibits immunologically mediated inflammatory responses **Dose:** 1 g PO bid; use with steroids and cyclosporine; ↓ in renal insufficiency or neutropenia; take on empty stomach **Caution/Contra:** [C, ?/–] **Supplied:** Caps 250, 500 mg; inj 500 mg **Notes/SE:** Pain, fever, HA, infection, HTN, diarrhea, anemia, leukopenia, edema **Interactions:** ↑ effects with acyclovir, ganciclovir, probenecid; ↑ effects of acyclovir, ganciclovir; ↓ effects with antacids, cholestyramine, cyclosporine, iron, food; ↓ effects of oral contraceptives, phenytoin, theophylline **Labs:** ↑ LFTs **NIPE:** Use barrier contraception during and 6 wk >drug therapy, ⊘ exposure to infection; take w/o food

Nabumetone (Relafen)
Uses: Arthritis and pain **Action:** NSAID; inhibits prostaglandin synthesis **Dose:** 1000–2000 mg/d qd–bid with food **Caution/Contra:** [C (D 3rd trimester), +] Peptic ulcer, NSAID sensitivity **Supplied:** Tabs 500, 750 mg **Notes/SE:** Dizziness, rash, GI upset, edema, peptic ulcer **Interactions:** ↑ effects with aminoglycosides; ↑ effects of anticoagulants, hypoglycemics, lithium, methotrexate, thrombolytics; ↑ GI effects with ASA, corticosteroids, K^+ supplements, NSAIDs, alcohol; ↓ effects of antihypertensives,

diuretics **Labs:** ↑ LFTs, BUN, serum creatinine; ↓ serum glucose, HMG, HCT, platelets **NIPE:** Photosensitivity - use sunscreen

Nadolol (Corgard) **Uses:** HTN and angina **Action:** Competitively blocks β-adrenergic receptors, β₁, β₂ **Dose:** 40–80 mg/d; ↑ to 240 mg/d (angina) or 320 mg/d (HTN) may be needed; ↓ dose in renal insufficiency and elderly **Caution/Contra:** [C (1st trimester; D if 2nd or 3rd trimester); +] Uncompensated CHF, shock, heart block, asthma **Supplied:** Tabs 20, 40, 80, 120, 160 mg **Notes/ SE:** Nightmares, paresthesias, hypotension, bradycardia, fatigue **Interactions:** ↑ effects with antihypertensives, diuretics, nitrates, alcohol; ↑ effects of aminophylline, lidocaine; ↑ risk of HTN with clonidine, ephedrine, epinephrine, MAOIs, phenylephrine, pseudoephedrine; ↑ bradycardia with digitalis glycosides, ephedrine, epinephrine, phenylephrine, pseudoephedrine; ↓ effects with ampicillin, antacids, clonidine, NSAIDs, thyroid meds; ↓ effects of glucagon, theophylline **Labs:** ↑ K⁺, cholesterol, triglycerides, BUN, uric acid **NIPE:** May ↑ cold sensitivity; ⊘ d/c abruptly

Nafcillin (Nallpen) **Uses:** Infections caused by susceptible strains of *Staphylococcus* and *Streptococcus* **Action:** Bactericidal; inhibits cell wall synthesis **Dose:** *Adults.* 1–2 g IV q4–6h. *Peds.* 50–200 mg/kg/d ÷ q4–6h **Caution/Contra:** [B, ?] Penicillin allergy **Supplied:** Inj **Notes/SE:** No adjustments for renal function; interstitial nephritis, diarrhea, fever, nausea **Interactions:** ↑ effects of methotrexate; ↓ effects with chloramphenicol, macrolides, tetracyclines; ↓ effects of cyclosporine, oral contraceptives, tacrolimus, warfarin **Labs:** ↑ serum protein **NIPE:** Aminoglycosides not compatible, risk of drug inactivation with fruit juice/carbonated drinks; monitor for superinfection

Naftifine (Naftin) **Uses:** Tinea cruris and tinea corporis **Action:** Antifungal antibiotic **Dose:** Apply bid **Caution/Contra:** [B, ?] **Supplied:** 1% cream; gel **Notes/SE:** Local irritation

Nalbuphine (Nubain) **Uses:** Moderate–severe pain; preop and obstetric analgesia **Action:** Narcotic agonist–antagonist; inhibits ascending pain pathways **Dose:** *Adults.* 10–20 mg IM or IV q4–6h PRN; max of 160 mg/d; single max dose, 20 mg. *Peds.* 0.2 mg/kg IV or IM to a max dose of 20 mg; ↓ in hepatic insufficiency **Supplied:** Inj 10, 20 mg/mL **Caution/Contra:** [B (D if prolonged or high doses at term), ?] Sulfite sensitivity **Notes/SE:** Causes CNS depression and drowsiness; caution in patients receiving opiates **Interactions:** ↑ CNS depression with cimetidine, CNS depressants; alcohol ↑ effects of digitoxin, phenytoin, rifampin **Labs:** ↑ serum amylase, lipase

Naloxone (Narcan) **Uses:** Reversal of narcotics **Action:** Competitive narcotic antagonist **Dose:** *Adults.* 0.4–2.0 mg IV, IM, or SC q5min; max total dose, 10 mg. *Peds.* 0.01–1.0 mg/kg/dose IV, IM, or SC; repeat IV q3min ×3 doses PRN **Caution/Contra:** [B, ?] May precipitate acute withdrawal in addicts **Supplied:** Inj 0.4, 1.0 mg/mL; neonatal inj 0.02 mg/mL **Notes/SE:** If no response after 10 mg, suspect nonnarcotic cause; hypotension, tachycardia, irritability, GI upset, pulmonary edema **Interactions:** ↓ effects of opioids

Naltrexone (ReVia)   Uses: Alcohol and narcotic addiction **Action:** Competitively binds to opioid receptors **Dose:** 50 mg/d PO; do not give until opioid-free for 7–10 d **Caution/Contra:** [C, M] Acute hepatitis, liver failure; opioid use **Supplied:** Tabs 50 mg **Notes/SE:** May cause hepatotoxicity; insomnia, GI upset, joint pain, HA, fatigue **Interactions:** ↑ lethargy & somnolence with thioridazine; ↓ effects of opioids

Naphazoline and Antazoline (Albalon-A Ophthalmic, others), Naphazoline and Pheniramine Acetate (Naphcon A)
Uses: Temporary relief from ocular redness and itching caused by allergy **Action:** Vasoconstrictor and antihistamine **Dose:** 1–2 gtt up to 4×/d **Caution/Contra:** [C, +] Contra in glaucoma, children <6 y, and with contact lenses **Supplied:** Soln 15 mL **Notes/SE:** Cardiovascular stimulation, dizziness, local irritation **Interactions:** ↑ risk of HTN crisis with MAOIs, TCAs

Naproxen (Aleve, Naprosyn, Anaprox)   Uses: Arthritis and pain **Action:** NSAID; inhibits prostaglandin synthesis **Dose:** *Adults & Peds >12 y.* 200–500 mg bid–tid to a max of 1500 mg/d; ↓ dose in hepatic impairment **Caution/Contra:** [B (D 3rd trimester), +] NSAID sensitivity, peptic ulcer **Supplied:** Tabs 200, 250, 375, 500 mg; delayed-release (EC) tabs 375, 500 mg; susp 125 mg/5 mL **Notes/SE:** Dizziness, pruritus, GI upset, peptic ulcer, edema **Interactions:** ↑ effects with aminoglycosides; ↑ effects of anticoagulants, hypoglycemics, lithium, methotrexate, thrombolytics; ↑ GI effects with ASA, corticosteroids, K⁺ supplements, NSAIDs, alcohol; ↓ effects of antihypertensives, diuretics **Labs:** ↑ urine 5-HIAA **NIPE:** Take with food

Naratriptan (Amerge)   Uses: Acute migraine attacks **Action:** Serotonin 5-HT₁ receptor antagonist **Dose:** 1–2.5 mg PO once; repeat PRN in 4 h; ↓ dose in mild renal/hepatic insufficiency **Caution/Contra:** [C, M] Contra in severe renal/hepatic impairment, avoid in angina, ischemic heart disease, uncontrolled HTN, and ergot use **Supplied:** Tabs 1, 2.5 mg **Notes/SE:** Dizziness, sedation, GI upset, paresthesias, ECG changes, coronary vasospasm, arrhythmias **Interactions:** ↑ effects with MAOIs, SSRIs; ↑ effects of ergot drugs; ↓ effects with nicotine

Nateglinide (Starlix)   Uses: Type 2 DM **Action:** ↑ Pancreatic release of insulin **Dose:** 120 mg PO tid 1–30 min pc; ↓ to 60 mg tid if near target HbA₁c **Caution/Contra:** [C, –]. Caution with drugs metabolized by CYP2C9/3A4 **Supplied:** Tabs 60, 120 mg **Notes/SE:** Hypoglycemia; URI; salicylates, nonselective β-blockers may enhance hypoglycemia **Interactions:** ↑ effects with nonselective BBs, MAOIs, NSAIDs, salicylates, ↓ effects with corticosteroids, niacin, sympathomimetics, thiazide diuretics, thyroid meds **Labs:** ↑ uric acid

Nedocromil (Tilade)   Uses: Mild–moderate asthma **Action:** Antiinflammatory agent **Dose:** 2 inhal 4×/d **Caution/Contra:** [B, ?/–] **Supplied:** Met-dose inhaler **Notes/SE:** Chest pain, dizziness, dysphonia, rash, GI upset, infection **NIPE:** May take 2–4 wk for full therapeutic effect

Nefazodone (Serzone) WARNING: Fatal hepatitis and liver failure possible; DC if LFT >3× ULN; do not re-treat Uses: Depression Action: Inhibits neuronal uptake of serotonin and norepinephrine Dose: Initially, 100 mg PO bid; usual 300–600 mg/d in 2 ÷ doses Caution/Contra: [C, ?] MAOIs, pimozide Supplied: Tabs 100, 150, 200, 250 mg Notes/SE: Orthostatic hypotension and allergic reactions; HA, drowsiness, xerostomia, constipation, GI upset Interactions: ↑ effects with benzodiazepines, buspirone; ↑ effects of alprazolam, buspirone, carbamazepine, cyclosporine, digoxin, triazolam; ↑ risk of QT prolongation with astemizole, cisapride, pimozide; ↑ risk of serious and/or fatal reaction with MAOIs; ↓ effects of propranolol Labs: ↑ LFTs, cholesterol; ↓ HCT NIPE: Take w/o food; may take 2–4 wk for full therapeutic effects

Nelfinavir (Viracept) Uses: HIV infection Action: Protease inhibitor; results in formation of immature, noninfectious virion Dose: *Adults.* 750 mg PO tid or 1250 mg PO bid. *Peds.* 20–30 mg/kg PO tid; with food Caution/Contra: [B, ?] Phenylketonuria, or triazolam/midazolam use Supplied: Tabs 250 mg; oral powder Notes/SE: Food ↑ absorption; interacts with St. John's Wort; dyslipidemia, lipodystrophy, diarrhea, rash Interactions: ↑ effects with erythromycin, ketoconazole, indinavir, ritonavir; ↑ effects of barbiturates, carbamazepine, cisapride, ergot alkaloids, erythromycin, lovastatin, midazolam, phenytoin, saquinavir, simvastatin, triazolam; ↓ effects with barbiturates, carbamazepine, phenytoin, rifabutin, rifampin; ↓ effects of oral contraceptives Labs: ↑ LFTs NIPE: Take with food; use barrier contraception

Neomycin, Bacitracin, and Polymyxin B (Neosporin Ointment) (See Bacitracin, Neomycin, and Polymyxin B, page 47); Neomycin, Colistin, and Hydrocortisone (Cortisporin-TC Otic Drops), Neomycin, Colistin, Hydrocortisone, and Thonzonium (Cortisporin-TC Otic Suspension) Uses: External otitis, infections of mastoidectomy and fenestration cavities Action: Antibiotic and antiinflammatory Dose: *Adults.* 4–5 gtt in ear(s) tid–qid. *Peds.* 3–4 gtt in ear(s) tid–qid Caution/Contra: [C, ?] Supplied: Otic gtt and susp Notes/SE: Local irritation

Neomycin and Dexamethasone (AK-Neo-Dex Ophthalmic, NeoDecadron Ophthalmic) Uses: Steroid-responsive inflammatory conditions of the cornea, conjunctiva, lid, and anterior segment Action: Antibiotic with antiinflammatory corticosteroid Dose: 1–2 gtt in eye(s) q3–4h or thin coat tid–qid until response, then ↓ to qd Caution/Contra: [C, ?] Supplied: Cream neomycin 0.5%/dexamethasone 0.1%; oint neomycin 0.35%/dexamethasone 0.05%; soln neomycin 0.35%/dexamethasone 0.1% Notes/SE: Use under supervision of ophthalmologist; local irritation

Neomycin and Polymyxin B (Neosporin Cream) Uses: Infection in minor cuts, scrapes, and burns Action: Bactericidal antibiotic Dose: Apply bid–qid Caution/Contra: [C, ?] Supplied: Cream neomycin

3.5 mg/polymyxin B 10,000 U/g **Notes/SE:** Different from Neosporin oint; local irritation

Neomycin, Polymyxin B, and Dexamethasone (Maxitrol)

Uses: Steroid-responsive ocular conditions with bacterial infection **Action:** Antibiotic with antiinflammatory corticosteroid **Dose:** 1–2 gtt in eye(s) q4–6h; apply oint in eye(s) 3–4×/d **Caution/Contra:** [C, ?] **Supplied:** Oint neomycin sulfate 3.5 mg/polymyxin B sulfate 10,000 U/dexamethasone 0.1%/g; susp identical/5 mL **Notes/SE:** Use under supervision of ophthalmologist; local irritation

Neomycin-Polymyxin Bladder Irrigant [GU Irrigant] Uses:

Continuous irrigant for prophylaxis against bacteriuria and gram– bacteremia associated with indwelling catheter use **Action:** Bactericidal antibiotic **Dose:** 1 mL irrigant added to 1 L of 0.9% NaCl; continuous bladder irrigation with 1–2 L of soln/24 h **Caution/Contra:** [C (D if GU irrigant), ?] **Supplied:** Amp 1, 20 mL **Notes/SE:** Potential for bacterial or fungal superinfection; slight possibility for neomycin-induced ototoxicity or nephrotoxicity

Neomycin, Polymyxin, and Hydrocortisone (Cortisporin Ophthalmic and Otic) Uses: Ocular and otic bacterial infections Ac-

tion: Antibiotic and antiinflammatory *Otic:* 3–4 gtt in the ear(s) 3–4×/d. *Ophth:* Apply a thin layer to the eye(s) or 1 gt 1–4×/d **Caution/Contra:** [C, ?] **Supplied:** Otic susp; ophth soln; ophth oint **Notes/SE:** Local irritation

Neomycin, Polymyxin B, and Prednisolone (Poly-Pred Ophthalmic) Uses: Steroid-responsive ocular conditions with bacterial in-

fection **Action:** Antibiotic and antiinflammatory **Dose:** 1–2 gtt in eye(s) q4–6h; apply oint in eye(s) 3–4×/d **Caution/Contra:** [C, ?] **Supplied:** Susp neomycin 0.35%/polymyxin B 10,000 U/prednisolone 0.5%/mL **Notes/SE:** Use under supervision of ophthalmologist

Neomycin Sulfate

Uses: Hepatic coma and preoperative bowel preparation **Action:** Aminoglycoside, poorly absorbed orally; suppresses GI bacterial flora **Dose:** *Adults.* 3–12 g/24 h PO in 3–4 ÷ doses. *Peds.* 50–100 mg/kg/24 h PO in 3–4 ÷ doses **Caution/Contra:** [C, ?/–] Caution in renal failure, neuromuscular disorders, hearing impairment. Do not use parenterally. **Supplied:** Tabs 500 mg; oral soln 125 mg/5 mL **Notes/SE:** Part of the Condon bowel prep; hearing loss with long-term use; rash, N/V **Interactions:** ↑ effects of anticoagulants, warfarin; ↓ effects of digoxin, methotrexate, penicillin V **NIPE:** Maintain adequate hydration

Nesiritide (Natrecor)

Uses: Acutely decompensated CHF **Action:** Human B-type natriuretic peptide **Dose:** 2-μg/kg IV bolus, then 0.01-μg/kg/min IV **Caution/Contra:** [C, ?/–] BP <90, cardiogenic shock; low cardiac filling pressures; patients in whom vasodilators are not appropriate **Supplied:** Vials 1.5 mg **Notes/SE:** Hypotension, requires continuous BP monitoring; HA, back pain, GI upset, arrhythmias, ↑ Cr **Interactions:** ↑ hypotension with ACEIs, nitrates **Labs:** ↑ creatinine

Nevirapine (Viramune)

WARNING: Reports of fatal hepatotoxicity even after short-term use; severe life-threatening skin reactions (Stevens–Johnson syndrome, toxic epidermal necrolysis, and hypersensitivity reactions); monitor closely during 1st 8 wk of treatment **Uses:** HIV infection **Action:** Nonnucleoside reverse transcriptase inhibitor **Dose:** *Adults.* Initially 200 mg/d for 14 d, then 200 mg bid. *Peds.* <8 y: 4 mg/kg/d for 14 d, then 7 mg/kg bid. >8 y: 4 mg/kg/d for 14 d, then 4 mg/kg bid; give w/o regard to food **Caution/Contra:** [C, +/–] Oral contraceptive use **Supplied:** Tabs 200 mg; susp 50 mg/5 mL **Notes/SE:** May cause life-threatening rash; HA, fever, diarrhea, neutropenia, hepatitis **Interactions:** ↑ effects with clarithromycin, erythromycin; ↓ effects with rifabutin, rifampin, St. John's Wort; ↓ effects of clarithromycin, indinavir, ketaconazole, methadone, oral contraceptives, protease inhibitors, warfarin **NIPE:** Use barrier contraception

Niacin (Nicolar, Niaspan) **Uses:** Adjunctive therapy in patients with significant hyperlipidemia **Action:** Inhibits lipolysis; decreases esterification of triglycerides; increases lipoprotein lipase activity **Dose:** 1–6 g tid; max of 9 g/d **Caution/Contra:** [A (C if does >RDA), +] Liver disease, peptic ulcer, arterial hemorrhage **Supplied:** SR caps 125, 250, 300, 400, 500 mg; tabs 25, 50, 100, 250, 500 mg; SR tabs 150, 250, 500, 750 mg; elixir 50 mg/5 mL **Notes/SE:** Upper body and facial flushing and warmth following dose; may cause GI upset; HA, flatulence, paresthesias, liver damage **Interactions:** ↑ effects of antihypertensives, anticoagulants; ↓ effects of hypoglycemics, probenecid, sulfinpyrazone **Labs:** False ↑ urinary catecholamines, false + urine glucose, ↑ LFTs, uric acid **NIPE:** Alcohol & hot beverages ↑ flushing

Nicardipine (Cardene) **Uses:** Chronic stable angina and HTN; prophylaxis of migraine **Action:** Ca channel blocker **Dose:** *Oral:* 20–40 mg PO tid. *SR:* 30–60 mg PO bid. *IV:* 5 mg/h IV cont inf; ↑ by 2.5 mg/h q15min to max 15 mg/h; take with food (not high fat); ↓ dose in renal/hepatic impairment **Caution/Contra:** [C, ?/–] Heart disease, cardiogenic shock **Supplied:** Caps 20, 30 mg; SR caps 30, 45, 60 mg; inj 2.5 mg/mL **Notes/SE:** *Oral-to-IV conversion:* 20 mg tid = 0.5 mg/h, 30 mg tid = 1.2 mg/h, 40 mg tid = 2.2 mg/h; flushing, tachycardia, hypotension, edema, HA **Interactions:** ↑ effects with azole antifungals, cimetidine, ranitidine, grapefruit juice; ↑ effects of cyclosporine, carbamazpine, prazosin, quinidine, tacrolimus; ↑ hypotension with antihypertensives, fentanyl, nitrates, quinidine, alcohol; ↑ dysrhythmias with digoxin, disopyramide, phenytoin; ↓ effects with NSAIDs, rifampin **Labs:** ↑ LFTs **NIPE:** ↑ risk of photosensitivity

Nicotine Gum (Nicorette, Nicorette DS) **Uses and Action:** See Nicotine Nasal Spray **Dose:** Chew 9–12 pieces/d PRN; max 30 pieces/d **Caution/Contra:** [C, ?] Life-threatening arrhythmias, unstable angina **Supplied:** 2 mg (96 pieces/box); Nicorette DS has 4 mg/piece **Notes/SE:** Patients must stop smoking and perform behavior modification for max effect; tachycardia, HA, GI upset **Interactions:** ↑ effects with cimetidine; ↑ effects of catecholamines, cortisol; ↑ hemodynamic & A-V blocking effects of adenosine; ↓ effects with coffee, cola **NIPE:** Chew 30 min for full dose of nicotine; ↓ absorption with coffee, soda, juices, wine w/n 15 min

Nicotine Nasal Spray (Nicotrol NS) **Uses:** Aid to smoking cessation for the relief of nicotine withdrawal **Action:** Provides systemic delivery of nicotine **Dose:** 0.5 mg/actuation; 1–2 sprays/h, not to exceed 10 sprays/h **Caution/Contra:** [D, M] Life-threatening arrhythmias, unstable angina **Supplied:** Nasal inhaler 10 mg/mL **Notes/SE:** Patients must stop smoking and perform behavior modification for max effect; local irritation, tachycardia, HA, taste perversion **Interactions:** ↑ effects with cimetidine, blue cohash; ↑ effects of catecholamines, cortisol; ↑ hemodynamic & A-V blocking effects of adenosine **NIPE:** Avoid in pts with chronic nasal disorders or severe reactive airway disease; ↑ incidence of cough

Nicotine Transdermal (Habitrol, Nicoderm, Nicotrol, ProStep) **Uses:** Aid to smoking cessation for the relief of nicotine withdrawal **Action:** Provides systemic delivery of nicotine **Dose:** Individualized to the patient's needs; apply 1 patch (14–22 mg/d), and taper over 6 wk **Caution/Contra:** [D, M] Life-threatening arrhythmias, unstable angina **Supplied:** Habitrol and Nicoderm 7, 14, 21 mg of nicotine/24 h; Nicotrol 5, 10, 15 mg/24 h; ProStep 11, 22 mg/24 h **Notes/SE:** Nicotrol to be worn for 16 h to mimic smoking patterns; others worn for 24 h; patients must stop smoking and perform behavior modification for max effect; insomnia, pruritus, erythema, local site reaction, tachycardia **Interactions:** ↑ effects with cimetidine, blue cohash; ↑ effects of catecholamines, cortisol; ↑ hemodynamic & A-V blocking effects of adenosine; ↑ HTN with bupropion **NIPE:** Change application site daily

Nifedipine (Procardia, Procardia XL, Adalat, Adalat CC) **Uses:** Vasospastic or chronic stable angina and HTN; tocolytic **Action:** Ca channel blocker **Dose:** *Adults.* SR tabs 30–90 mg/d. *Tocolysis:* 10–20 mg PO q4–6h. *Peds.* 0.6–0.9 mg/kg/24 h ÷ tid–qid **Caution/Contra:** [C, +] Heart block, aortic stenosis **Supplied:** Caps 10, 20 mg; SR tabs 30, 60, 90 mg **Notes/SE:** Adalat CC and Procardia XL not interchangeable; SL administration not recommended; HAs common on initial treatment; reflex tachycardia may occur with regular release dosage forms; edema, hypotension, flushing, dizziness **Interactions:** ↑ effects with antihypertensives, azole antifungals, cimetidine, cisapride, CCBs, diltiazem, famotidine, nitrates, quinidine, ranitidine, alcohol, grapefruit juice; ↑ effects of digitalis glycosides, phenytoin, vincristine; ↓ effects with barbiturates, nafcillin, NSAIDs, phenobarbital, rifampin, St. John's Wort, tobacco; ↓ effects of quinidine **Labs:** ↑ LFTs **NIPE:** Take w/o regard to food; ↑ risk of photosensitivity; use sunscreen

Nilutamide (Nilandron) **WARNING:** Interstitial pneumonitis possible; most cases in 1st 3 mon; follow CXR before Rx **Uses:** Combination with surgical castration for metastatic prostate CA **Action:** Nonsteroidal antiandrogen **Dose:** 300 mg/d in ÷ doses for 30 d, then 150 mg/d **Caution/Contra:** [N/A] Severe hepatic impairment or respiratory insufficiency **Supplied:** Tabs 50 (phased out), 150 mg **Notes/SE:** Hot flashes, loss of libido, impotence, N/V/D, gynecomastia, hepatic dysfunction (follow LFTs), interstitial pneumonitis **Interactions:** ↑ effects of phenytoin, theophylline, warfarin **Labs:** ↑ LFTs **NIPE:** Take w/o regard to food; visual adaptation may be delayed

Nimodipine (Nimotop)
Uses: Prevent vasospasm following subarachnoid hemorrhage **Action:** Ca channel blocker **Dose:** 60 mg PO q4h for 21 d; ↓ dose in hepatic failure **Caution/Contra:** [C, ?] **Supplied:** Caps 30 mg **Notes/SE:** Contents of caps may be administered via NG tube if caps cannot be swallowed whole; hypotension, HA, constipation **Interactions:** ↑ effects with antihypertensives, cimetidine, nitrates, omeprazole, protease inhibitors, quinidine, valproic acid, alcohol, grapefruit juice; ↓ effects of phenytoin **Labs:** ↑ LFTs **NIPE:** ↑ risk of photosensitivity - use sunscreen

Nisoldipine (Sular)
Uses: HTN **Action:** Ca channel blocker **Dose:** 10–60 mg/d PO; do not take with grapefruit juice or high-fat meal; ↓ starting doses in elderly or hepatic impairment **Caution/Contra:** [C, ?] **Supplied:** ER tabs 10, 20, 30, 40 mg **Notes/SE:** Edema, HA, flushing **Interactions:** ↑ effects with antihypertensives, azole antifungals, cimetidine, famotidine, nitrates, ranitidine, alcohol, high-fat foods; ↑ effects of tacrolimus; ↓ effects with NSAIDs, phenytoin, rifampin **Labs:** ↑ serum creatine kinase, BUN, creatinine

Nitazoxanide (Alinia)
Uses: *Cryptosporidium*- or *Giardia*-induced diarrhea in patients 1–11 y **Action:** Antiprotozoal **Dose:** *Peds. 12–47 mon:* 5 mL (11 mg) PO q12h × 3 days. *4–11 y:* 10 mL (200 mg) PO q12h × 3 days; take with food **Caution/Contra:** [B, ?] **Supplied:** 100 mg/5 mL oral susp **Notes/SE:** Suspension contains sucrose; likely to interact with highly protein-bound drugs; abdominal pain

Nitrofurantoin (Macrodantin, Furadantin, Macrobid)
WARNING: Pulmonary reactions possible **Uses:** Prevention and Rx UTI **Action:** Bacteriostatic; interferes with carbohydrate metabolism **Dose:** *Adults. Suppression:* 50–100 mg/d PO. *Rx:* 50–100 mg PO qid. *Peds.* 5–7 mg/kg/24 h in 4 ÷ doses; take with food, milk, or antacid **Caution/Contra:** [B, +] Avoid if CrCl <50 mL/min, pregnant at term, infants <1 mon (hemolytic anemia risk) **Supplied:** Caps and tabs 50, 100 mg; SR caps 100 mg; susp 25 mg/5 mL **Notes/SE:** Macrocrystals (Macrodantin) cause less nausea than other forms of the drug; GI side effects common; dyspnea and a variety of acute and chronic pulmonary reactions, peripheral neuropathy **Interactions:** ↑ effects with anticholinergics, probenecid, sulfinpyrazone; ↓ effects with antacids, quinolones **Labs:** False + urine glucose; false ↑ serum bilirubin, creatinine **NIPE:** Take with food; may discolor urine

Nitroglycerin (Nitrostat, Nitrolingual, Nitro-Bid Ointment, Nitro-Bid IV, Nitrodisc, Transderm-Nitro, others)
Uses: Angina pectoris, acute and prophylactic therapy, CHF, BP control **Action:** Relaxation of vascular smooth muscle **Dose:** *Adults. SL:* 1 tab q5min SL PRN for 3 doses. *Translingual:* 1–2 met-doses sprayed onto oral mucosa q3–5min, max 3 doses. *Oral:* 2.5–9 mg tid. *IV:* 5–20 μg/min, titrated to effect. *Topical:* Apply 1 in. of oint to the chest wall tid, wipe off at night. *TD:* 5–20 cm patch qd. *Peds.* 1

μg/kg/min IV, titrated to effect **Caution/Contra:** [B, ?] Pericardial tamponade, restrictive cardiomyopathy, constrictive pericarditis **Supplied:** SL tabs 0.3, 0.4, 0.6 mg; translingual spray 0.4 mg/dose; SR caps 2.5, 6.5, 9, 13 mg; SR tabs 2.6, 6.5, 9.0 mg; inj 0.5, 5, 10 mg/mL; oint 2%; TD patches 2.5, 5, 7.5, 10, 15 mg/24 h; buccal CR 1, 2, 3 mg **Notes/SE:** Tolerance to nitrates develops with chronic use after 1–2 wk; can be avoided by providing a nitrate-free period each day, using shorter-acting nitrates tid, and removing long-acting patches and oint before hs to prevent development of tolerance; HA, hypotension, lightheadedness, GI upset **Interactions:** ↑ hypotensive effects with antihypertensives, phenothiazines, sildenafil, alcohol; ↓ effects with ergot alkaloids; ↓ effects of SL tabs & spray with antihistamines, phenothiazines, TCAs **Labs:** False ↑ cholesterol, triglycerides **NIPE:** Replace SL tabs q6 mon & keep in original container

Nitroprusside (Nipride, Nitropress)   **Uses:** Hypertensive emergency, aortic dissection, pulmonary edema **Action:** ↓ SVR **Dose:** *Adults & Peds.* 0.5–10 μg/kg/min IV inf, titrated to effect; usual dose 3 μg/kg/min **Caution/Contra:** [C, ?] Decreased cerebral perfusion, compensatory HTN **Supplied:** Inj 10 mg/mL, 25 mg/mL **Notes/SE:** Thiocyanate, the metabolite, excreted by the kidney; thiocyanate toxicity at levels of 5–10 mg/dL; if used to treat aortic dissection, use β-blocker concomitantly; excessive hypotensive effects, palpitations, HA **Interactions:** ↑ effects with antihypertensives, anesthetics, guanabenz, guanfacine, sildenafil; ↓ effects with estrogens, sympathomimetics **NIPE:** Discard colored soln other than fluid light brown

Nizatidine (Axid)   **Uses:** Duodenal ulcers, GERD, heartburn **Action:** H_2-receptor antagonist **Dose:** *Active ulcer:* 150 mg PO bid or 300 mg PO hs; maint 150 mg PO hs. *GERD:* 300 mg PO bid; maint 75 mg PO bid; *Heartburn:* 75 mg PO bid; ↓ dose in renal impairment **Caution/Contra:** [B, +] H_2-antagonist sensitivity **Supplied:** Caps 75, 150, 300 mg **Notes/SE:** Dizziness, HA, constipation, diarrhea **Interactions:** ↑ effects of glipizide, glyburide, nifedipine, nitrendipine, nisoldipine, salicylates, tolbutamide; ↓ effects with antacids, tomato/mixed veg juice; ↓ effects of azole antifungals, delavirdine, didanosine **Labs:** False + urobilinogen **NIPE:** Smoking ↑ gastric acid secretion

Norepinephrine (Levophed)   **Uses:** Acute hypotensive states **Action:** Peripheral vasoconstrictor acting on both the arterial and venous beds **Dose:** *Adults.* 8–12 μg/min IV, titrate to effect. *Peds.* 0.05–0.1 mg/min IV, titrate to effect **Caution/Contra:** [C, ?] **Supplied:** Inj 1 mg/mL **Notes/SE:** Correct blood volume depletion as much as possible prior to vasopressor therapy; interaction with TCAs leads to severe HTN; infuse into large vein to avoid extravasation; phentolamine 5–10 mg/10 mL NS injected locally for extravasation **Interactions:** ↑ HTN with antihistamines, BBs, ergot alkloids, guanethidine, MAOIs, methyldopa, oxytocic meds, TCAs; ↑ risk of arrhythmias with cyclopropane, halothane

Norfloxacin (Noroxin)   **Uses:** Complicated and uncomplicated UTI due to gram– bacteria, prostatitis, and infectious diarrhea **Action:** Quinolone, inhibits

DNA gyrase **Dose:** *Adults.* 400 mg PO bid. *Gonorrhea:* 800 mg single dose. *Conjunctivitis:* 1–2 gtt qid **Caution/Contra:** [X, –] Do not use in PRG; quinolone sensitivity **Supplied:** Tabs 400 mg; ophth soln 0.3%; ↓ in renal impairment **Notes/SE:** Photosensitivity; drug interactions with antacids, theophylline, and caffeine; good concs in the kidney and urine, poor blood levels; do not use for urosepsis **Interactions:** ↑ effects with probenecid; ↑ effects of diazepam, theophylline, caffeine, metoprolol, propranolol, phenytoin, warfarin; ↓ effects with antacids, didanosine, iron salts, magnesium, sucralfate, sodium bicarbonate, zinc; ↓ effects with food; **Labs:** ↑ LFTs, BUN, serum creatinine **NIPE:** ⊘ give to children <18 y; ↑ fluids to 2–3 L/d; may cause photosensitivity - use sunscreen

Norgestrel (Ovrette) **Uses:** Contraceptive **Action:** Prevent follicular maturation and ovulation **Dose:** 1 tab/d; begin day 1 of menses **Caution/Contra:** [X, ?] Thromboembolism, severe hepatic disease, breast CA **Supplied:** Tabs 0.075 mg **Notes/SE:** Progestin-only products have higher risk of failure in prevention of PRG; edema, breakthrough bleeding, thromboembolism **Interactions:** ↓ effects with barbiturates, carbamazepine, hydantoins, griseofulvin, penicillins, rifampin, tetracyclines, St. John's Wort **NIPE:** Photosensitivity – use sunscreen; d/c drug if suspect PRG - use barrier contraception until confirmed

Nortriptyline (Aventyl, Pamelor) **Uses:** Endogenous depression **Action:** TCA; increases the synaptic CNS concs of serotonin and/or norepinephrine **Dose:** *Adults.* 25 mg PO tid–qid; doses >150 mg/d not recommended. *Elderly.* 10–25 mg hs. *Peds. 6–7 y:* 10 mg/d. *8–11 y:* 10–20 mg/d. *>11 y:* 25–35 mg/d; ↓ dose with hepatic insufficiency **Caution/Contra:** [D, +/–] Narrow-angle glaucoma, TCA hypersensitivity **Supplied:** Caps 10, 25, 50, 75 mg; soln 10 mg/5 mL **Notes/SE:** Max effect seen after 2 wk of therapy. Many anticholinergic side effects (blurred vision, urinary retention, xerostomia) **Interactions:** ↑ effects with antihistamines, CNS depressants, cimetidine, fluoxetine, oral contraceptives, phenothiazines, quinidine, alcohol; ↑ effects of anticoagulants; ↑ risk of HTN with clonidine, levodopa, sympathomimetics; ↓ effects with barbiturates, carbamazepine, rifampin **Labs:** ↑ serum bilirubin, alkaline phosphatase **NIPE:** Concurrent use with MAOIs have resulted in HTN, seizures, death; ↑ risk of photosensitivity - use sunscreen

Nystatin (Mycostatin) **Uses:** Mucocutaneous *Candida* infections (thrush, vaginitis) **Action:** Alters membrane permeability **Dose:** *Adults.* Oral: 400,000–600,000 U PO "swish and swallow" qid. *Vaginal:* 1 tab vaginally hs for 2 wk. *Topical:* Apply bid–tid to affected area. *Peds. Infants:* 200,000 U PO q6h. *Children:* See adult dosage **Caution/Contra:** [B (C oral), +] **Supplied:** Oral susp 100,000 U/mL; oral tabs 500,000 U; troches 200,000 U; vaginal tabs 100,000 U; topical cream and oint 100,000 U/g **Notes/SE:** Not absorbed orally; not effective for systemic infections; GI upset, Stevens-Johnson syndrome **NIPE:** Store susp up to 10 d in refrig

Octreotide (Sandostatin, Sandostatin LAR) **Uses:** Suppresses/ inhibits severe diarrhea associated with carcinoid and neuroendocrine GI tumors (ie, VIPoma, ZE syndrome); bleeding esophageal varices **Action:** Long-acting peptide; mimics natural hormone somatostatin **Dose:** *Adults*. 100–600 µg/d SC in 2–4 ÷ doses; initiate at 50 µg qd–bid. *Sandostatin LAR (depot):* 10–30 mg IM q4wk. *Peds*. 1–10 µg/kg/24 h SC in 2–4 ÷ doses **Caution/Contra:** [B, +] **Supplied:** Inj 0.05, 0.1, 0.2, 0.5, 1 mg/mL; 10, 20, 30 mg/5 mL depot **Notes/SE:** N/V, abdominal discomfort, flushing, edema, fatigue, cholelithiasis, hyper-/hypo-glycemia, hepatitis **Interactions:** ↓ effects of cyclosporine **Labs:** Small ↑ LFTs, ↓ serum thyroxine **NIPE:** May alter effects of hypoglycemics

Ofloxacin (Floxin, Ocuflox Ophthalmic) **Uses:** Lower respiratory tract, skin and skin structure, and UTIs, prostatitis, uncomplicated gonorrhea, and *Chlamydia* infections; topical for bacterial conjunctivitis; acute otitis media in children >1 y with tympanostomy tubes; otitis externa in adults and children >1 y; IV perforated ear drum >12 y **Action:** Bactericidal; inhibits DNA gyrase **Dose:** *Adults*. 200–400 mg PO bid or IV q12h. *Adults & Peds >1 y.* Ophth 1–2 gtt in eye(s) q2–4h for 2 d, then qid for =5 d. *Peds*. Do not administer systemically in children <18 y. *Peds 1–12 y.* Otic 5 gtt in ear(s) bid for 10 d. *Adults & Peds >12 y.* Otic 10 gtt in ear(s) bid for 10 d; ↓ dose in renal impairment; take on empty stomach **Caution/Contra:** [C, –] Quinolone sensitivity; drug interactions with antacids, sucralfate, and Al^{2+}-. Ca^{2+}-, Mg^{2+}-, Fe^{2+}-, or Zn^{2+}-containing products, which ↓ absorption **Supplied:** Tabs 200, 300, 400 mg; inj 20, 40 mg/mL; ophth and otic 0.3% **Notes/SE:** Ophth form can be used in ears; N/V/D, photosensitivity, insomnia, and HA **Interactions:** ↑ effects with cimetidine, probenecid, St. John's Wort; ↑ effects of cyclosporine, procainamide, theophylline, warfarin, caffeine; ↓ effects with antacids, antineoplastics, calcium, didanosine, iron, sodium bicarbonate, sucralfate, zinc **NIPE:** Take w/o food; use sunscreen; ↑ fluids to 2–3 L/d

Olanzapine (Zyprexa) **Uses:** Psychotic disorders, acute mania **Action:** Dopamine and serotonin antagonist **Dose:** 5–10 mg/d, ↑ weekly PRN to 20 mg/d max **Caution/Contra:** [C, –] **Supplied:** Tabs 2.5, 5, 7.5, 10, 15, 20 mg; oral disintegrating tabs 5, 10, 15, 20 mg **Notes/SE:** Takes wks to titrate to therapeutic dose; cigarette smoking decreases levels; HA, somnolence, orthostatic hypotension, tachycardia, dystonia, xerostomia, constipation **Interactions:** ↑ effects with fluvoxamine, probenecid; ↑ sedation with CNS depressants, alcohol; ↑ seizures with anticholinergic, CNS depressants; ↑ hypotension with antihypertensives, diazepam; ↓ effects with activated charcoal, carbamazepine, omeprazole, rifampin, St. John's Wort, tobacco; ↓ effects of dopamine agonists, levodopa **Labs:** ↑ LFTs **NIPE:** ↑ risk of tardive dyskinesia, photosensitivity, body temp impairment

Olmesartan (Benicar) **Uses:** HTN **Action:** Angiotensin II antagonist **Dose:** 20–40 mg PO qd **Caution/Contra:** [C (1st trimester, D 2nd and 3rd trimesters), ?/–] **Supplied:** Tabs 5, 20, 40 mg **Notes/SE:** Use lower dose with depleted intravascular volume **NIPE:** Take w/o regard to food; maintain hydration; ⊘ PRG, breast-feeding

Olopatadine (Patanol) Uses: Allergic conjunctivitis Action: H_1-receptor antagonist Dose: 1–2 gtt in eye(s) bid q6–8h Caution/Contra: [C, ?] Supplied: Soln 0.1% 5 mL Notes/SE: Do not instill if wearing contact lenses; local irritation, HA, rhinitis

Olsalazine (Dipentum) Uses: Maint of remission of ulcerative colitis Action: Topical antiinflammatory activity Dose: 500 mg PO bid; take with food Caution/Contra: [C, M] Salicylate sensitivity Supplied: Caps 250 mg Notes/SE: May cause diarrhea, HA, blood dyscrasias, hepatitis Labs: ↑ LFTs

Omalizumab (Xolair) Uses: Mod/sev asthma in pts (>)12 y, who have allergen reactivity & whose symptoms are inadequately controlled with inhaled corticosteroids Action: Anti-IgE antibody Dose: 150–375 mg sq q 2–4 wk (dose/frequency determined by total serum IgE level and BW; see labeling for dosing charts) Caution: [B,?/–] Contra: N/A Supplied: 150 mg in single-use 5-cc vial SE: Inj site reaction, sinusitis, HA, anaphylaxis (noted in 3 patients w/n 2 h of dose) Notes: Continue other asthma medications Interactions: No drug interaction studies done NIPE: ⊘ d/c abruptly; not for acute bronchospasm; admin w/n 8 h of reconstitution and store in refrigerator

Omeprazole (Prilosec) Uses: Duodenal and gastric ulcers, Zollinger–Ellison syndrome, GERD, and *H. pylori* infections Action: Proton-pump inhibitor Dose: 20–40 mg PO qd–bid Caution/Contra: [C, –] Supplied: Caps 10, 20, 40 mg Notes/SE: Combination (ie, antibiotic) therapy necessary for *H. pylori* infection; HA, diarrhea Interactions: ↑ effects of carbamazepine, diazepam, digoxin, glipizide, glyburide, nifedipine, nimodipine, nisoldipine, nitrendipine, phenytoin, tolbutamide, warfarin; ↓ effects with sucralfate; ↓ effects of ampicillin, cefpodoxime, cefuroxime, enoxacin, cyanocobalamin, ketoconazole Labs: ↑ LFTs; NIPE: Take w/o food

Ondansetron (Zofran) Uses: Prevent chemotherapy-associated and postop N/V Action: Serotonin receptor antagonist Dose: *Adults & Peds.* *Chemotherapy:* 0.15 mg/kg/dose IV prior to chemotherapy, then repeat 4 and 8 h after 1st dose or 4–8 mg PO tid; give 1st dose 30 min prior to chemotherapy. *Adults. Postop:* 4 mg IV immediately before induction of anesthesia or postop; ↓ dose with hepatic impairment; administer on a schedule, not PRN Caution/Contra: [B, +/–] Supplied: Tabs 4, 8 mg; inj 2 mg/mL Notes/SE: Diarrhea, HA, constipation, dizziness Interactions: ↓ effects with rifampin; Labs: ↑ fibrinogen, AST, ALT, serum bilirubin, ↓ HMG, serum albumin, transferrin, gamma globulin NIPE: Food increases absorption

Oprelvekin (Neumega) Uses: Prevent severe thrombocytopenia due to chemotherapy Action: Promotes proliferation and maturation of megakaryocytes (interleukin-11) Dose: *Adults.* 50 μg/kg/d SC for 10–21 d. *Peds.* 75–100 μg/kg/d SC for 10–21 d; *<12y:* Use only in clinical trials Caution/Contra: [C, ?/–] Supplied: Inj Notes/SE: Tachycardia, palpitations, arrhythmias, edema, HA, dizziness, insomnia, fatigue, fever, nausea, anemia, dyspnea [**Interactions:** None noted **Labs:** ↓ HMG, albumin **NIPE:** Monitor for peripheral edema; use med w/n 3 h of reconstitution

Oral Contraceptives, Biphasic, Monophasic, Triphasic, Progestin Only (Table 7, pages 253–255) **Uses:** Birth control and regulation of anovulatory bleeding **Action:** *Birth control:* Suppresses LH surge, prevents ovulation; progestins thicken cervical mucus; inhibits fallopian tubule cilia, ↓ endometrial thickness to ↓ chances of fertilization. *Anovulatory bleeding:* Cyclic hormones mimic body's natural cycle and help regulate endometrial lining, resulting in regular bleeding q28d; may also reduce uterine bleeding and dysmenorrhea **Dose:** 28-d cycle pills taken qd; 21-d cycle pills taken qd, no pills taken during the last 7 d of the cycle (during menses) **Caution/Contra:** [X, +] *Absolute contraindications:* Undiagnosed abnormal vaginal bleeding, PRG, estrogen-dependent malignancy, hypercoagulation disorders, liver disease, hemiplegic migraine, and smokers >35 y. *Relative caution/contra:* Migraine HAs, HTN, diabetes, sickle cell disease, and gallbladder disease **Supplied:** 28-d cycle pills (21 hormonally active pills + 7 placebo/Fe supplementation); 21-d cycle pills (21 hormonally active pills). Table 7, page 253 **Notes/SE:** Taken correctly, 99.9% effective for preventing PRG; not protective against STDs; encourage additional barrier contraceptive. Long term, can ↓ risk of ectopic PRG, benign breast disease, ovarian and uterine CA. *Rx for menstrual cycle control:* Start with a monophasic pill. Pill must be taken for 3 mon before switching to another brand. If abnormal bleeding continues, change to pill with higher estrogen dose. *Rx for birth control:* Choose pill with most beneficial side effect profile for particular patient. Side effects numerous and due to symptoms of estrogen excess or progesterone deficiency. Each pill's side effect profile is unique (found in package insert); tailor Rx to specific patient. *Common SE:* Intermenstrual bleeding, oligomenorrhea, amenorrhea, ↑ appetite/weight gain, loss of libido, fatigue, depression, mood swings, mastalgia, HAs, melasma, ↑ vaginal discharge, acne/greasy skin, corneal edema, nausea

Orphenadrine (Norflex) **Uses:** Muscle spasms **Action:** Central atropine-like effects cause indirect skeletal muscle relaxation, euphoria, and analgesia **Dose:** 100 mg PO bid, 60 mg IM/IV q12h **Caution/Contra:** [C, +] Glaucoma, GI obstruction, cardiospasm, MyG **Supplied:** Tabs 100 mg; SR tabs 100 mg; inj 30 mg/mL **Notes/SE:** Drowsiness, dizziness, blurred vision, flushing, tachycardia, constipation **Interactions:** ↑ CNS depression with anxiolytics, butorphanol, hypnotics, MAOIs, nalbuphine, opioids, pentazocine, phenothiazines, tramadol, TCA, kava kava, valerian, alcohol; ↑ effects with anticholinergics **NIPE:** Body heat impairment

Oseltamivir (Tamiflu) **Uses:** Prevention and Rx of influenza A and B **Action:** Inhibits viral neuraminidase **Dose:** *Adults.* Rx 75 mg bid for 5 d. *Peds. PO bid dosing: <15 kg:* 30 mg. *16–23 kg:* 45 mg. *24–40 kg:* 60 mg. *>41 kg:* as adult

↓ dose in renal impairment **Caution/Contra:** [C, ?/–] **Supplied:** Caps 75 mg, powder 12 mg/mL **Notes/SE:** Initiate w/n 48 h of symptom onset or exposure; N/V, insomnia **Interaction:** ↑ effects with probenecid **NIPE:** Take w/o regard to food

Oxacillin (Bactocill, Prostaphlin) **Uses:** Infections caused by susceptible strains of *S. aureus* and *Streptococcus* **Action:** Bactericidal; inhibits cell wall synthesis **Dose:** *Adults.* 250–500 mg (1 g severe) IM/IV q4–6h. *Peds.* 150–200 mg/kg/d IV ÷ q4–6h; ↓ dose in significant renal disease **Caution/Contra:** [B, M] Penicillin sensitivity **Supplied:** Inj; caps 250, 500 mg; soln 250 mg/5 mL **Notes/SE:** GI upset, interstitial nephritis, blood dyscrasias **Interactions:** ↑ effects with disulfiram, probenecid; ↑ effects of anticoagulants, methotrexate; ↓ effects with chloramphenicol, tetracyclines, carbonated drinks, fruit juice, food; ↓ effects of oral contraceptives **Labs:** False + urine and serum protein **NIPE:** Take w/o food

Oxaprozin (Daypro) **Uses:** Arthritis and pain **Action:** NSAID; inhibits prostaglandin synthesis **Dose:** 600–1200 mg/d; ↓ dose in renal/hepatic impairment **Caution/Contra:** [C (D in 3rd trimester or near term), ?] ASA/NSAID sensitivity, peptic ulcer, bleeding disorders **Supplied:** Caplets 600 mg **Notes/SE:** CNS inhibition, sleep disturbance, rash, GI upset, peptic ulcer, edema, renal failure **Interactions:** ↑ effects of aminoglycosides, anticoagulants, ASA, diuretics, lithium, methotrexate; ↓ effects of antihypertensives **NIPE:** ↑ risk of photosensitivity – use sunscreen; take with food

Oxazepam (Serax) [C-IV] **Uses:** Anxiety, acute alcohol withdrawal, anxiety with depressive symptoms **Action:** Benzodiazepine **Dose:** *Adults.* 10–15 mg PO tid–qid; severe anxiety and alcohol withdrawal may require up to 30 mg qid. *Peds.* 1 mg/kg/d in ÷ doses; avoid abrupt DC **Caution/Contra:** [D, ?] **Supplied:** Caps 10, 15, 30 mg; tabs 15 mg **Notes/SE:** One of the metabolites of diazepam (Valium); sedation, ataxia, dizziness, rash, blood dyscrasias, dependence **Interactions:** ↑ CNS effects with anticonvulsants, antidepressants, antihistamines, barbiturates, MAOIs, opioids, phenothiazines, kava kava, lemon balm, sassafras, valerian, alcohol; ↑ effects with cimetidine; ↓ effects with oral contraceptives, phenytoin, theophylline, tobacco; ↓ effects of levodopa **Labs:** False ↑ serum glucose **NIPE:** ⊘ d/c abruptly

Oxcarbazepine (Trileptal) **Uses:** Partial seizures **Action:** Blocks voltage-sensitive Na^+ channels, resulting in stabilization of hyperexcited neural membranes **Dose:** *Adults.* 300 mg bid, ↑ dose weekly; usual dose of 1200–2400 mg/d. *Peds.* 8–10 mg/kg bid, 600 mg/d max; ↑ dose weekly to target maint dose; ↓ dose in renal insufficiency **Caution/Contra:** [C, –] Possible cross-sensitivity to carbamazepine **Supplied:** Tabs 150, 300, 600 mg **Notes/SE:** Hyponatremia; HA, dizziness, fatigue, somnolence, GI upset, diplopia, mental conc difficulties; do not abruptly DC **Interactions:** ↑ effects with benzodiazepines, alcohol; ↑ effects of phenobarbital, phenytoin; ↓ effects with barbiturates, carbamazepine, phenobarbital, valproic acid, verapamil; ↓ effects of CCBs, oral contraceptives **Labs:** ↓ thyroid levels, serum sodium **NIPE:** Take w/o regard to food; use barrier contraception

Oxiconazole (Oxistat)   **Uses:** Tinea pedis, tinea cruris, and tinea corporis **Action:** Antifungal antibiotic **Dose:** Apply bid **Caution/Contra:** [B, M] **Supplied:** Cream 1%; lotion **SE:** Local irritation

Oxybutynin (Ditropan, Ditropan XL)   **Uses:** Symptomatic relief of urgency, nocturia, and incontinence associated with urgency or reflex neurogenic bladder **Action:** Direct smooth-muscle antispasmodic; ↑ bladder capacity **Dose:** *Adults & Peds >5 y.* 5 mg PO tid–qid. *Adults.* XL 5 mg PO qd; ↑ to 30 mg PO (5 and 10 mg/tab). *Peds 1–5 y.* 0.02 mg/kg/dose bid–qid (syrup 5 mg/5 mL); ↓ dose in elderly; periodic drug holidays recommended **Caution/Contra:** [B, ? (use with caution)] Glaucoma, MyG, GI or GU obstruction, ulcerative colitis, megacolon **Supplied:** Tabs 5 mg; XL tabs 5, 10, 15 mg; syrup 5 mg/5 mL **Notes/SE:** Anticholinergic side effects; drowsiness, xerostomia, constipation, tachycardia **Interactions:** ↑ effects with CNS depressants, alcohol; ↑ effects of atenolol, digoxin, nitrofurantoin; ↑ anticholinergic effects with antihistamines, anticholinergics; ↓ effects of haloperidol, levodopa **NIPE:** Impaired temperature regulation; ↑ photosensitivity

Oxybutynin transdermal system (Oxytrol) Uses: Treatment of overactive bladder **Action:** Direct smooth-muscle antispasmodic; increase bladder capacity **Dose:** One 3.9 mg/d system applied 2×/wk to abdomen, hip, or buttock **Caution:** [B, ?/–] **Contra:** Urinary retention, gastric retention, or uncontrolled narrow-angle glaucoma **Supplied:** 3.9 mg/d transdermal system **SE:** Anticholinergic side effects, itching/redness at application site **Notes:** Avoid reapplication to the same site w/n 7 d **Interactions:** ↑ effects with anticholinergics **NIPE:** Metabolized by the cytochrome P450 CYP3A4 enzyme system

Oxycodone   [Dihydrohydroxycodeinone]   (OxyContin, OxyIR, Roxicodone) [C-II]   **WARNING:** Swallow whole, do not crush **Uses:** Moderate–severe pain, normally used in combination with nonnarcotic analgesics **Action:** Narcotic analgesic **Dose:** *Adults.* 5 mg PO q6h PRN. *Peds. 6–12 y:* 1.25 mg PO q6h PRN. *>12 y:* 2.5 mg q6h PRN; ↓ in severe liver disease **Caution/Contra:** [B (D if prolonged use or near term), M] **Supplied:** Immediate-release caps (OxyIR) 5 mg; tabs (Percolone) 5 mg; CR (OxyContin) 10, 20, 40, 80 mg; liq 5 mg/5 mL; soln conc 20 mg/mL **Notes/SE:** Usually prescribed in combination with APAP or ASA; OxyContin used for chronic CA pain; hypotension, sedation, dizziness, GI upset, constipation, risk of abuse **Interactions:** ↑ CNS & resp. depression with amitriptylline, barbiturates, cimetidine, clomipramine, MAOIs, nortriptylline, protease inhibitors, TCAs **Labs:** False ↑ serum amylase, lipase **NIPE:** Take with food

Oxycodone and Acetaminophen (Percocet, Tylox) [C-II]   **Uses:** Moderate–severe pain **Action:** Narcotic analgesic **Dose:** *Adults.* 1–2 tabs/caps PO q4–6h PRN (acetaminophen max dose 4 g/d). *Peds.* Oxycodone 0.05–0.15

mg/kg/dose q4–6h PRN; up to 5 mg/dose **Caution/Contra:** [B (D if prolonged use or near term), M] **Supplied:** Percocet tabs, (mg oxycodone/mg APAP): 2.5/325, 5/325, 7.5/325, 10/325, 7.5/500, 10/650; Tylox caps 5 mg of oxycodone, 500 mg of APAP; soln 5 mg of oxycodone and 325 mg of APAP/5 mL **Notes/SE:** Hypotension, sedation, dizziness, GI upset, constipation **Interactions:** ↑ CNS & resp. depression with amitriptyline, barbiturates, cimetidine, clomipramine, MAOIs, nortriptyline, protease inhibitors, TCAs **Labs:** False ↑ serum amylase, lipase **NIPE:** Take with food

Oxycodone and Aspirin (Percodan, Percodan-Demi) [C-II]
Uses: Moderate–moderately severe pain **Action:** Narcotic analgesic with NSAID **Dose:** *Adults.* 1–2 tabs/caps PO q4–6h PRN. *Peds.* 0.05–0.15 mg/kg/dose q4–6h, max 5 mg/dose (based on oxycodone); ↓ dose in severe hepatic failure **Caution/Contra:** [B (D if prolonged use or near term), M] Peptic ulcer **Supplied:** Percodan 4.5 mg oxycodone HCl/0.38 mg oxycodone terephthalate/325 mg ASA; Percodan-Demi 2.25 mg oxycodone HCl/0.19 mg oxycodone terephthalate/325 mg ASA **Notes/SE:** Sedation, dizziness, GI upset, constipation **Interactions:** ↑ CNS & resp. depression with amitriptyline, barbiturates, cimetidine, clomipramine, MAOIs, nortriptyline, protease inhibitors, TCAs; ↑ effects of anticoagulants **Labs:** False ↑ serum amylase, lipase **NIPE:** Take with food

Oxymorphone (Numorphan) [C-II]
Uses: Moderate–severe pain, sedative **Action:** Narcotic analgesic **Dose:** 0.5 mg IM, SC, IV initially, 1–1.5 mg q4–6h PRN. *PR:* 5 mg q4–6h PRN **Caution/Contra:** [B, ?] **Supplied:** Inj 1, 1.5 mg/mL; supp 5 mg **Notes/SE:** Chemically related to hydromorphone; hypotension, sedation, GI upset, constipation, histamine release **Interactions:** ↑ effects with CNS depressants, cimetidine, neuroleptics, alcohol; ↓ effects with phenothiazines **Labs:** False ↑ amylase, lipase

Oxytocin (Pitocin)
Uses: Induction of labor and control of postpartum hemorrhage; promote milk letdown in lactating woman **Action:** Stimulates muscular contractions of the uterus; stimulates milk flow during nursing **Dose:** 0.001–0.002 U/min IV inf; titrate to desired effect to a max of 0.02 U/min. *Breast-feeding:* 1 spray in both nostrils 2–3 min before feeding **Caution/Contra:** [Uncategorized, no anomalies expected, +/–] **Supplied:** Inj 10 U/mL; nasal soln 40 U/mL **Notes/ SE:** Monitor vital signs closely; nasal form for breast-feeding only; can cause uterine rupture and fetal death; arrhythmias, anaphylaxis, water intoxication **Interactions:** ↑ pressor effects with sympathomimetics

Paclitaxel (Taxol)
Uses: Ovarian and breast CA **Action:** Mitotic spindle poison promotes microtubule assembly and stabilization against depolymerization **Dose:** 135–250 mg/m² as a 3–24 h IV inf; glass or polyolefin containers using polyethylene-lined nitroglycerin tubing sets; PVC inf sets result in leaching of plasticizer; ↓ dose in hepatic failure; maintain adequate hydration **Caution/Contra:** [D, – (unknown excretion, but nursing must be stopped)] **Supplied:** Inj 6 mg/mL **Notes/SE:** Hypersensitivity reactions (dyspnea, hypotension, urticaria,

rash) usually w/n 10 min of starting inf; minimize with corticosteroid, antihistamine (H₁- and H₂-antagonist) pretreatment. Myelosuppression, peripheral neuropathy, transient ileus, myalgia, bradycardia, hypotension, mucositis, N/V/D, fever, rash, HA, and phlebitis; hematologic toxicity schedule-dependent; leukopenia dose-limiting by 24-h inf; neurotoxicity dose-limiting by short (1–3 h) inf **Interactions:** ↑ effects with BBs, cyclosporine, dexamethasone, diazepam, digoxin, etoposide, ketoconazole, midazolam, quinidine, teniposide, troleandomycine, verapamil, vincristine; ↑ risk of bleeding with anticoagulants, platelet inhibitors, thrombolytics; ↑ mylosuppression when cisplatin is admin <paclitaxel; ↓ effects with carbamazepine, phenobarbital; ↓ effects of live virus vaccines **Labs:** ↑ ALT, AST, serum bilirubin, alkaline phosphatase **NIPE:** ⊘ PRG, breast-feeding, live virus vaccines; use barrier contraception

Palivizumab (Synagis)   **Uses:** Prevents RSV **Action:** RSV fusion protein monoclonal antibody **Dose:** *Peds.* 15 mg/kg IM monthly, typically Nov–Apr **Caution/Contra:** [C, ?] Caution in renal or hepatic dysfunction **Supplied:** Vials 50, 100 mg **Notes/SE:** URI, rhinitis, cough, ↑ LFT, local irritation **NIPE:** Use drug w/n 6 h >reconstitution; ⊘ inj in gluteal site; for prophylaxis

Palonosetron (Aloxi)   **WARNING:** May prolong QTc interval **Uses:** Prevent acute/delayed N&V with moderately/highly emetogenic chemotherapy **Action:** 5HT3 serotonin receptor antagonist **Dose:** *Adults.* 0.25 mg IV 30 min <chemo; do not repeat w/n 7 d **Caution:** [B, ?] **Contra:** N/A **Supplied:** 0.25 mg/5 mL **SE:** HA, constipation, dizziness, abdominal pain, anxiety **Notes:** N/A **Interactions:** potential for drug interactions low

Pamidronate (Aredia)   **Uses:** Hypercalcemia of malignancy and Paget's disease; palliation of symptomatic bone metastases **Action:** Inhibition of normal and abnormal bone resorption **Dose:** *Hypercalcemia:* 60 mg IV over 4 h or 90 mg IV over 24 h. *Paget's disease:* 30 mg/d IV for 3 d; slow inf rate necessary **Caution/Contra:** [C, ?/–] **Supplied:** Powder for inj 30, 60, 90 mg **Notes/SE:** Fever, tissue irritation at inj site, uveitis, fluid overload, HTN, abdominal pain, N/V, constipation, UTI, bone pain, hypokalemia, hypocalcemia, hypomagnesemia, and hypophosphatemia **Interactions:** ↓ serum calcium levels with foscarnet; ↓ effects with calcium, vitamin D **NIPE:** ⊘ ingest food with calcium or vitamins with minerals < or 2–3 h > admin of drug

Pancrelipase (Pancrease, Cotazym, Creon, Ultrase)   **Uses:** Exocrine pancreatic secretion deficiency (CF, chronic pancreatitis, other pancreatic insufficiency) and for steatorrhea of malabsorption syndrome **Action:** Pancreatic enzyme supplementation **Dose:** *Adults & Peds.* 1–3 caps (tabs) with meals and snacks; dosage ↑ to 8 caps (tabs); do not crush or chew EC products; dosage is dependent on digestive requirements of patient; avoid antacids. **Caution/Contra:** [C, ?/–] **Supplied:** Caps, tabs **Notes/SE:** N/V, abdominal cramps **Interactions:** ↓ effects with antacids with calcium or magnesium; ↓ effects of iron **Labs:** ↑ serum and urine uric acid **NIPE:** Take with food; stress adherence to diet (usually low-fat, high-protein, high-calorie)

Pancuronium (Pavulon) Uses: Rx of patients on mechanical ventilation **Action:** Nondepolarizing neuromuscular blocker **Dose:** *Adults.* 2–4 mg IV q2–4h PRN. *Peds.* 0.02–0.10 mg/kg/dose q2–4h PRN; ↓ dose for renal/hepatic impairment; intubate patient and keep on controlled ventilation; use an adequate amount of sedation or analgesia **Caution/Contra:** [C, ?/–] **Supplied:** Inj 1, 2 mg/mL **Notes/SE:** Tachycardia, HTN, pruritus, other histamine reactions **Interactions:** ↑ effects with aminoglycosides, bacitracin, clindamycin, enflurane, K+-depleting diuretics, isoflurane, lidocaine, lithium, metocurine, quinine, sodium colistimethate, succinylcholine, tetracycline, trimethaphan, tubocurarine, verapamil; ↓ effects with carbamazepine, phenytoin, theophylline

Pantoprazole (Protonix) Uses: GERD, PUD, erosive gastritis, ZE syndrome **Action:** Proton-pump inhibitor **Dose:** 40 mg/d PO; do not crush or chew tablets; 40 mg IV/d (not >3 mg/min and use Protonix filter) **Caution/Contra:** [B, ?/–] **Supplied:** Tabs 40 mg; inj **Notes/SE:** Chest pain, anxiety, GI upset, ↑ levels on LFTs

Paregoric [Camphorated Tincture of Opium] [C-III] Uses: Diarrhea, pain, and neonatal opiate withdrawal syndrome **Action:** Narcotic **Dose:** *Adults.* 5–10 mL PO qd–qid PRN. *Peds.* 0.25–0.5 mL/kg qd–qid. *Neonatal withdrawal syndrome:* 3–6 mL/kg PO q3–6h PRN to relieve symptoms for 3–5 d, then taper over 2–4 wk **Caution/Contra:** [B (D if prolonged use or high dose near term), +] **Supplied:** Liq 2 mg morphine = 20 mg opium/5 mL **Notes/SE:** Contains anhydrous morphine from opium; short-term use only; hypotension, sedation, constipation **Interactions:** ↓ effects of ampicillin esters, azole antifungals, iron salts **Labs:** ↑ LFTs, serum creatinine **NIPE:** Take w/o regard to food

Paroxetine (Paxil, Paxil CR) Uses: Depression, OCD, panic disorder, social anxiety disorder, PMDD **Action:** Serotonin reuptake inhibitor **Dose:** 10–60 mg PO single daily dose in AM; CR 25 mg/d PO; ↑ 12.5 mg/wk (max range 26–62.5 mg/d) **Caution/Contra:** [B, ?/–] DDI, MAOI **Supplied:** Tabs 10, 20, 30, 40 mg; susp 10 mg/5 mL; CR 12.5, 25 mg **Notes/SE:** Sexual dysfunction, HA, somnolence, dizziness, GI upset, diarrhea, xerostomia, tachycardia **Interactions:** ↑ effects with cimetidine; ↑ effects of BBs, dexfenfluramine, dextromethorphan, fenfluramine, haloperidol, MAOIs, theophylline, thioridazine, TCAs, warfarin, St. John's Wort, alcohol; ↓ effects with cyproheptadine, phenobarbital, phenytoin; ↓ effects of digoxin, phenytoin **Labs:** ↑ LFTs **NIPE:** Take w/o regard to food, may take up to 4 wk for full effect

Pegfilgrastim (Neulasta) Uses: ↓ Frequency of infection in patients with nonmyeloid malignancies receiving myelosuppressive anticancer drugs that cause febrile neutropenia **Actions:** Colony-stimulating factor **Dose:** *Adults.* 6 mg SC × 1/chemo cycle; never give between 14 d before and 24 h after dose of cytotoxic chemotherapy **Contra/Caution:** [C, M] Contra in patients hypersensitive to drugs used to treat *E. coli* or filgrastim, caution in sickle cell **Supplied:** Syringes 6 mg/0.6 mL **Notes/SE:** HA, fever weakness, fatigue, dizziness, insomnia, edema, N/V/D, stomatitis, anorexia, constipation, taste perversion, dyspepsia, abdominal pain, granulocytopenia, neutropenic fever, ↑ LFT, uric acid, arthralgia, myalgia, bone pain, ARDS, alopecia, splenic rupture, aggravation of sickle cell disease **Interactions:** ↑ effects with lithium **Labs:** ↑ alkaline phosphatase, LDH, uric acid **NIPE:** ⊘ exposure to infection

Peg Interferon Alfa-2a (Pegasys)
Uses: Chronic hepatitis C with compensated liver disease **Action:** BRM **Dose:** 180 mcg (1 mL) SQ once weekly × 48 wk; ↓ dose in renal impairment **Caution/Contra:** [C, ?/–] Autoimmune hepatitis, decompensated liver disease **Supplied:** 180-µg/mL inj **Notes/SE:** May aggravate neuropsychiatric, autoimmune, ischemic, and infectious disorders **NIPE:** ⊘ exposure to infection, use barrier contraception

Peg Interferon Alfa-2b (PEG-Intron)
Uses: Rx hepatitis C **Action:** Immune modulation **Dose:** 1 µg/kg/wk SC; 1.5 µg/kg/wk combined with ribavirin **Caution/Contra:** [C, ?/–] Contra in hemoglobinopathy; caution in patients with psychiatric Hx **Supplied:** Vials 50, 80, 120, 150 µg/0.5 mL **Notes/SE:** ↓ Flu-like symptoms by giving hs or with APAP; neutropenia and thrombocytopenia may require DC; follow CBC and platelets; depression, insomnia, suicidal behavior, GI upset, alopecia, pruritus **Interactions:** ↑ myelosuppression with antineoplastics; ↑ effects of doxorubicin, theophylline; ↑ neurotoxicity with vinblastine **Labs:** ↑ ALT, ↓ neutrophils, platelets **NIPE:** Maintain hydration; use barrier contraception

Pemirolast (Alamast)
Uses: Allergic conjunctivitis **Action:** Mast cell stabilizer **Dose:** 1–2 gtt in each eye qid **Caution/Contra:** [C, ?/–] **Supplied:** 1 mg/mL **Notes/SE:** HA, rhinitis, cold/flu symptoms, local irritation; wait 10 min after instilling before inserting contacts

Penbutolol (Levatol)
Uses: HTN **Action:** Competitively blocks β-adrenergic receptors, β₁, β₂ **Dose:** 20–40 mg/d; ↓ dose in hepatic insufficiency **Caution/Contra:** [C (1st trimester); D if 2nd or 3rd trimester), M] Asthma, cardiogenic shock, cardiac failure, heart block, bradycardia **Supplied:** Tabs 20 mg **Notes/SE:** Flushing, hypotension, fatigue, hyperglycemia, GI upset, sexual dysfunction, bronchospasm **Interactions:** ↑ effects with CCBs, fluoroquinolones; ↑ bradycardia with adenosine, amiodarone, digitalis, dipyridamole, epinephrine, neuroleptics, phenylephrine, physostigmine, tacrine; ↑ effects of lidocaine, verapamil; ↓ effects with antacids, NSAIDs; ↓ effects of insulin, hypoglycemics, theophylline **Labs:** ↑ serum glucose, BUN, K⁺, lipoprotein, triglycerides, uric acid **NIPE:** ↑ cold sensitivity

Penciclovir (Denavir)
Uses: Herpes simplex (herpes labialis/cold sores) **Action:** Competitive inhibitor of DNA polymerase **Dose:** Apply topically at 1st sign of lesions, then q2h for 4 d **Caution/Contra:** [B, ?/–] **Supplied:** Cream 1% **Notes/SE:** Erythema, HA

Penicillin G, Aqueous (Potassium or Sodium) (Pfizerpen, Pentids)
Uses: Most gram+ infections (except staphylococci), including

streptococci; *N. meningitidis*, syphilis, clostridia, and anaerobes (except *Bacteroides*) **Action:** Bactericidal; inhibits cell wall synthesis **Dose:** *Adults.* 400,000–800,000 U PO qid; IV doses vary greatly depending on indications; range 0.6–24 MU/d in ÷ doses q4h *Peds. Newborns <1 wk:* 25,000–50,000 U/kg/dose IV q12h. *Infants 1 wk–<1 mon:* 25,000–50,000 U/kg/dose IV q8h. *Children:* 100,000–300,000 U/kg/24 h IV ÷ q4h; ↓ in renal impairment **Caution/Contra:** [B, M] **Supplied:** Tabs 200,000, 250,000, 400,000, 800,000 U; susp 200,000, 400,000 U/5 mL; powder for inj **Notes/SE:** Beware of hypersensitivity reactions; interstitial nephritis, diarrhea, hypersensitivity, seizures **Interactions:** ↑ effects with probenecid; ↑ effects of methotrexate; ↑ risk of bleeding with anticoagulants; ↓ effects with chloramphenicol, macrolides, tetracyclines; ↓ effects of oral contraceptives **Labs:** ↑ LFTs, ↓ serum albumin, folate **NIPE:** Monitor for superinfection; use barrier contraception

Penicillin G Benzathine (Bicillin)
Uses: Useful as a single-dose treatment regimen for streptococcal pharyngitis, rheumatic fever, and glomerulonephritis prophylaxis, and syphilis **Action:** Bactericidal; inhibits cell wall synthesis **Dose:** *Adults.* 1.2–2.4 MU deep IM inj q2–4wk. *Peds.* 50,000 U/kg/dose to a max of 2.4 MU/dose deep IM inj q2–4wk **Caution/Contra:** [B, M] **Supplied:** Inj 300,000, 600,000 U/mL **Notes/SE:** Sustained action with detectable levels up to 4 wk; considered drug of choice for treatment of noncongenital syphilis; Bicillin L-A contains the benzathine salt only; Bicillin C-R contains a combination of benzathine and procaine (300,000 U procaine with 300,000 U benzathine/mL or 900,000 U benzathine with 300,000 U procaine/2 mL); pain at inj site, acute interstitial nephritis, anaphylaxis **Interactions:** see Penicillin G

Penicillin G Procaine (Wycillin, others)
Uses: Moderately severe infections caused by penicillin G–sensitive organisms that respond to low, persistent serum levels **Action:** Bactericidal; inhibits cell wall synthesis **Dose:** *Adults.* 0.6–4.8 MU/d in ÷ doses q12–24h. *Peds.* 25,000–50,000 U/kg/d IM ÷ qd–bid; give probenecid at least 30 min prior to penicillin to prolong action. **Caution/Contra:** [B, M] **Supplied:** Inj 300,000, 500,000, 600,000 U/mL **Notes/SE:** Long-acting parenteral penicillin; blood levels up to 15 h; pain at inj site, interstitial nephritis, anaphylaxis; **Interactions:** see Penicillin G, Aqueous

Penicillin V (Pen-Vee K, Veetids, others)
Uses: Most gram+ infections, including streptococci **Action:** Bactericidal; inhibits cell wall synthesis **Dose:** *Adults.* 250–500 mg PO q6h, q8h, q12h. *Peds.* 25–50 mg/kg/24 h PO in 4 ÷ doses; ↓ in severe renal disease; take on empty stomach **Caution/Contra:** [B, M] **Supplied:** Tabs 125, 250, 500 mg; susp 125, 250 mg/5 mL **Notes/SE:** Well-tolerated oral penicillin; 250 mg = 400,000 U of penicillin G; GI upset, interstitial nephritis, anaphylaxis, convulsions **Interactions:** see Penicillin G, Aqueous

Pentamidine (Pentam 300, NebuPent)
Uses: Rx and prevention of PCP **Action:** Inhibits DNA, RNA, phospholipid, and protein synthesis **Dose:** *Adults & Peds.* 4 mg/kg/24 h IV qd for 14–21 d. *Adults & Peds >5 y. Prevention:*

300 mg once q4wk, administered via Respiragard II neb; IV requires ↓ dose in renal impairment. **Caution/Contra:** [C, ?] **Supplied:** Inj 300 mg/vial; aerosol 300 mg **Notes/SE:** Follow CBC (leukopenia and thrombocytopenia); monitor glucose and pancreatic function monthly for the 1st 3 mon; monitor for hypotension following IV administration; associated with pancreatic islet cell necrosis leading to hyperglycemia; chest pain, fatigue, dizziness, rash, GI upset, pancreatitis, renal impairment, blood dyscrasias **Interactions:** ↑ nephrotoxic effects with aminoglycosides, amphotericin B, capreomycin, cidofovir, cisplatin, cyclosporine, colistin, ganciclovir, methoxyflurane, polymyxin B, vancomycin; ↑ bone marrow suppression with antineoplastics, radiation therapy **Labs:** ↑ LFTs, serum K⁺ **NIPE:** Reconstitute with sterile H_2O only, inhalation may cause metallic taste; ↑ fluids to 2–3 L/d

Pentazocine (Talwin) [C-IV]   **Uses:** Moderate–severe pain **Action:** Partial narcotic agonist–antagonist **Dose:** *Adults.* 30 mg IM or IV; 50–100 mg PO q3–4h PRN. *Peds. 5–8 y:* 15 mg IM q4h PRN. *8–14 y:* 30 mg IM q4h PRN; ↓ dose in renal/hepatic impairment **Caution/Contra:** [C (1st trimester, D if prolonged use or high doses near term), +/–] **Supplied:** Tabs 50 mg (+ naloxone 0.5 mg); inj 30 mg/mL **Notes/SE:** 30–60 mg IM equianalgesic to 10 mg of morphine IM; associated with considerable dysphoria; drowsiness, GI upset, xerostomia, seizures **Interactions:** ↑ CNS depression with antihistamines, barbiturates, hypnotics, phenothiazines, alcohol; ↑ effects with cimetidine; ↑ effects of digitoxin, phenytoin, rifampin; ↓ effects of opioids **Labs:** ↑ serum amylase, lipase **NIPE:** May cause withdrawal in pts using opioids

Pentobarbital (Nembutal, others) [C-II]   **Uses:** Insomnia, convulsions, and induced coma following severe head injury **Action:** Barbiturate **Dose:** *Adults. Sedative:* 20–40 mg PO or PR q6–12h. *Hypnotic:* 100–200 mg PO or PR hs PRN. *Induced coma:* Load 5–10 mg/kg IV, then maint 1–3 mg/kg/h IV cont inf to keep the serum level between 20 and 50 mg/mL. *Peds. Hypnotic:* 2–6 mg/kg/dose PO hs PRN. *Induced coma:* See adult dosage **Caution/Contra:** [D, +/–] Significant hepatic impairment **Supplied:** Caps 50, 100 mg; elixir 18.2 mg/5 mL (= 20 mg pentobarbital); supp 30, 60, 120, 200 mg; inj 50 mg/mL **Notes/ SE:** Tolerance to sedative-hypnotic effect acquired w/n 1–2 wk; can cause respiratory depression, hypotension when used aggressively IV for cerebral edema; bradycardia, hypotension, sedation, lethargy, hangover, rash, Stevens–Johnson syndrome, blood dyscrasias, respiratory depression **Interactions:** ↑ effects with chloramphenicol, MAOIs, narcotic analgesics, kava kava, valerian, alcohol; ↓ effects of BBs, CCBs, corticosteroids, cyclosporine, digitoxin, disopyramide, doxycycline, estrogen, griseofulvin, neuroleptics, oral anticoagulants, oral contraceptives, propafenone, quinidine, tacrolimus, theophylline, TCAs **Labs:** ↑ ammonia; ↓ bilirubin

Pentosan Polysulfate Sodium (Elmiron)   **Uses:** Relief of pain/discomfort associated with interstitial cystitis **Action:** Acts as buffer on bladder wal

Dose: 100 mg PO tid on empty stomach with water 1 h ac or 2 h pc **Caution/Contra:** [B, ?/–] **Supplied:** Caps 100 mg **Notes/SE:** Alopecia, diarrhea, nausea, HAs, ↑ LFTs, anticoagulant effects, thrombocytopenia **Interactions:** Risk of ↑ anticoagulation with anticoagulants, ASA, thrombolytics

Pentostatin (Nipent) **WARNING:** Fatal, acute pulmonary toxicity with concomitant administration of other chemotherapeutic agents **Uses:** Hairy cell leukemia, CLL, mycosis fungoides, ALL, and adult T-cell leukemia **Action:** Irreversible inhibitor of adenosine deaminase **Dose:** 4–5 mg/m²/wk for 3 consecutive wk; ↓ dose in renal/hepatic impairment **Caution/Contra:** [D, ?/–] Leukopenia **Supplied:** Inj 10 mg **Notes/SE:** Renal dysfunction; myelosuppression (especially leukopenia), lymphocytopenia, fever, and infection possible; neurologic toxicity symptoms (lethargy and fatigue), dry skin, keratoconjunctivitis, N/V **Interactions:** ↑ effects with allopurinol, fludarabine, vidarabine

Pentoxifylline (Trental) **Uses:** Symptomatic management of peripheral vascular disease **Action:** Lowers blood cell viscosity by restoring erythrocyte flexibility **Dose:** 400 mg PO tid pc; treat for at least 8 wk to see full effect; ↓ to bid if GI or CNS effects occur **Caution/Contra:** [C, +/–] Cerebral or retinal hemorrhage **Supplied:** Tabs 400 mg **Notes/SE:** Dizziness, HA, GI upset **Interactions:** ↑ effects with cimetidine, fluoroquinolones, H₂ antagonists, warfarin; ↑ effects of antihypertensives, theophyllin **Labs:** ↓ serum calcium, magnesium **NIPE:** Take with food

Pergolide (Permax) **Uses:** Parkinson's disease **Action:** Centrally active dopamine receptor agonist **Dose:** Initially, 0.05 mg PO tid, titrated q2–3d to desired effect; usual maint 2–3 mg/d in ÷ doses **Caution/Contra:** [B, ?/–] Ergot sensitivity **Supplied:** Tabs 0.05, 0.25, 1.0 mg **Notes/SE:** May cause hypotension during initiation of therapy; dizziness, somnolence, confusion, nausea, constipation, dyskinesia, rhinitis, MI **Interactions:** ↑ risk of dyskinesia with levodopa; ↑ hypotension with antihypertensives; ↓ effects with antipsychotics, butyrophenones, haloperidol, metoclopramide, phenothiazines, thioxanthenes **Labs:** ↓ prolactin **NIPE:** Take with food

Perindopril Erbumine (Aceon) **Uses:** HTN, CHF, DN, post-MI **Action:** ACE inhibitor **Dose:** 4–8 mg/d; avoid taking with food; ↓ dose in elderly/renal impairment **Caution/Contra:** [C (1st trimester, D 2nd and 3rd trimesters), ?/–] ACE-inhibitor-induced angioedema, bilateral renal artery stenosis, primary hyperaldosteronism **Supplied:** Tabs 2, 4, 8 mg **Notes/SE:** HA, hypotension, dizziness, GI upset, cough **Interactions:** ↑ effects with antihypertensives, diuretics; ↑ effects of cyclosporine, insulin, lithium, sulfonylureas, tacrolimus; ↓ effects with NSAIDs **Labs:** ↑ serum K⁺, LFTs, uric acid, cholesterol, creatinine **NIPE:** ↓ effects if taken with food; risk of persistant cough

Permethrin (Nix, Elimite) **Uses:** Eradication of lice and scabies **Action:** Pediculicide **Dose:** *Adults & Peds.* Saturate hair and scalp; allow 10 min before rinsing **Caution/Contra:** [B, ?/–] **Supplied:** Topical liq 1%; cream 5%

Notes/SE: Local irritation **NIPE:** Drug remains on hair up to 2 wk, reapply in 1 wk if live lice

Perphenazine (Trilafon)
Uses: Psychotic disorders, intractable hiccups, severe nausea **Action:** Phenothiazine; blocks dopaminergic receptors in the brain **Dose:** *Adults. Antipsychotic:* 4–16 mg PO tid; max 64 mg/d. *Hiccups:* 5 mg IM q6h PRN or 1 mg IV at intervals not <1–2 mg/min to a max of 5 mg. *Peds. 1–6 y:* 4–6 mg/d in ÷ doses. *6–12 y:* 6 mg/d in ÷ doses. *>12 y:* 4–16 mg 2–4×/d; ↓ dose in hepatic insufficiency **Caution/Contra:** [C, ?/–] Phenothiazine sensitivity, narrow-angle glaucoma, bone marrow depression, severe liver or cardiac disease; severe hyper-/hypotension **Supplied:** Tabs 2, 4, 8, 16 mg; oral conc 16 mg/5 mL; inj 5 mg/mL **Notes/SE:** Hypotension, tachycardia, bradycardia, extrapyramidal symptoms, drowsiness, seizures, photosensitivity, skin discoloration, blood dyscrasias, constipation **Interactions:** ↑ effects with antidepressants; ↑ effects of anticholinergics, antidepressants, propranolol, phenytoin; ↑ CNS effects with CNS depressants, alcohol; ↓ effects with antacids, lithium, phenobarbital, caffeine, tobacco; ↓ effects of levodopa, lithium **Labs:** ↑ serum cholesterol, glucose, ↓ uric acid, false + urine PRG test **NIPE:** Take oral dose with food; risk of photosensitivity—use sunscreen

Phenazopyridine (Pyridium, others)
Uses: Lower urinary tract irritation **Action:** Local anesthetic on urinary tract mucosa **Dose:** *Adults.* 100–200 mg PO tid. *Peds 6–12 y.* 12 mg/kg/24 h PO in 3 ÷ doses; ↓ in renal insufficiency **Caution/Contra:** [B, ?] Renal/hepatic disease **Supplied:** Tabs 100, 200 mg **Notes/SE:** GI disturbances; causes red-orange urine color, which can stain clothing; HA, dizziness, acute renal failure, methemoglobinemia **Labs:** Interferes with urinary tests for glucose, ketones, bilirubin, protein, steroids **NIPE:** Urine may turn red; take >meals

Phenelzine (Nardil)
Uses: Depression **Action:** MAOI **Dose:** *Adults.* 15 mg tid. *Elderly:* 15–60 mg/d in ÷ doses; avoid tyramine-containing foods **Caution/Contra:** [C, –] Interactions with SSRI, ergots, tripans **Supplied:** Tabs 15 mg **Notes/SE:** May cause orthostatic hypotension; edema, dizziness, sedation, rash, sexual dysfunction, xerostomia, constipation, urinary retention; may take 2–4 wk to see therapeutic effect **Interactions:** ↑ HTN reaction with amphetamines, fluoxetine, levodopa, metaraminol, phenylephrine, phenylpropanolamine, pseudoephedrine, reserpine, sertraline, tyramine, alcohol, foods with tyramine, caffeine, tryptophan; ↑ effects of barbiturates, narcotics, sedatives, sumatriptan, TCAs, ephedra, ginseng **Labs:** ↓ glucose, false + increase in bilirubin & uric acid

Phenobarbital [C-IV]
Uses: Seizure disorders, insomnia, and anxiety **Action:** Barbiturate **Dose:** *Adults. Sedative-hypnotic:* 30–120 mg PO or IM PRN. *Anticonvulsant:* Loading dose of 10–12 mg/kg in 3 ÷ doses, then 1–3 mg/kg/24 h PO, IM, or IV. *Peds. Sedative-hypnotic:* 2–3 mg/kg/24 h PO or IM hs PRN. *Anticonvulsant:* Loading dose of 15–20 mg/kg ÷ into 2 equal doses 4 h apart, then 3–5 mg/kg/24 h PO ÷ in 2–3 doses **Caution/Contra:** [D, M] Porphyria **Supplied:** Tabs

8, 15, 16, 30, 32, 60, 65, 100 mg; elixir 15, 20 mg/5 mL; inj 30, 60, 65, 130 mg/mL **Notes/SE:** Tolerance develops to sedation; paradoxic hyperactivity seen in pediatric patients; long half-life allows single daily dosing (Table 2, page 243); bradycardia, hypotension, hangover, Stevens–Johnson syndrome, blood dyscrasias, respiratory depression **Interactions:** ↑ CNS depression with CNS depressants, anesthetics, antianxiety meds, antihistamines, narcotic analgesics, alcohol, Indian snakeroot, kava kava; ↑ effects with chloramphenicol, MAOIs, procarbazine, valproic acid; ↓ effects with rifampin; ↓ effects of anticoagulants, BBs, carbamazepine, clozapine, corticosteroids, doxorubicin, doxycycline, estrogens, felodipine, griseofulvin, haloperidol, methadone, metronidazole, oral contraceptives, phenothiazines, quinidine, theophylline, TCAs, verapamil **Lab:** ↑ LFTs, creatinine, ↑ or ↓ bilirubin **NIPE:** May take 2–3 wk for full effects, ⊘ d/c abruptly

Phenylephrine (Neo-Synephrine)
Uses: Vascular failure in shock, hypersensitivity, or drug-induced hypotension; nasal congestion; mydriatic **Action:** α-Adrenergic agonist **Dose:** *Adults. Mild–moderate hypotension:* 2–5 mg IM or SC elevates BP for 2 h; 0.1–0.5 mg IV elevates BP for 15 min. *Severe hypotension/shock:* Initiate cont inf @ 100–180 mg/min; after BP is stabilized, maint rate of 40–60 mg/min. *Nasal congestion:* 1–2 sprays/nostril PRN. *Ophth:* 1 gt 15–30 min before exam. *Peds. Hypotension:* 5–20 μg/kg/dose IV q10–15 min or 0.1–0.5 mg/kg/min IV inf, titrated to desired effect. *Nasal congestion:* 1 spray/nostril q3–4h PRN **Caution/Contra:** [C, +/–] HTN, bradycardia, arrhythmias, acute pancreatitis, hepatitis, coronary disease, narrow-angle glaucoma **Supplied:** Inj 10 mg/mL; nasal soln 0.125, 0.16, 0.25, 0.5, 1%; ophth soln 0.12, 2.5, 10% **Notes/SE:** Promptly restore blood volume if loss has occurred; use large veins for inf to avoid extravasation; phentolamine 10 mg in 10–15 mL of NS for local inj as antidote for extravasation; arrhythmias, HTN, peripheral vasoconstriction activity potentiated by oxytocin, MAOIs, and TCAs; HA, weakness, necrosis, ↓ renal perfusion **Interactions:** ↑ HTN with BBs, MAOIs; ↑ pressor response with guanethidine, methyldopa, reserpine, TCAs

Phenytoin (Dilantin)
Uses: Seizure disorders **Action:** Inhibits seizure spread in the motor cortex **Dose:** *Adults & Peds. Load:* 15–20 mg/kg IV, max inf rate 25 mg/min or PO in 400-mg doses at 4-h intervals. *Adults. Maint:* Initially, 200 mg PO or IV bid or 300 mg hs; then follow serum conc. *Peds. Maint:* 4–7 mg/kg/24 h PO or IV ÷ qd–bid; avoid oral susp if possible due to erratic absorption **Caution/Contra:** [D, +] Heart block, sinus bradycardia **Supplied:** Caps 30, 100 mg; chew tabs 50 mg; oral susp 30, 125 mg/5 mL; inj 50 mg/mL **Notes/SE:** Follow levels (Table 2, Page 243); note: Phenytoin is bound to albumin, and levels reflect both bound and free phenytoin; in the presence of ↓ albumin and azotemia, low phenytoin levels may be therapeutic (normal free levels); nystagmus and ataxia early signs of toxicity; gum hyperplasia with long-term use. *IV:* Hypotension, bradycardia, arrhythmias, phlebitis; peripheral neuropathy, rash, blood dyscrasias, Stevens–Johnson syndrome **Interactions:** ↑ effects with amiodarone, allopurinol, chloramphenicol,

disulfiram, isoniazid, omeprazole, sulfonamides, quinolones, trimethoprim; ↑ effects of lithium; ↓ effects with cimetidine, cisplatin, diazoxide, folate, pyridoxine, rifampin; ↓ effects of azole antifungals, benzodiazepines, carbamazepine, corticosteroids, cyclosporine, digitalis glycosides, doxycycline, furosemide, levodopa, oral contraceptives, quinidine, tacrolimus, theophylline, thyroid meds, valproic acid **Labs:** ↑ serum cholesterol, glucose, alkaline phosphatase **NIPE:** Take with food; may alter urine color; use barrier contraception; ⊘ d/c abruptly

Physostigmine (Antilirium) **Uses:** Antidote for TCA, atropine, and scopolamine overdose; glaucoma **Action:** Reversible cholinesterase inhibitor **Dose:** *Adults.* 2 mg IV or IM q20min. *Peds.* 0.01–0.03 mg/kg/dose IV q15–30 min to total of 2 mg if necessary **Caution/Contra:** [C, ?] GI or GU obstruction **Supplied:** Inj 1 mg/mL; ophth oint 0.25% **Notes/SE:** Rapid IV administration associated with convulsions; cholinergic side effects; may cause asystole sweating, salivation, lacrimation, GI upset, changes in heart rate **Interactions:** ↑ respiratory depression with succinylcholine, ↑ effects with cholinergics, jahoranki tree, pill-bearing spurge **Labs:** ↑ ALT, AST, serum amylase

Phytonadione [Vitamin K] (AquaMEPHYTON, others) **Uses:** Coagulation disorders caused by faulty formation of factors II, VII, IX, and X; hyperalimentation **Action:** Needed for the production of factors II, VII, IX, and X **Dose:** *Children and Adults.* *Anticoagulant-induced prothrombin deficiency:* 1.0–10.0 mg PO or IV slowly. *Hyperalimentation:* 10 mg IM or IV qwk. *Infants.* 0.5–1.0 mg/dose IM, SC, or PO **Caution/Contra:** [C, +] **Supplied:** Tabs 5 mg; inj 2, 10 mg/mL **Notes/SE:** With parenteral Rx, the 1st change in prothrombin usually seen in 12–24 h; anaphylaxis can result from IV dosage; administer IV slowly; GI upset (oral), inj site reactions **Interactions:** ↓ effects with antibiotics, cholestyramine, colestipol, salicylates, sucralfate; ↓ effects of oral anticoagulants **Labs:** Falsely ↑ urine steroids

Pimecrolimus (Elidel) **Uses:** Atopic dermatitis **Action:** T-lymphocyte inhibition **Dose:** Apply bid for at least 1 wk resolution; apply to dry skin only; wash hands after **Caution/Contra:** [C, ?/–] Caution with local infection, lymphadenopathy **Supplied:** Ointment 0.03%, 0.1%; 30-g, 60-g tubes **Notes/SE:** Phototoxicity, local irritation/burning, flu-like symptoms

Pindolol (Visken) **Uses:** HTN **Action:** Competitively blocks β-adrenergic receptors, $β_1$, $β_2$, ISA **Dose:** 5–10 mg bid, 60 mg/d max; ↓ dose in hepatic/renal failure **Caution/Contra:** [B (1st trimester); D if 2nd or 3rd trimester), +/–] Uncompensated CHF, cardiogenic shock, bradycardia, heart block, asthma, COPD **Supplied:** Tabs 5, 10 mg **Notes/SE:** Insomnia, dizziness, fatigue, edema, GI upset, dyspnea; fluid retention may exacerbate CHF **Interactions:** ↑ effects with amiodarone, antihypertensives, diuretics; ↓ effects with NSAIDs; ↓ effect of hypoglycemics **Labs:** ↑ LFTs, uric acid **NIPE:** ⊘ d/c abruptly; ↑ cold sensitivity

Pioglitazone (Actos) **Uses:** Type 2 DM **Action:** Increases insulin sensitivity **Dose:** 15–45 mg/d **Caution/Contra:** [C, –] Contra in hepatic impairment

Supplied: Tabs 15, 30, 45 mg **Notes/SE:** Weight gain, URI, HA, hypoglycemia, edema **Interactions:** ↑ effects with ketoconazole; ↓ effects of oral contraceptives **Labs:** ↑ LFTs, ↓ HMG, HCT **NIPE:** Take w/o regard to food; use barrier contraception

Pipecuronium (Arduan)
Uses: Adjunct to general anesthesia **Action:** Nondepolarizing neuromuscular blocker **Dose:** *Adults & Peds.* 0.05–0.085 mg/kg initially, then 0.5–2 μg/kg/min (ICU); ↓ dose in renal failure **Supplied:** Inj 10 mg; **Caution/Contra:** [C, ?] **Notes/SE:** Hypotension, bradycardia **Interactions:** ↑ effects with aminoglycosides, bacitracin, BBs, CCBs, clindamycin, colistin, cyclosporine, enflurane, furosemide, halothane, isoflurane, lithium, magnesium salts, manitol, polymyxin B, quinidine, tetracyclines, vancomycin; ↓ effects with calcium, carbamazepine, steroids, theophylline, caffeine **NIPE:** Does not affect pain perception or anxiety

Piperacillin (Pipracil)
Uses: Infections caused by gram– bacteria (including *Klebsiella, Proteus, E. coli, Enterobacter, P. aeruginosa,* and *Serratia*) of skin, bone, respiratory tract, urinary tract, and abdomen, and septicemia **Action:** Bactericidal; inhibits cell wall synthesis **Dose:** *Adults.* 3 g IV q4–6h. *Peds.* 200–300 mg/kg/d IV ÷ q4–6h; ↓ dose in renal failure **Caution/Contra:** [B, M] Penicillin sensitivity **Supplied:** Inj **Notes/SE:** Often used in combination with aminoglycoside; ↓ platelet aggregation, interstitial nephritis, renal failure, anaphylaxis, hemolytic anemia **Interactions:** ↑ effects with probenecid; ↑ effects of anticoagulants, methotrexate; ↓ effects with macrolides, tetracyclines; ↓ effects of oral contraceptives **Labs:** ↑ LFTs, BUN, creatinine, positive direct Coombs test, ↓ K+ **NIPE:** Inactivation of aminoglycosides if drugs given together – admin at least 1 h apart

Piperacillin-Tazobactam (Zosyn)
Uses: Infections caused by gram– bacteria (including *Klebsiella, Proteus, E. coli, Enterobacter, P. aeruginosa,* and *Serratia*) involving skin, bone, respiratory tract, urinary tract, and abdomen, and septicemia **Action:** Bactericidal; inhibits cell wall synthesis **Dose:** *Adults.* 3.375–4.5 g IV q6h; ↓ dose in renal failure **Caution/Contra:** [B, M] Penicillin or β-lactam sensitivity **Supplied:** Inj **Notes/SE:** Often used in combination with aminoglycoside; diarrhea, HA, insomnia, GI upset, serum sickness-like reaction, pseudomembranous colitis; **see Piperacillin Interactions; Additional Labs:** ↓ HMG, HCT, protein, albumin

Pirbuterol (Maxair)
Uses: Prevention and Rx of reversible bronchospasm **Action:** β₂-Adrenergic agonists **Dose:** *Adults & Peds >12 y.* 2 inhal q4–6h; max 12 inhal/d **Caution/Contra:** [C, ?/–] **Supplied:** Aerosol 0.2 mg/actuation; Autohaler dry powder 0.2 mg/actuation **Notes/SE:** Nervousness, restlessness, trembling, HA, taste changes, tachycardia **Interactions:** ↑ effects with epinephrine, sympathomimetics; ↑ vascular effects with MAOIs, TCAs; ↓ effects with BBs **NIPE:** Rinse mouth after use; shake well before use

Piroxicam (Feldene)
Uses: Arthritis and pain **Action:** NSAID; inhibits prostaglandin synthesis **Dose:** 10–20 mg/d **Caution/Contra:** [B (1st trimester; D if

3rd trimester or near term), +] GI bleeding, ASA or NSAID sensitivity **Supplied:** Caps 10, 20 mg **Notes/SE:** Dizziness, rash, GI upset, edema, acute renal failure, peptic ulcer **Interactions:** ↑ effects with probenecid; ↑ effects of aminoglycosides, anticoagulants, hypoglycemics, lithium, methotrexate; ↑ risk of bleeding with ASA, corticosteroids, NSAIDs, feverfew, garlic, ginger, ginkgo biloba, alcohol; ↓ effect with BBs, antacids, cholestyramine; ↓ effect of BBs, diuretics **Labs:** ↑ BUN, LFTs, serum chloride, serum sodium, PT **NIPE:** Take with food, full effect >2 wk admin, ↑ risk of photosensitivity

Plasma Protein Fraction (Plasmanate, others)   **Uses:** Shock
and hypotension **Action:** Plasma volume expansion **Dose:** *Adults.* Initially, 250–500 mL IV (not >10 mL/min); subsequent inf depends on clinical response. *Peds.* 10–15 mL/kg/dose IV; subsequent inf depend on clinical response **Caution/Contra:** [C, +] **Supplied:** Inj 5% **Notes/SE:** 130–160 mEq Na/L; not substitute for RBC; hypotension associated with rapid inf; hypocoagulability, metabolic acidosis, PE

Plicamycin (Mithracin)   **Uses:** Hypercalcemia of malignancy; dissemi-
nated embryonal cell carcinoma or germ cell tumors of the testis **Action:** Antibiotic; binds to the outside of the DNA molecule, interrupting DNA-directed RNA synthesis, DNA intercalation **Dose:** *Hypercalcemia:* 25 μg/kg/d IV qod for 3–8 doses. *CA:* 25–30 μg/kg/d for 8–10 d; ↓ dose in renal failure **Caution/Contra:** [D, ?] Thrombocytopenia, coagulation disorders, bone marrow impairment **Supplied:** Inj **Notes/SE:** Thrombocytopenia; drug-induced deficiency of clotting factors II, V, VII, and X, resulting in bleeding and bruising **Interactions:** ↑ risk of bleeding with anticoagulants, ASA, cephalosporines, NSAIDs, thrombolytics; ↑ hypocalcemia with bisphosphonates, calcitonin, foscarnet, glucagons **Labs:** ↑ LFTs, BUN, creatinine, ↓ serum calcium, K+, phosphorus **NIPE:** ⊘ immunizations, exposure to infections; use birth control

Pneumococcal Vaccine, Polyvalent (Pneumovax-23)   **Uses:**
Immunization against pneumococcal infections in patients predisposed to or at high risk **Action:** Active immunization **Dose:** *Adults & Peds >2 y.* 0.5 mL IM **Caution/Contra:** [C, M] Do not vaccinate during immunosuppressive therapy, active infection, Hodgkin's disease, children <2 y. **Supplied:** Inj 25 mg each of polysaccharide isolates/0.5-mL dose **Notes/SE:** Local reactions, arthralgia, fever, myalgia **Interactions:** ↓ effects with corticosteroids, immunosuppressants

Pneumococcal 7-Valent Conjugate Vaccine (Prevnar)   **Uses:**
Immunization against pneumococcal infections in infants and children **Action:** Active immunization **Dose:** 0.5 mL IM/dose; series of 3 doses; 1st dose at 2 mon of age with subsequent doses q2mon **Caution/Contra:** [C, +] Diphtheria toxoid sensitivity, febrile illness, thrombocytopenia **Supplied:** Inj **Notes/SE:** Local reactions, arthralgia, fever, myalgia

Podophyllin (Podocon-25, Condylox Gel 0.5%, Condylox)
Uses: Topical therapy of benign growths (genital and perianal warts [condylomata

acuminata], papillomas, fibroids) **Action:** Direct antimitotic effect; exact mecha-...ism unknown **Dose:** Apply Condylox gel and Condylox 3 consecutive d/wk for 4 ... ...-25 ...aringly on the lesion, leave on for 1–4 h, then thoroughly ...plied: Podocon-25 (w/benzoin) ... bleeding lesions, immunocompromise **Sup-**Condylox soln 0.5% 35 g (clear) ... 0.5% 35 g (clear) **Notes/SE:** Podocon-25 applied only by ... ...cian; do not dispense; local reactions, significant absorption; anemias, tachycardia, paresthesias, GI upset, renal/hepatic damage

Polyethylene Glycol [PEG]-Electrolyte Solution (GoLYTELY, CoLyte)
Uses: Bowel prep prior to examination or surgery **Action:** Osmotic cathartic **Dose:** *Adults.* Following 3–4 h fast, drink 240 mL of soln until 4 L is consumed. *Peds.* 25–40 mL/kg/h for 4–10 h **Caution/Contra:** [C, ?] GI obstruction, bowel perforation, megacolon, ulcerative colitis **Supplied:** Powder for reconstitution to 4 L in container **Notes/SE:** 1st BM should occur in approximately 1 h; cramping or nausea, bloating

Polymyxin B and Hydrocortisone (Otobiotic Otic)
Uses: Superficial bacterial infections of external ear canal **Action:** Antibiotic antiinflammatory combination **Dose:** 4 gtt in ear(s) tid–qid **Caution/Contra:** [B, ?] **Supplied:** Soln polymyxin B 10,000 U/hydrocortisone 0.5%/mL **Notes/SE:** Useful in neomycin allergy, local irritation

Potassium Citrate (Urocit-K)
Uses: Alkalinizes urine, prevention of urinary stones (uric acid, Ca stones if hypocitraturic) **Action:** Urinary alkalinizer **Caution/Contra:** [A, +] Severe renal impairment, dehydration, hyperkalemia, peptic ulcer; use of K-sparing diuretics or salt substitutes **Dose:** 10–20 mEq PO tid with meals, max 100 mEq/d **Notes/SE:** Tabs 540 mg = 5 mEq, 1080 mg = 10 mEq; GI upset, hypocalcemia, hyperkalemia, metabolic alkalosis; **Interactions:** ↑ risk of hyperkalemia with ACEIs, K⁺-sparing diuretics

Potassium Citrate and Citric Acid (Polycitra-K)
Uses: Alkalinize urine, prevention of urinary stones (uric acid, Ca stones if hypocitraturic) **Action:** Urinary alkalinizer **Dose:** 10–20 mEq PO tid with meals, max 100 mEq/d **Caution/Contra:** [A, +] Severe renal impairment, dehydration, hyperkalemia, peptic ulcer; use of K-sparing diuretics or salt substitutes **Notes/SE:** Soln 10 mEq/5 mL; powder 30 mEq/packet; GI upset, hypocalcemia, hyperkalemia, metabolic alkalosis **Interactions:** ↑ risk of hyperkalemia with ACEIs, K⁺-sparing diuretics

Potassium Iodide [Lugol's Solution] (SSKI, Thyro-Block)
Uses: Thyroid storm, reduction of vascularity before thyroid surgery, blocks thyroid uptake of radioactive isotopes of iodine, thins bronchial secretions **Action:** Iodine supplement **Dose:** *Adults & Peds. Preop thyroidectomy:* 50–250 mg PO tid (2–6 gtt strong iodine soln); administer 10 d preop. *Peds 1 y. Thyroid crisis:* 300 mg (6 gtt SSKI q8h). *<1 y.* 1/2 adult dose **Caution/Contra:** [D, +] Iodine sensitivity, hyperkalemia, tuberculosis, PE, bronchitis, renal impairment **Supplied:** Tabs

130 mg; soln (SSKI) 1 g/mL; Lugol's soln, strong iodine 100 mg/mL; syr... .25 mg/5 mL **Notes/SE:** Fever, HA, urticaria, angioedema, goiter, GI upset, eosinophilia **Interactions:** ↑ risk of hypothyroidism with antithyroid drugs and lithium; ↑ risk of hyperkalemia with ACEIs, K⁺-sparing diuretics, K⁺ supplements **Labs:** May alter thyroid function tests **NIPE:** Take >meals with food or milk

Potassium Supplements (Kaon, Kaochlor, K-Lor, Slow-K, Micro-K, Klorvess, others) **Uses:** Prevention or Rx of hypokalemia
(often related to diuretic use) **Action:** Supplementation of K **Dose: Adults.** 20–10 mEq/d PO ÷ qd–bid; IV 10–20 mEq/h, max 40 mEq/h and 150 mEq/d; *Peds.* mEq/kg/d PO ÷ qd–qid; *IV max dose 0.5–1 mEq/kg/h Caution/Contra:* [A, +] *Use cautiously in renal insufficiency* as well as with NSAIDs and ACE inhibitors **Supplied:** Oral forms (Table 8, page 256); injectable forms **Notes/SE:** Can cause GI irritation; mix powder and liq with beverage (unsalted tomato juice, etc); follow serum K⁺; Cl⁻ salt recommended in coexisting alkalosis; for coexisting acidosis use acetate, bicarbonate, citrate, or gluconate salt; bradycardia, hyperkalemia, heart block **Interactions:** ↑ effects with ACEI, K⁺-sparing diuretics, salt substitutes **NIPE:** Take with food

Pramipexole (Mirapex) **Uses:** Parkinson's disease **Action:** Dopamine agonist **Dose:** 1.5–4.5 mg/d, beginning with 0.375 mg/d in 3 ÷ doses; titrate dosage slowly **Caution/Contra:** [C, ?/–] **Supplied:** Tabs 0.125, 0.25, 1, 1.5 mg **Notes/SE:** Orthostatic hypotension, asthenia, somnolence, abnormal dreams, GI upset, EPS **Interactions:** ↑ effects with cimetidine, diltiazem, quinidine, quinine, ranitidine, triamterene, verapamil; ↑ effects of levodopa; ↑ CNS depression with CNS depressants, alcohol; ↓ effects with antipsychotics, butyrophenones, metoclopramide, phenothiazines, thioxanthenes **NIPE:** May take with food; ⊘ d/c abruptly

Pramoxine (Anusol Ointment, Proctofoam-NS, others) **Uses:** Relief of pain and itching from external and internal hemorrhoids and anorectal surgery; topical for burns and dermatosis **Action:** Topical anesthetic **Dose:** Apply cream, oint, gel, or spray freely to anal area q3h **Caution/Contra:** [C, ?] **Supplied:** [OTC] All 1%; foam (Proctofoam-NS), cream, oint, lotion, gel, pads, spray **Notes/SE:** Contact dermatitis **NIPE:** ⊘ use on large areas

Pramoxine + Hydrocortisone (Enzone, Proctofoam-HC) **Uses:** Relief of pain and itching from hemorrhoids **Action:** Topical anesthetic, antiinflammatory **Dose:** Apply freely to anal area tid–qid **Caution/Contra:** [C, ?/–] **Supplied:** Cream pramoxine 1%, acetate 0.5/1%; foam pramoxine 1%, hydrocortisone 1%; lotion pramoxine 1%, hydrocortisone 0.25/1/2.5%, pramoxine 2.5%, hydrocortisone 1% **Notes/SE:** Contact dermatitis **NIPE:** ⊘ use on large areas

Pravastatin (Pravachol) **Uses:** Reduction of ↑ cholesterol levels **Action:** HMG-CoA reductase inhibitor **Dose:** 10–40 mg PO hs; ↓ dose with significant renal/hepatic insufficiency **Caution/Contra:** [X, –] Liver disease or persistent

LFT ↑ **Supplied:** Tabs 10, 20, 40 mg **Notes/SE:** Use caution with concurrent gemfibrozil; HA, GI upset, hepatitis, myopathy, renal failure **Interactions:** ↑ risk of myopathy & rhabdomyolysis with clarithromycin, clofibrate, cyclosporine, danazol, erythromycin, fluoxetine, gemfibrozil, niacin, nefazodone, troleandomycin; ↑ effects with azole antifungals, cimetidine, grapefruit juice; ↓ effects with cholestyramine, isradipine **Labs:** ↑ LFTs **NIPE:** ⊘ PRG, breast-feeding; take w/o regard to food; full effect may take up to 4 wks; ↑ risk of photosensitivity - use sunscreen

Prazosin (Minipress)   **Uses:** HTN **Action:** Peripherally acting α-adrenergic blocker **Dose:** *Adults.* 1 mg PO tid; can ↑ to max daily dose of up to 20 mg/d. *Peds.* 5–25 µg/kg/dose q6h, up to 25 µg/kg/dose **Caution/Contra:** [C, ?] **Supplied:** Caps 1, 2, 5 mg **Notes/SE:** Can cause orthostatic hypotension, take the 1st dose hs; tolerance develops to this effect; tachyphylaxis may result; dizziness, edema, palpitations, fatigue, GI upset **Interactions:** ↑ hypotension with antihypertensives, diuretics, nitrates, alcohol; ↓ effects with NSAIDs, butcher's broom **Labs:** ↑ serum sodium levels, vanillylmandelic acid level; alters test for pheochromocytoma **NIPE:** ⊘ d/c abruptly

Prednisolone See **Steroids, Systemic,** page 209, and Table 4, page 248, and **Steroids, Topical,** page 210, and Table 5, page 249 **Interactions:** ↑ effects with clarithromycin, erythromycin, estrogen, ketoconazole, oral contraceptives, troleandomycin; ↓ effects with antacids, aminoglutethamide, barbiturates, cholestyramine, colestipol, phenytoin, rifampin; ↓ effects of anticoagulants, hypoglycemics, isoniazid, salicylates, vaccine toxoids **Labs:** False neg skin allergy tests; false ↑ cortisol, digoxin, theophylline **NIPE:** ⊘ use live virus vaccines, ⊘ d/c abruptly; take with food.

Prednisone See **Steroids, Systemic,** page 209, and Table 4, page 248, and **Steroids, Topical,** page 210, and Table 5, page 249; **Interactions:** ↑ effects with clarithromycin, cyclosporine, erythromycin, estrogen, ketoconazole, oral contraceptives, troleandomycin; ↓ effects with antacids, aminoglutethamide, barbiturates, carbamazepine, cholestyramine, colestipol, phenytoin, rifampin; ↓ effects of anticoagulants, hypoglycemics, isoniazid, salicylates, vaccine toxoids **Labs:** False neg skin allergy tests, false ↑ cortisol, digoxin, theophylline **NIPE:** Take with food; ⊘ use live virus vaccine, ⊘ d/c abruptly, infection may be masked

Probenecid (Benemid, others)   **Uses:** Prevention of gout and hyperuricemia; prolongs serum levels of penicillins or cephalosporins **Action:** Renal tube blocking agent **Dose:** *Adults.* *Gout:* 250 mg bid for >1 wk, then 0.5 g PO bid; can ↑ by 500 mg/mon up to 2–3 g/d. *Antibiotic effect:* 1–2 g PO 30 min <antibiotic dose. *Peds >2 y.* 25 mg/kg, then 40 mg/kg/d PO ÷ qid **Caution/Contra:** [B, ?] High-dose ASA, moderate/severe renal impairment, age <2 y **Supplied:** Tabs 500 mg **Notes/SE:** Do not use during acute gout attack; HA, GI upset, rash, pruritus, dizziness, blood dyscrasias **Interactions:** ↑ effects of acyclovir, allopurinol; ↑ effects of benzodiazepines, cephalosporins, ciprofloxacin, clofibrate, dapsone, dyphylline, methotrexate, NSAIDs, olanzapine, rifampin, sulfonamides, sulfonylureas zidovudine; ↓ effects with niacin, alcohol; ↓ effects of penicillamine **Labs:** ↑ urine glucose; false ↑ level of theophylline **NIPE:** Take with food, ↑ fluids to 2–3 L/d; ⊘ ASA, NSAIDs, salicylates

Procainamide (Pronestyl, Procan)   Uses: Supraventricular and ventricular arrhythmias **Action:** Class 1A antiarrhythmic **Dose:** *Adults. Recurrent VF/VT:* 20 mg/min IV (max total 17 mg/kg). *Maint:* 1–4 mg/min. *Stable wide-complex tachycardia of unknown origin, AF with rapid rate in WPW syndrome:* 20 mg/min IV until arrhythmia suppression, hypotension, QRS widens >50%, then 1–4 mg/min. *Chronic dosing:* 50 mg/kg/d PO in ÷ doses q4–6h. *Peds. Chronic maint:* 15–50 mg/kg/24 h PO ÷ q3–6h; ↓ dose in renal/hepatic impairment **Caution/Contra:** [C, +] CHB, 2nd- or 3rd-degree heart block w/o pacemaker, torsades de pointes, SLE **Supplied:** Tabs and caps 250, 375, 500 mg; SR tabs 250, 500, 750, 1000 mg; inj 100, 500 mg/mL **Notes/SE:** Follow levels (Table 2, page 245); can cause hypotension and a lupus-like syndrome; GI upset, taste perversion, arrhythmias, tachycardia, heart block, angioneurotic edema **Interactions:** ↑ effects with acetazolamide, amiodarone, cimetidine, ranitidine, trimethoprim; ↑ effects of anticholinergics, antihypertensives; ↓ effects with procaine, alcohol **Labs:** ↑ LFTs, + Coombs test **NIPE:** Take with food if GI upset, ⊘ crush sustained release tab

Procarbazine (Matulane)   WARNING: Highly toxic; handle with care
Uses: Hodgkin's disease, NHL, brain tumors **Action:** Alkylating agent; inhibits DNA and RNA synthesis **Dose:** 2–4 mg/kg/d ×7 d, then 4–6 mg/kg/d until response; maint 1–2 mg/kg/d in combination, 60–100 mg/m²/d ×10–14 d **Caution/Contra:** [D, ?] Alcohol ingestion **Supplied:** Caps 50 mg **Notes/SE:** Myelosuppression, hemolytic reactions (with G6PD deficiency), N/V/D; disulfiram-like reaction; cutaneous reactions; constitutional symptoms, myalgia, and arthralgia; CNS effects, azoospermia, and cessation of menses **Interactions:** ↑ CNS depression with antihistamines, antihypertensives, barbiturates, CNS depressants, narcotics, phenothiazines; ↑ effects of hypoglycemics; ↑ risk of HTN with guanethidine, levodopa, MAOIs, methyldopa, sympathomimetics, TCAs, tyramine-containing foods; ↓ effects of digoxin **NIPE:** Disulfiram-like reaction with alcohol; ↑ fluids to 2–3 L/d; ↑ risk of photosensitivity – use sunscreen; ⊘ exposure to infection

Prochlorperazine (Compazine)   Uses: N/V, agitation, and psychotic disorders **Action:** Phenothiazine; blocks postsynaptic dopaminergic CNS receptors **Dose:** *Adults. Antiemetic:* 5–10 mg PO tid–qid or 25 mg PR bid or 5–10 mg deep IM q4–6h. *Antipsychotic:* 10–20 mg IM acutely or 5–10 mg PO tid–qid for maint. *Peds.* 0.1–0.15 mg/kg/dose IM q4–6h or 0.4 mg/kg/24 h PO ÷ tid–qid; ↑ doses may be required for antipsychotic effect **Caution/Contra:** [C, +/–] Phenothiazine sensitivity, narrow-angle glaucoma, bone marrow suppression, severe liver/cardiac disease **Supplied:** Tabs 5, 10, 25 mg; SR caps 10, 15, 30 mg; syrup 5 mg/5 mL; supp 2.5, 5, 25 mg; inj 5 mg/mL **Notes/SE:** Extrapyramidal side effects common; treat with diphenhydramine **Interactions:** ↑ effects with chloroquine, indomethacin, narcotics, procarbazine, SSRIs, pyrimethamine; ↑ effects of antidepressants, BBs, alcohol; ↓ effects with antacids, anticholinergics, barbiturates, tobacco; ↓ effects of guanethidine, levodopa, lithium **Labs:** False + urine bilirubin, amylase, phenylketonuria, ↑ serum prolactin **NIPE:** ⊘ d/c abruptly; ↑ risk of photosensitivity – use sunscreen; urine may turn pink/red

Procyclidine (Kemadrin) **Uses:** Parkinson's syndrome **Action:** Blocks excess acetylcholine **Dose:** 2.5 mg PO tid, up to 20 mg/d **Caution/Contra:** [C, ?] Contra in glaucoma **Supplied:** Tabs 5 mg **Notes/SE:** Anticholinergic side effects **Interactions:** ↑ CNS effects of amantadine; ↑ effects of digoxin; ↑ anticholinergic effects with anticholinergics, antipsychotics, amantadine, phenothiazines, rimantadine, quinidine, TCAs; ↓ effects of levodopa **NIPE:** Take >meals, ⊘ d/c abruptly; may cause heat intolerance

Promethazine (Phenergan) **Uses:** N/V, motion sickness **Action:** Phenothiazine; blocks postsynaptic mesolimbic dopaminergic receptors in the brain **Dose:** *Adults.* 12.5–50 mg PO, PR, or IM bid–qid PRN. *Peds.* 0.1–0.5 mg/kg/dose PO or IM q12–6h PRN **Caution/Contra:** [C, +/–] **Supplied:** Tabs 12.5, 25, 50 mg; syrup 6.25 mg/5 mL, 25 mg/5 mL; supp 12.5, 25, 50 mg; inj 25, 50 mg/mL **Notes/SE:** Drowsiness, tardive dyskinesia, EPS, lowered seizure threshold, hypotension, GI upset, blood dyscrasias, photosensitivity **Interactions:** ↑ effects with CNS depressants, MAOIs, alcohol; ↑ effects of antihypertensives; ↓ effects with anticholinergics, barbiturates, tobacco; ↓ effect of levodopa **NIPE:** Effects skin allergy tests; use sunscreen for photosensitivity

Propafenone (Rythmol) **Uses:** Life-threatening ventricular arrhythmias and AF **Action:** Class IC antiarrhythmic **Dose:** 150–300 mg PO q8h **Caution/Contra:** [C, ?] Uncontrolled CHF, bronchospasm, cardiogenic shock, conduction disorders, amprenavir or ritonavir use **Supplied:** Tabs 150, 225, 300 mg **Notes/SE:** Dizziness, unusual taste, 1st-degree heart block, arrhythmias, prolongation of QRS and QT intervals; fatigue, GI upset, blood dyscrasias **Interactions:** ↑ effects with cimetidine, quinidine; ↑ effects of anticoagulants, BBs, digitalis glycosides, theophylline; ↓ effects with rifampin, phenobarbital, rifabutin **Labs:** ↑ ANA titers **NIPE:** Take w/o regard to food

Propantheline (Pro-Banthine) **Uses:** Symptomatic treatment of small intestine hypermotility, spastic colon, ureteral spasm, bladder spasm, pylorospasm **Action:** Antimuscarinic agent **Dose:** *Adults.* 15 mg PO ac and 30 mg PO hs. *Peds.* 1–3 mg/kg/24 h PO ÷ tid–qid; ↓ dose in elderly **Caution/Contra:** [C, ?] Narrow-angle glaucoma, ulcerative colitis, toxic megacolon, GI or GU obstruction **Supplied:** Tabs 7.5, 15 mg **Notes/SE:** Anticholinergic side effects (xerostomia and blurred vision) common **Interactions:** ↑ anticholinergic effects with antihistamines, antidepressants, atropine, haloperidol, phenothiazines, quinidine, TCAs; ↑

effects of atenolol, digoxin; ↓ effects with antacids **NIPE:** May cause heat intolerance, ↑ risk of photosensitivity - use sunscreen

Propofol (Diprivan) Uses: Induction or maint of anesthesia; continuous sedation in intubated patients **Action:** Sedative hypnotic; mechanism unknown **Dose:** *Adults. Anesthesia:* 2–2.5 mg/kg induction, then 0.1–0.2 mg/kg/min inf. *ICU sedation:* 5–50 μg/kg/min cont inf. *Peds. Anesthesia:* 2.5–3.5 mg/kg induction, then 125–300 μg/kg/min; ↓ dose in elderly, debilitated, or ASA II or IV patients **Caution/Contra:** Inj 10 mg/mL **Notes/SE:** 1 mL of propofol contains 0.1 g fat; may ↑ triglycerides with extended dosing; hypotension, pain at inj site, apnea, anaphylaxis **Interactions:** ↑ effects with antihistamines, opioids, hypnotics, alcohol **Labs:** ↓ serum cortisol levels

Propoxyphene (Darvon), Propoxyphene and Acetaminophen (Darvocet), and Propoxyphene and Aspirin (Darvon Compound-65, Darvon-N + Aspirin) [C-IV] Uses: Mild–moderate pain **Action:** Narcotic analgesic **Dose:** 1–2 PO q4h PRN; ↓ dose in hepatic impairment, elderly **Caution/Contra:** [C (D if prolonged use), M] Hepatic impairment (APAP), peptic ulcer (ASA); severe renal impairment **Supplied:** *Darvon:* Propoxyphene HCl caps 65 mg. *Darvon-N:* Propoxyphene napsylate 100-mg tabs. *Darvocet-N:* Propoxyphene napsylate 50 mg/APAP 325 mg. *Darvocet-N 100:* Propoxyphene napsylate 100 mg/APAP 650 mg. *Darvon Compound-65:* Propoxyphene HCl 65 mg/ASA 389 mg/caffeine 32 mg in caps. *Darvon-N with ASA:* Propoxyphene napsylate 100 mg/ASA 325 mg. **Notes/SE:** Overdose can be lethal; hypotension, dizziness, sedation, GI upset, ↑ levels on LFTs **Interactions:** ↑ CNS depression with antidepressants, antihistamines, barbiturates, glutethimide, methocarbamol, protease inhibitors, alcohol, St. John's Wort; ↑ effects of BBs, carbamazepine, MAOIs, phenobarbital, TCAs, warfarin; ↓ effects with tobacco **Labs:** ↑ LFTs, serum amylase, lipase **NIPE:** Take with food if GI upset

Propranolol (Inderal) Uses: HTN, angina, MI, hyperthyroidism; prevents migraines and atrial arrhythmias **Action:** Competitively blocks β-adrenergic receptors, β₁, β₂; only β-blocker to block conversion of T_4 to T_3 **Dose:** *Adults. Angina:* 80–320 mg/d PO ÷ bid–qid or 80–160 mg/d SR. *Arrhythmia:* 10–80 mg PO tid–qid or 1 mg IV slowly, repeat q5min up to 5 mg. *HTN:* 40 mg PO bid or 60–80 mg/d SR, ↑ weekly to max 640 mg/d. *Hypertrophic subaortic stenosis:* 20–40 mg PO tid–qid. *MI:* 180–240 mg PO ÷ tid–qid. *Migraine prophylaxis:* 80 mg/d ÷ qid–tid, ↑ weekly to max 160–240 mg/d ÷ tid–qid; wean off if no response in 6 wk. *Pheochromocytoma:* 30–60 mg/d ÷ tid–qid. *Thyrotoxicosis:* 1–3 mg IV single dose; 10–40 mg PO q6h. *Tremor:* 40 mg PO bid, ↑ as needed to max 320 mg/d. *Peds. Arrhythmia:* 0.5–1.0 mg/kg ÷ tid–qid, ↑ as needed q3–7d to max 60 mg/d; 0.01–0.1 mg/kg IV over 10 min, max dose 1 mg. *HTN:* 0.5–1.0 mg/kg ÷ bid–qid, ↑ as needed q3–7d to 2 mg/kg/d max; ↓ dose in renal impairment **Caution/Contra:** [C (1st trimester, D if 2nd or 3rd trimester), +] Uncompensated CHF, cardiogenic shock, bradycardia, heart block, PE, severe respiratory disease **Sup-**

plied: Tabs 10, 20, 40, 60, 80 mg; SR caps 60, 80, 120, 160 mg; oral soln 4, 8, 80 mg/mL; inj 1 mg/mL **Notes/SE:** Bradycardia, hypotension, fatigue, GI upset, erectile dysfunction, hypoglycemia **Interactions:** ↑ effects with antihypertensives, cimetidine, fluvoxamine, flecainide, hydralazine, methimazole, neuroleptics, nitrates, propylthiouracil, quinidine, quinolones, theophylline, alcohol; ↑ effects of digitalis, glycosides, hypoglycemics, hydralazine, lidocaine, neuroleptics, rizatripton; ↓ effects with NSAIDs, phenobarbital, phenytoin, rifampin, tobacco **Labs:** ↑ LFTs, BUN, K+, serum lipoprotein, triglycerides, uric acid; ↑ or ↓ serum glucose **NIPE:** ⊘ d/c abruptly; ↑ cold sensitivity

Propylthiouracil [PTU]
Uses: Hyperthyroidism **Action:** Inhibits production of T_3 and T_4 and conversion of T_4 to T_3 **Dose:** *Adults.* **Initial:** 100 mg PO q8h (may need up to 1200 mg/d); after patient euthyroid (6–8 wk), taper dose by 1/2 q4–6wk. *Maint:* 50–150 mg/24 h; can usually be DC in 2–3 y. *Peds.* **Initial:** 5–7 mg/kg/24 h PO ÷ q8h. *Maint:* 1/3–2/3 of initial dose; ↓ dose in elderly **Caution/Contra:** [D, –] **Supplied:** Tabs 50 mg **Notes/SE:** Monitor patient clinically; monitor TFT, fever, rash, leukopenia, dizziness, GI upset, taste perversion, SLE-like syndrome **Interactions:** ↑ effects with iodinated glycerol, lithium, potassium iodide, sodium iodide **Labs:** ↑ LFTs, PT; ↑ effects of anticoagulants **NIPE:** Take with food for GI upset; omit dietary sources of iodine; full effects take 6–12 wk

Protamine (generic)
Uses: Reversal of heparin effect **Action:** Neutralizes heparin by forming a stable complex **Dose:** *Adults & Peds.* Based on amount of heparin reversal desired; give IV slowly; 1 mg reverses approximately 100 U of heparin given in the preceding 3–4 h, 50 mg max dose **Caution/Contra:** [C, ?] **Supplied:** Inj 10 mg/mL **Notes/SE:** Follow coagulation studies; may have anticoagulant effect if given w/o heparin; hypotension, bradycardia, dyspnea, hemorrhage

Pseudoephedrine (Sudafed, Novafed, Afrinol, others)
Uses: Decongestant **Action:** Stimulates α-adrenergic receptors, resulting in vasoconstriction **Dose:** *Adults.* 30–60 mg PO q6–8h; SR caps 120 mg PO q12h. *Peds.* 4 mg/kg/24 h PO ÷ qid **Caution/Contra:** [C, +] Contra in poorly controlled HTN or CAD disease and in MAOIs **Supplied:** Tabs 30, 60 mg; caps 60 mg; SR tabs 120, 240 mg; SR caps 120 mg; liq 7.5 mg/0.8 mL, 15, 30 mg/5 mL; ↓ dose in renal insufficiency **Notes/SE:** Ingredient in many cough and cold preparations; HTN, insomnia, tachycardia, arrhythmias, nervousness, tremor **Interactions:** ↑ risk of HTN crisis with MAOIs; ↑ effects with BBs, sympathomimetics; ↓ effects with TCAs; ↓ effect of methyldopa, reserpine

Psyllium (Metamucil, Serutan, Effer-Syllium)
Uses: Constipation and diverticular disease of the colon **Action:** Bulk laxative **Dose:** 1 tsp (7 g) in a glass of water qd–tid **Caution/Contra:** [B, ?] Do not use if suspected bowel obstruction; psyllium in effervescent (Effer-Syllium) form usually contains K+; use caution in patients with renal failure; phenylketonuria (in products with aspartame) **Supplied:** Granules 4, 25 g/tsp; powder 3.5 g/packet **Notes/SE:** Diarrhea, abdomi-

nal cramps, bowel obstruction, constipation, bronchospasm **Interactions:** ↓ effects of digitalis glycosides, K⁺-sparing diuretics, nitrofurantoin, salicylates, tetracyclines, warfarin **NIPE:** Psyllium dust inhalation may cause wheezing, runny nose, watery eyes

Pyrazinamide (generic)   **Uses:** Active TB in combination with other agents **Action:** Bacteriostatic; mechanism unknown **Dose:** *Adults.* 15–30 mg/kg/ 24 h PO ÷ tid–qid; max 2 g/d. *Peds.* 15–30 mg/kg/d PO ÷ qd–bid; dosage regimen differs for directly observed therapy; ↓ dose for renal/hepatic impairment **Caution/Contra:** [C, +/–] Severe hepatic damage, acute gout **Supplied:** Tabs 500 mg **Notes/SE:** Use in combination with other anti-TB drugs; consult *MMWR* for the latest TB recommendations; hepatotoxicity, malaise, GI upset, arthralgia, myalgia, gout, photosensitivity **Interactions:** ↓ effects of cyclosporine, tacrolimus **Labs:** False + urine ketones **NIPE:** ↑ risk of photosensitivity; ↑ fluids to 2 L/d

Pyridoxine [Vitamin B₆]   **Uses:** Rx and prevention of vitamin B₆ deficiency **Action:** Supplementation of vitamin B₆ **Dose:** *Adults. Deficiency:* 10–20 mg/d PO. *Drug-induced neuritis:* 100–200 mg/d; 25–100 mg/d prophylaxis. *Peds.* 5–25 mg/d ×3 wk **Caution/Contra:** [A (C if doses exceed RDA), +] **Supplied:** Tabs 25, 50, 100 mg; inj 100 mg/mL **Notes/SE:** Allergic reactions, HA, nausea **Interactions:** ↑ pyridoxine needs with chloramphenicol, cycloserine, hydralazine, immunosuppressant drugs, isoniazid, oral contraceptives, penicillamine, high-protein diet; ↓ effects of levodopa, phenobarbital, phenytoin **Labs:** False ↑ urobilinogen **NIPE:** Lactation suppressed with pyridoxine

Quazepam (Doral) [C-IV]   **Uses:** Insomnia **Action:** Benzodiazepine **Dose:** 7.5–15 mg PO hs PRN; ↓ dose in the elderly, hepatic failure **Caution/Contra:** [X, ?/–] Narrow-angle glaucoma **Supplied:** Tabs 7.5, 15 mg **Notes/SE:** Do not DC abruptly; sedation, hangover, somnolence, respiratory depression **Interactions:** ↑ effects with azole antifungals, cimetidine, digoxin, disulfiram, isoniazid, levodopa, macrolides, neuroleptics, phenytoin, quinolones, SSRIs, verapamil, grapefruit juice, alcohol; ↓ effects with carbamazepine, rifampin, rifabutin, tobacco **NIPE:** ⊘ breastfeed, PRG, d/c abruptly; use barrier contraception

Quetiapine (Seroquel)   **Uses:** Acute exacerbations of schizophrenia **Action:** Serotonin and dopamine antagonism **Dose:** 150–750 mg/d; initiate at 25–100 mg bid–tid; slowly ↑ dose; ↓ dose for hepatic and geriatric patients **Caution/Contra:** [C, –] **Supplied:** Tabs 25, 100, 200 mg **Notes/SE:** Multiple reports of confusion with Serzone (nefazodone); HA, somnolence, weight gain, orthostatic hypotension, dizziness, cataracts, neuroleptic malignant syndrome, tardive dyskinesia, QT prolongation **Interactions:** ↑ effects with azole antifungals, cimetidine, macrolides, alcohol; ↑ effects of antihypertensives, lorazepam; ↓ effects with barbiturates, carbamazepine, glucocorticoids, phenytoin, rifampin, thioridazine; ↓ effects of dopamine antagonists, levodopa **Labs:** ↑ LFTs, cholesterol, triglycerides **NIPE:** ↑ risk of cataract formation, tardive dyskinesia; take w/o regard to food; ↓ body temp regulation

Quinapril (Accupril) **Uses:** HTN, CHF, DN, post-MI **Action:** ACE inhibitor **Dose:** 10–80 mg PO qd in a single dose; ↓ dose in renal impairment **Caution/Contra:** [D, +] ACE inhibitor sensitivity or angioedema **Supplied:** Tabs 5, 10, 20, 40 mg **Notes/SE:** Dizziness, HA, hypotension, impaired renal function, angioedema, taste perversion, cough **Interactions:** ↑ effects with diuretics, antihypertensives; ↑ effects of insulin, lithium; ↓ effects with ASA, NSAIDs; ↓ effects of quinolones, tetracyclines **Labs:** ↑ BUN, serum creatinine **NIPE:** ↓ absorption with high-fat foods; ↑ risk of cough

Quinidine (Quinidex, Quinaglute) **Uses:** Prevention of tachydysrhythmias **Action:** Class 1A antiarrhythmic **Dose:** *Adults. Conversion of AF or flutter:* Use after digitalization. 200 mg q2–3h for 8 doses; then ↑ daily dose to a max of 3–4 g or until normal rhythm. *Peds.* 15–60 mg/kg/24 h PO in 4–5 + doses; ↓ dose in renal impairment **Caution/Contra:** [C, +] Contra in digitalis toxicity and AV block; conduction disorders; sparfloxacin or ritonavir use **Supplied:** *Sulfate:* Tabs 200, 300 mg; SR tabs 300 mg. *Gluconate:* SR tabs 324 mg; inj 80 mg/mL **Notes/SE:** Follow serum levels (Table 2, Page 245); extreme hypotension may be seen with IV administration. Sulfate salt is 83% quinidine; gluconate salt is 62% quinidine; syncope, QT prolongation, GI upset, arrhythmias, fatigue, cinchonism (tinnitus, hearing loss, delirium, visual changes), fever, hemolytic anemia, thrombocytopenia, rash **Interactions:** ↑ effects with acetazolamide, antacids, amiodarone, azole antifungals, cimetidine, K+, macrolides, sodium bicarbonate, thiazide diuretics, lily-of-the-valley, pheasant's eye herb, scopolia root, squill; ↑ effects of anticoagulants, dextromethorphan, digitalis glycosides, disopyramide, haloperidol, metoprolol, nifedipine, procainamide, propafenone, propranolol, TCAs, verapamil; ↓ effects with barbiturates, disopyramide, nifedipine, phenobarbital, phenytoin, rifampin, sucralfate **NIPE:** Take with food, ↑ risk of photosensitivity

Quinupristin-Dalfopristin (Synercid) **Uses:** Infections caused by vancomycin-resistant *E. faecium* and other gram+ organisms **Action:** Inhibits both the early and late phases of protein synthesis at the ribosomes **Dose:** *Adults & Peds.* 7.5 mg/kg IV q8–12h (use central line if possible); not compatible with NS or heparin; therefore, flush IV lines with dextrose; ↓ in hepatic failure **Caution/Contra:** [B, M] **Supplied:** Inj 500 mg (150 mg quinupristin/350 mg dalfopristin) **Notes/SE:** Hyperbilirubinemia, inf site reactions and pain, arthralgia, myalgia **Interactions:** ↑ effects of CCBs, carbamazepine, cyclosporine, diazepam, disopyramide, docetaxel, lovastatin, methylprednisolone, midazolam, paclitaxel, protease inhibitors, quinidine, tacrolimus, vinblastine **Labs:** ↑ LFTs, BUN, creatinine, HCT; ↑ or ↓ serum glucose, K+

Rabeprazole (Aciphex) **Uses:** PUD, GERD, ZE **Action:** Proton-pump inhibitor **Dose:** 20 mg/d; may be ↑ to 60 mg/d; do not crush tabs **Caution/Contra:** [B, ?/–] **Supplied:** Tabs 60 mg **Notes/SE:** HA, fatigue, GI upset **Interactions:** ↑ effects of cyclosporine, digoxin; ↓ effects of ketoconazole **Labs:** ↑ LFTs, TSH **NIPE:** Take w/o regard to food; ↑ risk of photosensitivity

Raloxifene (Evista) **Uses:** Prevention of osteoporosis **Action:** Partial antagonist of estrogen that behaves like estrogen **Dose:** 60 mg/d **Caution/Contra:** [X, –] Thromboembolism **Supplied:** Tabs 60 mg **Notes/SE:** Chest pain, insomnia, rash, hot flashes, GI upset, hepatic dysfunction **Interactions:** ↓ effects with ampicillin, cholestyramine **NIPE:** ⊘ PRG, breast-feeding; take w/o regard to food; ↑ risk of venous thromboembolic use

Ramipril (Altace) **WARNING:** ACE inhibitors used during the 2nd and 3rd trimesters of PRG can cause injury and even death to the developing fetus **Uses:** HTN, CHF, DN, post-MI **Action:** ACE inhibitor **Dose:** 2.5–20 mg/d PO ÷ qd–bid; ↓ in renal failure **Caution/Contra:** [D, +] ACE-inhibitor-induced angioedema **Supplied:** Caps 1.25, 2.5, 5, 10 mg **Notes/SE:** May use in combination with diuretics; may cause cough; HA, dizziness, hypotension, renal impairment, angioedema **Interactions:** ↑ effects with α-adrenergic blockers, loop diuretics; ↑ effects of insulin, lithium; ↑ risk of hyperkalemia with K^+, K^+-sparing diuretics, K^+ salt substitutes, trimethoprim, ↓ effects with ASA, NSAIDs, food; **Labs:** ↑ BUN, creatinine, K^+, ↓ HMG, HCT, cholesterol **NIPE:** ↑ risk of photosensitivity; ↑ risk of cough esp with capsaicin; take w/o food

Ranitidine (Zantac) **Uses:** Duodenal ulcer, active benign ulcers, hypersecretory conditions, and GERD **Action:** H_2-receptor antagonist **Dose:** *Adults.* *Ulcer:* 150 mg PO bid, 300 mg PO hs, or 50 mg IV q6–8h; or 400 mg IV/d cont inf, then maint of 150 mg PO hs. *Hypersecretion:* 150 mg PO bid, up to 6 mg/d. *GERD:* 300 mg PO bid; maint 300 mg PO hs. *Peds.* 0.75–1.5 mg/kg/dose IV 6–h or 1.25–2.5 mg/kg/dose PO 1h; ↓ dose in renal failure **Caution/Contra:** [B, +] **Supplied:** Tabs 75, 150, 300 mg; syrup 15 mg/mL; inj 25 mg/mL **Notes/SE:** Oral and parenteral doses are different; dizziness, sedation, rash, GI upset **Interactions:** ↑ effects of glipizide, glyburide, lidocaine, nifedipine, nitrendipine, nisoldipine, procainamide, TCAs, theophylline, tolbutamide, warfarin; ↓ effects with antacids, tobacco; ↓ effects of cefuroxime, cefpodoxime, diazepam, enoxacin, ketoconazole, itraconazole, oxaprozin **Labs:** ↑ serum creatinine, LFTs, false + urine protein **NIPE:** ASA, NSAIDs, alcohol, caffeine increase stomach acid production

Rasburicase (Elitek) **Uses:** ↑ Plasma uric acid due to tumor lysis (pediatrics) **Action:** Catalyzes uric acid **Dose:** *Peds.* 0.15 or 0.20 mg/kg IV over 30 min, qd × 5 **Caution/Contra:** [C, ?/–] Anaphylaxis, screen for G6PD deficiency to avoid hemolysis, methemoglobinemia; falsely ↓ uric acid values **Supplied:** 1.5 mg inj **Notes/SE:** Fever, neutropenia, GI upset, HA, rash

Repaglinide (Prandin) **Uses:** Type 2 DM **Action:** Stimulates insulin release from pancreas **Dose:** 0.5–4 mg ac, start 1–2 mg, ↑ to 16 mg/d max; take pc **Caution/Contra:** [C, ?/–] DKA, type 1 DM **Supplied:** Tabs 0.5, 1, 2 mg **Notes/SE:** HA, hyper-/hypoglycemia, GI upset **Interactions:** ↑ effects with ASA, BBs, chloramphenicol, erythromycin, ketoconazole, miconazole, MAOIs, NSAIDs, probenecid, sulfa drugs, warfarin, celery, coriander, dandelion root, fenugreek, garlic, ginseing, juniper berries; ↓ effects with barbiturates, carbamazepine,

CCBs, corticosteroids, diuretics, estrogens, isoniazid, oral contraceptives, phenytoin, phenothiazines, rifampin, sympathomimetics, thiazide diuretics, thyroid drugs **NIPE:** Take 15 min <meal; skip drug if meal skipped

Reteplase (Retavase) **Uses:** Post-AMI **Action:** Thrombolytic agent **Dose:** 10 U IV over 2 min, 2nd dose in 30 min 10 U IV over 2 min **Caution/Contra:** [C, ?/–] Internal bleeding, spinal surgery or trauma, Hx CVA vascular malformations, uncontrolled hypotension, sensitivity to thrombolytics ↑ risk of bleeding **Supplied:** Inj 10.8 U/2 mL **Notes/SE:** Bleeding, allergic reactions **Interactions:** ↑ risk of bleeding with ASA, abciximab, dipyridamole, heparin, NSAIDs, oral anticoagulants, vitamin K antagonists **Labs:** ↓ fibrinogen, plasminogen **NIPE:** Monitor ECG during treatment for ↑ risk of reperfusion arrhythmias

Ribavirin (Virazole) **Uses:** RSV infection in infants and hepatitis C (in combination with interferon alfa-2b) **Action:** Unknown **Dose:** *RSV:* 6 g in 300 mL sterile water inhaled over 12–18 h. *Hep C:* 600 mg PO bid in combination with interferon alfa-2b (see Rebetron, page 132) **Caution/Contra:** [X, ?] Autoimmune hepatitis **Supplied:** Powder for aerosol 6 g; caps 200 mg **Notes/SE:** Aerosolized by a SPAG; may accumulate on soft contact lenses; monitor H/H frequently; PRG test monthly; fatigue, HA, GI upset, anemia, myalgia, alopecia, bronchospasm **Interactions:** ↓ effects with aluminum, magnesium, simethicone; ↓ effect of zidovudine **Labs:** ↑ bilirubin, uric acid, ↓ HMG **NIPE:** ⊘ PRG, breast-feeding; ↑ risk of photosensitivity; take w/o regard to food

Rifabutin (Mycobutin) **Uses:** Prevention of *M. avium* complex infection in AIDS patients with a CD4 count <100 **Action:** Inhibits DNA-dependent RNA polymerase activity **Dose:** 150–300 mg/d PO **Caution/Contra:** [B; ?/–] WBC <1000/mm³ or platelets <50,000/mm³; ritonavir **Supplied:** Caps 150 mg **Notes/SE:** Adverse effects/drug interactions similar to rifampin; discolored urine, rash, neutropenia, leukopenia, myalgia, ↑ LFTs **Interactions:** ↑ effects with ritonavir; ↓ effects of anticoagulants, anticonvulsants, barbiturates, benzodiazepines, BBs, clofibrate, corticosteroids, cyclosporine, dapsone, delavirdine, digoxin, eprosartan, fluconazole, hypoglycemics, ketoconazole, nifedipine, oral contraceptives, propafenone, protease inhibitors, quinidine, tacrolimus, theophylline **Labs:** ↑ ALT, AST, alkaline phosphatase **NIPE:** Urine and body fluids may turn reddish brown in color, discoloration of soft contact lenses, use barrier contraception, take w/o food

Rifampin (Rifadin) **Uses:** TB and Rx and prophylaxis of *N. meningitidis, H. influenzae,* or *S. aureus* carriers; adjunct for severe *S. aureus* **Action:** Inhibits DNA-dependent RNA polymerase activity **Dose:** *Adults.* *N. meningitidis and H. influenzae carrier:* 600 mg/d PO for 4 d. *TB:* 600 mg PO or IV qd or 2×/wk with combination therapy regimen. *Peds.* 10–20 mg/kg/dose PO or IV qd–bid; ↓ dose in hepatic failure **Caution/Contra:** [C, +] Amprenavir, multiple drug interactions **Supplied:** Caps 150, 300 mg; inj 600 mg **Notes/SE:** Never use as single agent for active TB; orange-red discoloration of bodily secretions; rash, GI upset, ↑ LFTs, flushing, HA; multiple drug interactions **Interactions:** ↓ effects with aminosalicylic acid; ↓ effects of acetaminophen, aminophylline, amiodarone, anticoagulants, barbiturates, BBs, CCBs, chloramphenicol, clofibrate, delaviridine, digoxin, disopyramide, doxycycline, enalapril, estrogens, haloperidol, hypoglycemics, hydantoins, methadone, morphine, nifedipine, ondansetron, oral contraceptives, phenytoin, protease inhibitors, quinidine, repaglinide, sertraline, sulfapyridine, sulfones, tacrolimus, theophylline, thyroid drugs, tocainide, TCAs, theophylline, verapamil, zidovudine, zolpidem **Labs:** ↑ LFTs, uric acid; affects serum folate and vit B$_{12}$ levels **NIPE:** Use barrier contraception, take w/o food, reddish brown color in urine and body fluids, stains soft contact lenses

Rifapentine (Priftin)   **Uses:** TB **Action:** Inhibits DNA-dependent RNA polymerase activity **Dose:** *Intensive phase:* 600 mg PO 2 ×/wk for 2 mon; separate doses by 3 or more days. *Continuation phase:* 600 mg/wk **Caution/Contra:** [C, ?/–] **Supplied:** Tabs 150 mg **Notes/SE:** Adverse effects/drug interactions similar to rifampin; hyperuricemia, HTN, HA, dizziness, rash, GI upset, blood dyscrasias, ↑ LFTs, hematuria, discolored secretions; **see Rifampin**

Rimantadine (Flumadine)   **Uses:** Prophylaxis and Rx of influenza A virus infections **Action:** Antiviral agent **Dose:** *Adults.* 100 mg PO bid. *Peds.* 5 mg/kg/d PO, 150 mg/d max; ↓ dose in severe renal/hepatic impairment, elderly; initiate w/in 48 h of symptom onset **Caution/Contra:** [C, –] **Supplied:** Tabs 100 mg; syrup 50 mg/5 mL **Notes/SE:** Orthostatic hypotension, edema, dizziness, GI upset, lowered seizure threshold; **Interactions:** ↑ effects with cimetidine; ↓ effects with acetaminophen, ASA

Rimexolone (Vexol Ophthalmic)   **Uses:** Postop inflammation and uveitis **Action:** Steroid **Dose:** *Adults & Peds >2 y.* Uveitis: 1–2 gtt/h daytime and q2h at night, taper to 1 gt q4h; postop 1–2 gtt qid up to 2 wk **Caution/Contra:** [C, ?/–] Ocular infections **Supplied:** Susp 1% **Notes/SE:** Taper dose to zero; blurred vision, local irritation **NIPE:** Shake well, ⊘ touch eye with dropper

Risedronate (Actonel)   **Uses:** Prevention and Rx of postmenopausal osteoporosis; Paget's disease **Action:** Bisphosphonate; inhibits osteoclast-mediated bone resorption **Dose:** 5 mg/d PO with 6–8 oz water; 30 mg/d for 2 mon for Paget's; take 30 min before 1st food/drink of the day; maintain upright position for at least 30 min after administration **Caution/Contra:** [C, ?/–] Not recommended in moderate–severe renal impairment; esophageal structural abnormality, inability to stand or sit upright; interaction with Ca supplements **Supplied:** Tabs 5, 30 mg **Notes/SE:** GI distress, arthralgia; rash, abdominal pain, esophagitis, arthralgia, diarrhea, bone pain **Interactions:** ↓ effects with antacids, calcium, food **Labs:** Interference with bone-imaging agents **NIPE:** Alcohol intake and cigarette smoking promote osteoporosis

Risperidone (Risperdal)   **Uses:** Psychotic disorders **Action:** Benzisoxazole antipsychotic agent **Dose:** 1–6 mg PO bid; ↓ starting doses in elderly, renal/hepatic impairment **Caution/Contra:** [C, –] **Supplied:** Tabs 1, 2, 3, 4 mg

Notes/SE: Orthostatic hypotension, extrapyramidal reactions with higher doses, tachycardia, arrhythmias, sedation, dystonias, neuroleptic malignant syndrome, sexual dysfunction, constipation, xerostomia, blood dyscrasias, cholestatic jaundice, weight gain **Interactions:** ↑ effects with clozapine, CNS depressants, alcohol; ↑ effects of antihypertensives; ↓ effects with carbamazepine; ↓ effects of levodopa **Labs:** ↑ LFTs, serum prolactin **NIPE:** ↑ risk photosensitivity, extrapyramidal effects; may alter body temp regulation

Ritonavir (Norvir) **Uses:** HIV infection **Actions:** Protease inhibitor; inhibits maturation of immature noninfectious virions to mature infectious virus **Dose:** 600 mg PO bid or 400 mg PO bid in combination with saquinavir; titrate over 1 wk to ↓ GI complications; take with food **Caution/Contra:** [B, +] Ergotamine, amiodarone, bepridil, flecainide, propafenone, quinidine, pimozide, midazolam, triazolam **Supplied:** Caps 100 mg; soln 80 mg/mL **Notes/SE:** Many drug interactions; store in refrigerator; perioral and peripheral paresthesias; dyslipidemia, lipodystrophy, hyperglycemia, GI upset, ↑ LFTs, decreased mentation, rash, blood dyscrasias **Interactions:** ↑ effects with erythromycin, interleukins, grapefruit juice, food; ↑ effects of amiodarone, astemizole, atorvastatin, barbiturates, bepridil, bupropion, cerivastatin, cisapride, clorazepate, clozapine, clarithromycin, despiramine, diazepam, encainide, ergot alkaloids, estazolam, flecainide, flurazepam, indinavir, ketoconazole, lovastatin, meperidine, midazolam, nelfinavir, phenytoin, pimozide, piroxicam, propafenone, propoxyphene, quinidine, rifabutin, saquinavir, sildenafil, simvastatin, SSRIs, TCAs, terfenadine, triazolam, troleandomycin, zolpidem; ↓ effects with barbiturates, carbamazepine, phenytoin, rifabutin, rifampin, St. John's Wort, tobacco; ↓ effects of didanosin, hypnotics, methadone, oral contraceptives, sedatives, theophylline, warfarin **Labs:** ↑ serum glucose, LFTs, triglycerides, uric acid **NIPE:** Food ↑ absorption; use barrier contraception; disulfiram-like reaction with disulfiram, metronidazole

Rivastigmine (Exelon) **Uses:** Mild–moderate dementia associated with Alzheimer's disease **Action:** Enhances cholinergic activity **Dose:** 1.5 mg bid; ↑ to 6 mg bid, with increases at 2-wk intervals **Caution/Contra:** [B, ?] **Supplied:** Caps 1.5, 3, 4.5, 6 mg; soln 2 mg/mL **Notes/SE:** Dose-related GI adverse effects; dizziness, somnolence, tremor, diaphoresis **Interactions:** ↑ risk of GI bleed with NSAIDs; ↓ effects with nicotine; ↓ effects of anticholinergics **NIPE:** Take with food

Rizatriptan (Maxalt) **Uses:** Acute migraine **Action:** Serotonin 5-HT$_1$ receptor antagonist **Dose:** 5–10 mg PO; may repeat once in 2 h **Caution/Contra:** [C, M] Ischemic heart disease, Prinzmetal's angina, uncontrolled HTN, w/n 2 wk of MAOI use, ergots **Supplied:** Tabs 5, 10 mg; disintegrating tabs 5, 10 mg **Notes/SE:** GI adverse effects (dose-related); ↑ BP, chest pain, dizziness, drowsiness, fatigue, flushing, dyspnea, coronary vasospasm **Interactions:** ↑ effects with MAOIs, propranolol; ↑ vasospastic reaction with ergot-containing drugs; ↑ risk of hyperreflexia, incoordination, weakness with SSRIs **NIPE:** Food delays drug action; ⊘ take >30 mg/24 h

Rofecoxib (Vioxx) Uses: Osteoarthritis, RA, acute pain, and primary dysmenorrhea **Action:** NSAID; COX-2 inhibitor **Dose:** 12.5–50 mg/d; ↓ dose in severe renal/hepatic impairment, elderly **Caution/Contra:** [C, ?/–] ASA or NSAID sensitivity **Supplied:** Tabs 12.5, 25 mg; susp 12.5, 25 mg/5 mL **Notes/SE:** Alert patients about GI ulceration or bleeding; dizziness, edema, HTN, HA, renal failure; no effect on bleeding parameters; may ↑ thromboembolism risk **Interactions:** ↑ risk of bleeding with ASA, NSAIDs, feverfew, garlic, ginger, horse chestnut, red clover, alcohol, tobacco; ↑ effects of amitriptyline, lithium, methotrexate, theophylline, warfarin; ↑ risk of photosensitivity with dong quai, St. John's Wort; ↓ effects with antacids, rifampin; ↓ effects of ACEIs, diuretics **Labs:** ↑ ALT, AST **NIPE:** Take with food

Rosiglitazone (Avandia) Uses: Type 2 DM **Action:** ↑ Insulin sensitivity **Dose:** 4–8 mg/d PO or in 2 ÷ doses w/o regard to meals **Caution/Contra:** [C, –] Contra in active liver disease **Supplied:** Tabs 2, 4, 8 mg **Notes/SE:** Weight gain, hyperlipidemia, HA, edema, fluid retention, exacerbate CHF, hyper-/hypoglycemia, hepatic damage **Interactions:** ↑ risk of hypoglycemia with insulin, ketoconazole, oral hypoglycemics, fenugreek, garlic, ginseng, glucomannan; ↓ effects of oral contraceptives **Labs:** ↑ ALT, total cholesterol, LDL, HDL, ↓ HMG, HCT **NIPE:** Use barrier contraception

Rosuvastatin (Crestor) Uses: Rx primary hypercholesterolemia and mixed dyslipidemia **Action:** HMG-CoA reductase inhibitor **Dose:** *Adults.* 5–40mg PO qd; 5 mg PO max daily with cyclosporine; 10 mg PO daily with gemfibrozil or CrCl <30 mL/min (avoid Al/Mg antacids for 2 h after dose) **Caution:** [X,?/–] **Contra:** Active liver disease or persistent unexplained elevations of transaminases **Supplied:** Tabs 5, 10, 20, 40 mg **SE:** Myalgia, constipation, asthenia, abdominal pain, nausea; may cause myopathy and in rare cases rhabdomyolysis **Notes:** May increase anticoagulant effect of warfarin; monitor LFTs at baseline, 12 wk, then q 6mon **Interactions:** ↑ effects of warfarin; ↑ risk of myopathy with cyclosporine, fibrates, niacin, statins **Labs:** ↑ ALT, AST, CK; + urine protein, HMG; **NIPE:** ⊘ PRG or breast feeding

Salmeterol (Serevent) Uses: Asthma, exercise-induced bronchospasm, COPD **Action:** Sympathomimetic bronchodilator **Dose:** 2 inhal bid **Caution/Contra:** [C, ?/–] Do not use w/n 14 d of MAOI use **Supplied:** Met-dose inhaler **Notes/SE:** Not for acute attacks; HA, pharyngitis, tachycardia, arrhythmias, nervousness, GI upset, tremors **Interactions:** ↑ effects with MAOIs, TCAs; ↓ effects with BBs **Labs:** ↓ serum K⁺ **NIPE:** Shake canister <use, inhale q12h, not for acute exacerbations

Saquinavir (Fortovase) Uses: HIV infection **Action:** HIV protease inhibitor **Dose:** 1200 mg PO tid w/n 2 h pc **Caution/Contra:** [B, +] Triazolam, midazolam, ergots **Supplied:** Caps 200 mg **Notes/SE:** Dyslipidemia, lipodystrophy, rash, hyperglycemia, GI upset, weakness, hepatic dysfunction **Interactions:** ↑ effects with clarithromycin, delavirdine, erythromycin, indinavir, ketoconazole, nelfinavir, ritonavir, grapefruit juice, food; ↑ effects of astemizole, cisapride, clarithromycin, ergot alkaloids, erythromycin, lovastatin, midazolam, phenytoin, sildenafil, simvastatin, terfenadine, triazolam; ↓ effects with barbiturates, carbamazepine, dexamethasone, efavirenz, phenytoin, rifabutin, rifampin, St. John's Wort; ↓ effects of oral contraceptives **Labs:** ↑ LFTs, ↓ neutrophils **NIPE:** Use barrier contraception; ↑ risk of photosensitivity

Sargramostim [GM-CSF] (Prokine, Leukine)
Uses: Myeloid recovery following BMT or CA chemotherapy **Action:** Activates mature granulocytes and macrophages **Dose:** *Adults & Peds.* 250 mg/m²/d IV for 21 d (BMT) **Caution/Contra:** [C, ?/–] > 10% blasts **Supplied:** Inj 250, 500 mg **Notes/SE:** Bone pain, fever, hypotension, tachycardia, flushing, GI upset, myalgia **Interactions:** ↑ effects with corticosteroids, lithium **Labs:** ↑ serum glucose, BUN, creatinine, LFTs; ↓ albumin, calcium **NIPE:** Avoid exposure to infection

Scopolamine, Scopolamine Transdermal (Scopace, Transderm-Scop)
Uses: Prevention of N/V associated with motion sickness, anesthesia, and opiates; mydriatic, cycloplegic, Rx iridocyclitis **Action:** Anticholinergic, antiemetic **Dose:** Apply 1 TD patch behind the ear q3d: 0.4–0.8 PO, repeat PRN q4–6h; apply at least 4 h before exposure; ↓ dose in elderly **Caution/Contra:** [C, +] Narrow-angle glaucoma, GI or GU obstruction, thyrotoxicosis, paralytic ileus **Supplied:** Patch 1.5 mg, tabs 0.4 mg, ophthalmic 0.25% **Notes/SE:** Xerostomia, drowsiness, blurred vision, tachycardia, constipation **Interactions:** ↑ effects with antihistamines, amantadine, antidepressants, disopyramide, opioids, procainamide, quinidine, TCAs, alcohol; ↓ effects of acetaminophen, digoxin, ketoconazole, levodopa, K⁺, phenothiazines, riboflavin **NIPE:** ⊘ d/c abruptly; wash hands after applying patch; may cause heat intolerance

Secobarbital (Seconal) [C-II]
Uses: Insomnia **Action:** Rapid-acting barbiturate **Dose:** *Adults.* 100–200 mg. *Peds.* 3–5 mg/kg/dose, up to 100 mg; ↓ dose in elderly **Caution/Contra:** [D, +] Porphyria **Supplied:** Caps 100 mg **Notes/SE:** Tolerance acquired in 1–2 wk; respiratory depression, CNS depression, porphyria, photosensitivity **Interactions:** ↑ effects with MAOIs, valproic acid, alcohol, kava kava, valerian; ↑ effects of meperidine; ↓ effects of anticoagulants, BBs, CCBs, CNS depressants, chloramphenicol, corticosteroids, cyclosporine, digitoxin, disopyramide, doxycycline, estrogen, griseofulvin, methadone, neuroleptics, oral contraceptives, propafenone, quinidine, tacrolimus, theophylline **NIPE:** ⊘ PRG, breast-feeding; use barrier contraception

Selegiline (Eldepryl)
Uses: Parkinson's disease **Action:** Inhibits MAO activity **Dose:** 5 mg PO bid; ↓ dose in elderly **Caution/Contra:** [C, ?] Meperidine, SSRI, and TCAs **Supplied:** Tabs 5 mg **Notes/SE:** Nausea, dizziness, orthostatic hypotension, arrhythmias, tachycardia, edema, confusion, xerostomia **Interactions:** ↑ risk of serotonin syndrome with dextroamphetamine, dextromethorphan, fenfluramine, meperidine, methylphenidate, sibutramine, venlafaxine; ↑ risk of hypertension with dextroamphetamine, levodopa, methylphenidate, SSRIs, tyra-

mine containing foods, alcohol, ephedra, ginseng, ma-huang, St. John's Wort **Labs:** False ↑ uric acid, urine protein; false + urine ketones, urine glucose

Selenium Sulfide (Exsel Shampoo, Selsun Blue Shampoo, Selsun Shampoo)
Uses: Scalp seborrheic dermatitis, itching and flaking of the scalp due to dandruff; treatment of tinea versicolor **Action:** Antiseborrheic **Dose:** *Dandruff, seborrhea:* Massage 5–10 mL into wet scalp, leave on 2–3 min, rinse, and repeat; use 2×/wk, then once q1–4wk PRN. *Tinea versicolor:* Apply 2.5% qd for 7 d on area and lather with small amounts of water; leave on skin for 10 min, then rinse **Caution/Contra:** [C, ?] **Supplied:** Shampoo 1, 2.5% **Notes/SE:** Dry or oily scalp, lethargy, hair discoloration, local irritation **NIPE:** ⊘ use on excoriated skin, avoid eyes; may cause reversible hair loss; rinse thoroughly after use

Serotonin 5-HT₁ Receptor Agonists (See Table 11, page 259)
Uses: Migraine w/wo aura **Action:** Serotonin receptor antagonism results in vasoconstriction **Dose:** See Table 11, Page 259 **Caution/Contra:** [C, ?, sumatriptan −] Contra in sumatriptan sensitivity, ischemic CAD, MI **Notes/SE:** Flushing, dizziness, pressure/heaviness

Sertraline (Zoloft)
Uses: Depression, panic disorders, obsessive–compulsive disorder, posttraumatic stress disorders (PTSD), social anxiety disorder **Action:** Inhibits neuronal uptake of serotonin **Dose:** *Depression:* 50–200 mg/d PO. *PTSD:* 25 mg PO qd ×1 wk, then 50 mg PO qd, max 200 mg/d **Caution/Contra:** [C, ?/–] MAOI use w/n 14 d; caution in hepatic impairment, concomitant pimozide **Supplied:** Tabs 25, 50, 100 mg **Notes/SE:** Can activate manic/hypomanic state; has caused weight loss in clinical trials; insomnia, somnolence, fatigue, tremor, xerostomia, nausea, dyspepsia, diarrhea, ejaculatory dysfunction, ↓ libido, hepatotoxicity **Interactions:** ↑ effects with cimetidine, MAOIs, tryptophan, St. John's Wort; ↑ effects of clozapine, diazepam, hydantoins, sumatriptan, tolbutamide, TCAs, warfarin, alcohol; ↓ effects with carbamazepine, rifampin **Labs:** ↑ LFTs, triglycerides, ↓ uric acid

Sibutramine (Meridia)
Uses: Obesity **Action:** Blocks uptake of norepinephrine, serotonin, and dopamine **Dose:** 10 mg/d, may ↓ to 5 mg after 4 wk **Caution/Contra:** [C, −] MAOI use w/n 14 d, uncontrolled HTN, arrhythmias **Supplied:** Caps 5, 10, 15 mg **Notes/SE:** Use with low-calorie diet, monitor BP and HR; HA, insomnia, xerostomia, constipation, rhinitis, tachycardia, HTN **Interactions:** ↑ risk of serotonin syndrome with dextromethorphan, ergots, fentanyl, lithium, meperidine, MAOIs, naratriptan, pentazocine, rizatriptan, sumatriptan, SSRIs, trometherophan, tryptophan, zolmitriptan, St. John's Wort; ↑ effects with cimetidine, erythromycin, ketoconazole; ↑ CNS depression with alcohol **NIPE:** Avoid alcohol; take early in the day to avoid insomnia

Sildenafil (Viagra)
Uses: Erectile dysfunction **Action:** Smooth-muscle relaxation and ↑ inflow of blood to the corpus cavernosum; inhibits phosphodiesterase type 5 responsible for cGMP breakdown; ↑ cGMP activity **Dose:** 25–100 mg 1 h before sexual activity, max dosing is once daily; ↓ dose if >65 y; avoid fatty

foods with dose **Caution/Contra:** [B, ?] Contra with nitrates of any form; retinitis pigmentosa; potent CYP3A4 inhibitors (ie, protease inhibitors); hepatic/severe renal impairment **Supplied:** Tabs 25, 50, 100 mg **Notes/SE:** HA, flushing, dizziness, blue haze visual disturbance, usually reversible; cardiac events in absence of nitrates debatable **Interactions:** ↑ effects with amlodipine, cimetidine, erythromycin, indinavir, itraconazole, ketoconazole, nelfinavir, protease inhibitors, ritonavir, saquinavir, grapefruit juice; ↑ risk of hypotension with antihypertensives, nitrates; ↓ effects with rifampin **NIPE:** High-fat food delays absorption; ↑ risk of cardiac arrest if used with nitrates

Silver Nitrate (Dey-Drop, others)
Uses: Prevent ophthalmia neonatorum due to GC; remove granulation tissue and warts and cauterize wounds **Action:** Caustic antiseptic and astringent **Dose:** *Adults & Peds.* Apply to moist surface 2–3×/wk for several wks or until effect. *Peds. Newborns:* Apply 2 gtt into conjunctival sac immediately after birth **Caution/Contra:** [C, ?] Do not use on broken skin **Supplied:** Topical impregnated applicator sticks, soln 10%, 25, 50%; ophth 1% amp **Notes/SE:** May stain tissue black, usually resolves; local irritation, methemoglobinemia

Silver Sulfadiazine (Silvadene)
Uses: Prevention of sepsis in 2nd- and 3rd-degree burns **Action:** Bactericidal **Dose:** *Adults & Peds.* Aseptically cover the affected area with 1/16-in. coating bid **Caution/Contra:** [B, ?/–] Age <2 mon **Supplied:** Cream 1% **Notes/SE:** Can have systemic absorption with extensive application; itching, rash, skin discoloration, blood dyscrasias, hepatitis, allergy **Interactions:** ↓ effects of topical proteolytic enzymes

Simethicone (Mylicon)
Uses: Flatulence **Action:** Defoaming action **Dose:** *Adults & Peds.* 40–125 mg PO pc and hs PRN **Caution/Contra:** [C, ?] Intestinal perforation or obstruction **Supplied:** Tabs 80, 125 mg; caps 125 mg; gtt 40 mg/0.6 mL **Notes/SE:** Diarrhea, nausea **NIPE:** Formation of gas not prevented by drug; ↑ belching and flatus

Simvastatin (Zocor)
Uses: ↓ elevated cholesterol levels **Action:** HMG-CoA reductase inhibitor **Dose:** 5–80 mg PO; with meals; ↓ dose in renal insufficiency **Caution/Contra:** [X, –] Avoid concurrent use of gemfibrozil; liver disease **Supplied:** Tabs 5, 10, 20, 40 mg **Notes/SE:** Use caution with concurrent use of gemfibrozil; HA, GI upset, myalgia, myopathy, hepatitis **Interactions:** ↑ effects with amprenavir, azole antifungals, cyclosporine, danazol, diltiazem, gemfibrozil, indinavir, macrolides, nefazadone, nelfinavir, ritonavir, saquinavir, verapamil, grapefruit juice; ↑ effects of digoxin, warfarin; ↓ effects with cholestyramine, colestipol, fluvastatin, isradipine **Labs:** ↑ LFTs **NIPE:** Take with food and in the evening; ⊘ PRG, breast-feeding

Sirolimus [Rapamycin] (Rapamune)
WARNING: Can cause immunosuppression and infections **Action:** Inhibits T-lymphocyte activation **Dose:** 2 mg/d PO; dilute in water or orange juice; do not drink grapefruit juice while on sirolimus; take 4 h after cyclosporin; ↓ dose

in hepatic impairment **Caution/Contra:** [C, ?/–] Grapefruit juice, ketoconazole **Supplied:** Soln 1 mg/mL **Notes/SE:** Routine blood levels not needed except in peds or liver failure (trough 9–17 ng/mL); HTN, edema, chest pain, fever, HA, insomnia, acne, rash, hypercholesterolemia, hyper-/hypokalemia, GI upset, infections, blood dyscrasias, arthralgia, tachycardia, renal impairment, hepatic artery thrombosis, graft loss and death in de novo liver transplant **Interactions:** ↑ effects with azole antifungals, cimetidine, cyclosporine, diltiazem, macrolides, nicardipine, protease inhibitors, verapamil, grapefruit juice; ↓ effects with carbamazepine, phenobarbital, phenytoin, rifabutin, rifapentin, rifampin; ↓ effects of live virus vaccines **Labs:** ↑ LFTs, BUN, creatinine, cholesterol, triglycerides **NIPE:** Take w/o regard to food; ⊘ PRG while taking drug and for 12 wk >drug d/c

Smallpox vaccine (Dryvax)   **Uses:** Active immunization against smallpox **Action:** Live vaccine **Dose:** *Adults.* Primary vaccination: 2–3 punctures (scarification w/bifurcated needle); re-vaccination – 15 punctures. **Caution:** [C, –] Caution if latex sensitivity or potential of contact transmission to contraindicated patients; contra in children <18 y, in febrile illness, immunosuppression, Hx of eczema and their household contacts; in emergency situations, no absolute contraindications **Supplied:** Vial for reconstitution ≅100 million pock-forming units/mL **Notes/SE:** Malaise, fever, regional lymphadenopathy, encephalopathy, rashes, spread of inoculation to other sites administered; Stevens–Johnson syndrome, eczema vaccinatum with severe disability

Sodium Bicarbonate [NaHCO₃]   **Uses:** Alkalinization of urine, RTA, metabolic acidosis **Dose:** *Adults.* *ECC:* Initiate adequate ventilation, 1 mEq/kg/dose IV; can repeat 0.5 mEq/kg in 10 min once or based on acid–base status. *Metabolic acidosis:* 2–5 mEq/kg IV over 8 h and PRN based on acid–base status. *Alkalinize urine:* 4 g (48 mEq) PO, then 1–2 g q4h; adjust based on urine pH; 2 amp in 1 L D_5 W @100–250 mL/h IV; monitor urine pH and serum bicarbonate. *Chronic renal failure:* 1–3 mEq/kg/d PO. *Distal RTA:* 1 mEq/kg/d PO. *Peds.* >1 y: *ECC:* See Adults. >1 y: *ECC:* Initiate adequate ventilation, 1:1 dilution 1 mEq/mL dosed 1 mEq/kg IV; can repeat with 0.5 mEq/kg in 10 min once or based on acid–base status. *Chronic renal failure:* See Adults. *Distal RTA:* 2–3 mEq/kg/d PO. *Proximal RTA:* 5–10 mEq/kg/d titrate based on serum bicarbonate levels. *Urine alkalinization:* 84–840 mg/kg/d (1–10 mEq/kg/d) ÷ doses; adjust based on urine pH **Caution/Contra:** [C, ?] **Supplied:** IV inf, powder, and tabs; 300 mg = 3.6 mEq; 325 mg = 3.8 mEq; 520 mg = 6.3 mEq; 600 mg = 7.3 mEq; 650 mg = 7.6 mEq **Notes/SE:** 1 g neutralizes 12 mEq of acid; in infants, do not exceed 10 mEq/min inf; belching, edema, flatulence, hypernatremia, metabolic alkalosis **Interactions:** ↑ effects of anorexiants, amphetamines, ephedrine, flecainide, mecamylamine, pseudoephedrine, quinidine, sympathomimetics; ↓ effects of BBs, cefpodoxime, cefuroxime, ketoconazole, lithium, methotrexate, quinolones, salicylates, sulfonylureas, tetracyclines **Labs:** False + urinary protein **NIPE:** ⊘ take w/n 2 h of other drugs; ↑ risk of milk-alkali syndrome with long-term use or when taken with milk

Sodium Citrate (Bicitra) Uses: Alkalinizes urine; dissolves uric acid and cysteine stones Action: Urinary alkalinizer Dose: *Adults.* 2–6 tsp (10–30 mL) diluted in 1–3 oz water pc and hs. *Peds.* 1–3 tsp (5–15 mL) diluted in 1–3 oz water pc and hs; best after meals Caution/Contra: [C, +] Do not give to patients on aluminum-based antacids. Contra in severe renal impairment or Na-restricted diets Supplied: 15- or 30-mL unit dose: 16 (473 mL) or 4 (118 mL) fl oz Notes/SE: Tetany, metabolic alkalosis, hyperkalemia, GI upset; avoid use of multiple 50-mL amps; can cause hypernatremia/hyperosmolarity Interactions: ↑ effects of amphetamines, ephedrine, flecainide, pseudoephedrine, quinidine; ↓ effects of barbiturates, chlorpropamide, lithium, salicylates NIPE: Dilute with water; take >meals to avoid laxative effect

Sodium Oxybate (Xyrem) [C-III] Uses: Narcolepsy-associated cataplexy Action: Inhibitory neurotransmitter Dose: 2.25 g PO qhs, second dose 2.5–4 h later; may increase to max of 9 g/d Caution/Contra: [B, ?/–] May lead to dependence; significant vomiting, respiratory depression, psychiatric symptoms; contra in succinic semialdehyde dehydrogenase deficiency; potentiates ethanol Supplied: 500 mg/mL 180 mL oral soln Notes/SE: Synonym for γ-hydroxybutyrate (GHB), a substance abused recreationally and as a "date rape drug"; controlled distribution requires prescriber and patient registration; must be administered when patient in bed; confusion, depression, diminished level of consciousness, incontinence Interactions: ↑ risk of CNS depression with sedatives, hypnotics, alcohol NIPE: Dilute with 2 oz water, do not eat w/n 2 h of taking this drug

Sodium Polystyrene Sulfonate (Kayexalate) Uses: Hyperkalemia Action: Na and K ion-exchange resin Dose: *Adults.* 15–60 g PO or 30–60 g PR q6h based on serum K⁺. *Peds.* 1 g/kg/dose PO or PR q6h based on serum K⁺; given with an agent, eg, sorbitol, to promote movement through the bowel Caution/Contra: [C, M] Hypernatremia Supplied: Powder; susp 15 g/60 mL sorbitol Notes/SE: Can cause hypernatremia, hypokalemia, Na⁺ retention, GI upset, fecal impaction; enema acts more quickly than PO Interactions: ↑ risk of systemic alkalosis with calcium- or magnesium-containing antacids NIPE: Mix with chilled fluid other than orange juice

Sorbitol (generic) Uses: Constipation Action: Laxative Dose: 30–60 mL of a 20–70% soln PRN Caution/Contra: [B, +] Anuria Supplied: Liq 70% Notes/SE: Edema, electrolyte losses, lactic acidosis, GI upset, xerostomia NIPE: ⊘ use unless clear solution

Sotalol (Betapace) WARNING: Monitor patients for 1st 3 d of therapy to reduce risks of induced arrhythmia Uses: Ventricular arrhythmias, AF Action: β-Adrenergic-blocking agent Dose: 80 mg PO bid; may be ↑ to 240–320 mg/d; ↓ dose in renal failure Caution/Contra: [B (1st trimester; D if 2nd or 3rd trimester), +] Asthma, bradycardia, prolonged QT interval, 2nd- or 3rd-degree heart block w/o pacemaker, cardiogenic shock, uncontrolled CHF, CrCl <40 mL/min Supplied: Tabs 80, 120, 160, 240 mg Notes/SE: Betapace should not be substituted for Betapace AF because of significant differences in labeling; bradycardia, chest pain, palpitations, fatigue, dizziness, weakness, dyspnea **Interactions:** ↑ effects with ASA, antihypertensives, nitrates, oral contraceptives, fluoxetine, prazosin, sulfinpyrazone, verapamil, alcohol; ↑ risk of prolonged QT interval with amiodarone, amitriptyline, bepridil, disopyramide, erythromycin, gatifloxacin, haloperidol, imipramine, moxifloxacin, quinidine, pimozide, procainamide, sparfloxacin, thioridazine; ↑ effects of lidocaine; ↓ effects with antacids, clonidine, NSAIDs, thyroid drugs; ↓ effects of hypoglycemics, terbutaline, theophylline **Labs:** ↑ BUN, serum glucose, lipoprotein, triglycerides, K⁺, uric acid **NIPE:** may ↑ sensitivity to cold; d/c MAOIs 14 d <drug; take w/o food

Sotalol (Betapace AF)

WARNING: To minimize risk of induced arrhythmia, patients initiated/reinitiated on Betapace AF should be placed for a minimum of 3 d (on their maint dose) in a facility that can provide cardiac resuscitation, continuous ECG monitoring, and calculations of CrCl; Betapace should not be substituted for Betapace AF because of differences in labeling **Uses:** Maintains sinus rhythm for symptomatic AF/flutter **Action:** β-Adrenergic-blocking agent **Dose:** *Initial CrCl >60 mL/min:* 80 mg PO q12h. *CrCl 40–60 mL/min:* 80 mg PO q2h; ↑ to 120 mg during hospitalization; monitor QT interval 2–4 h after each dose, with dose reduction or discontinuation if QT interval >500 ms **Caution/Contra:** [B (1st trimester); D if 2nd or 3rd trimester), +] Asthma, bradycardia, prolonged QT interval, 2nd- or 3rd-degree heart block w/o pacemaker, cardiogenic shock, uncontrolled CHF, CrCl <40 mL/min; caution if converting from previous antiarrhythmic therapy **Supplied:** Tabs 80, 120, 160 mg **Notes/SE:** Bradycardia, chest pain, palpitations, fatigue, dizziness, weakness, dyspnea; routinely evaluate renal function and QT interval; **see Sotalol**

Sparfloxacin (Zagam)

Uses: Community-acquired pneumonia, acute exacerbations of chronic bronchitis **Action:** Quinolone antibiotic; inhibits DNA gyrase **Dose:** 400 mg PO on day 1, then 200 mg q24h for 10 days; ↓ dose in renal dysfunction **Caution/Contra:** [C, ?/–] Significant phototoxicity (even from sunlight through windows); QT prolongation; do not administer w/drugs that prolong QT interval **Supplied:** Tabs 200 mg **Notes/SE:** Interactions with theophylline, caffeine, sucralfate, warfarin, and antacids; restlessness, N/V/D, rash, ruptured tendons, ↑ LFTs, sleep disorders, confusion, convulsions; must protect from sunlight up to 5 days after last dose **Interactions:** ↑ effects with cimetidine, probenecid; ↑ effects of cyclosporine, diazepam, metroprolol, theophylline, warfarin, caffeine; ↑ risk of prolonged QT interval with amiodarone, bepridil, disopyramide, erythromycin, pentamidine, phenothiazines, procainamide, propranolol, quinidine, sotalol, TCAs; ↓ effects with antacids, antineoplastics, didanosine, sucralfate **NIPE:** ↑ risk of tendon rupture & photosensitivity; take w/o regard to food; ↑ fluids to 2–3 L/d

Spironolactone (Aldactone)

Uses: Hyperaldosteronism, ascites from CHF or cirrhosis **Action:** Aldosterone antagonist; K⁺-sparing diuretic **Dose:** *Adults.* 25–100 mg PO qid; CHF (NYHA class III–IV) 25–50 mg/d. *Peds.* 1–3.3

mg/kg/24 h PO ÷ bid–qid. *Neonates:* 0.5–1 mg/kg/dose q8h; take with food **Caution/Contra:** [D, +] Hyperkalemia, renal failure, anuria **Supplied:** Tabs 25, 50, 100 mg **Notes/SE:** Hyperkalemia and gynecomastia, arrhythmia, sexual dysfunction, confusion, dizziness **Interactions:** ↑ risk of hyperkalemia with ACEIs, K⁺ supplements, K⁺-sparing diuretics, ↑ K⁺ diet; ↑ effects of lithium; ↓ effects with salicylates; ↓ effects of anticoagulants **Labs:** False ↑ of corticosteroids, digoxin **NIPE:** Take with food; ↑ risk of gynecomastia; maximum effects of drug may take 2–3 wk

Stavudine (Zerit)   WARNING: Lactic acidosis and severe hepatomegaly with steatosis and pancreatitis reported **Uses:** Advanced HIV disease **Action:** Reverse-transcriptase inhibitor **Dose:** *Adults.* >60 kg: 40 mg bid. <60 kg: 30 mg bid. *Peds.* Birth–13 d: 0.5 mg/kg q12h. >14 d and <30 kg: 1 mg/kg q12h. = 30 kg: Adult dose; ↓ dose in renal failure **Caution/Contra:** [C, +] **Supplied:** Caps 15, 20, 30, 40 mg; soln 1 mg/mL **Notes/SE:** May cause peripheral neuropathy, HA, chills, fever, malaise, rash, GI upset, anemias, lactic acidosis, ↑ levels on LFTs, pancreatitis **Interactions:** ↑ risk of pancreatitis with didanosine; ↑ effects with probenecid; ↓ effects with zidovudine **Labs:** ↑ LFTs **NIPE:** Take w/o regard to food

Steroids, Systemic   (Table 4, page 248) The following relates only to the commonly used systemic glucocorticoids **Uses:** Endocrine disorders (adrenal insufficiency), rheumatoid disorders, collagen-vascular diseases, dermatologic diseases, allergic states, cerebral edema, nephritis, nephrotic syndrome, immunosuppression for transplantation, hypercalcemia, malignancies (breast, lymphomas), preoperatively (in any patient who has been on steroids in the previous year, known hypoadrenalism, preop for adrenalectomy); inj into joints/tissue **Action:** Glucocorticoid **Dose:** Varies with use and institutional protocols. *Adrenal insufficiency, acute: Adults.* Hydrocortisone: 100 mg IV, then 300 mg/d ÷ q6h; convert to 50 mg PO q8h ×6 doses, taper to 30–50 mg/d ÷ bid. *Peds.* Hydrocortisone: 1–2 mg/kg IV, then 150–250 mg/d ÷ tid. *Adrenal insufficiency, chronic (physiologic replacement):* May need mineralocorticoid supplementation such as Florinef. *Adults.* Hydrocortisone 20 mg PO qAM, 10 mg PO qPM; cortisone 0.5–0.75 mg/kg/d ÷ bid; cortisone 0.25–0.35 mg/kg/d IM; dexamethasone 0.03–0.15 mg/kg/d or 0.6–0.75 mg/m²/d ÷ q6–12h PO, IM, IV. *Peds.* Hydrocortisone 0.5–0.75 mg/kg/d PO tid; hydrocortisone succinate 0.25–0.35 mg/kg/d IM. *Asthma, acute: Adults.* Methylprednisolone 60 mg q6h. *Peds.* Prednisolone 1–2 mg/kg/d or prednisone 1–2 mg/kg/d ÷ qd–bid for up to 5 d; prednisolone 2–4 mg/kg/d IV ÷ tid. *Congenital adrenal hyperplasia: Peds.* Initially, hydrocortisone 30–36 mg/m²/d PO ÷ 1/3 dose qAM, 2/3 dose qPM; maint 20–25 mg/m²/d ÷ bid. *Extubation/airway edema:* Dexamethasone 0.5–1 mg/kg/d IM/IV ÷ q6h, start beginning 24 h prior to extubation; continue for 4 additional doses. *Immunosuppressive/antiinflammatory: Adults & Older Peds.* Hydrocortisone 15–240 mg PO, IM, IV q12h; methylprednisolone: 4–48 mg/d PO, taper to lowest effective dose; methylprednisolone Na succinate 10–80 mg/d IM. *Adults.* Prednisone or prednisolone

5–60 mg/d PO ÷ qd–qid. *Infants & Younger Children.* Hydrocortisone 2.5–10 mg/kg/d PO ÷ q6–8h; 1–5 mg/kg/d IM/IV ÷ bid. *Nephrotic syndrome: Peds.* Prednisolone or prednisone 2 mg/kg/d PO ÷ tid–qid until urine is protein-free for 5 d, use up to 28 d; for persistent proteinuria, 4 mg/kg/dose PO qod max 120 mg/d for an additional 28 d; maint 2 mg/kg/dose qod for 28 d; taper over 4–6 wk (max 80 mg/d). *Septic shock* (controversial): *Adults.* Hydrocortisone 500 mg–1 g IM/IV q2–6h. *Peds.* Hydrocortisone 50 mg/kg IM/IV, repeat q4–24 h PRN. *Status asthmaticus: Adults & Peds.* Hydrocortisone 1–2 mg/kg/dose IV q6h, then decrease by 0.5–1 mg/kg q6h. *Rheumatic disease: Adults. Intraarticular:* Hydrocortisone acetate 25–37.5 mg large joint, 10–25 mg small joint; methylprednisolone acetate 20–80 mg large joint, 4–10 mg small joint. *Intrabursal:* Hydrocortisone acetate 25–37.5 mg. *Intraganglial:* Hydrocortisone acetate 25–37.5 mg. *Tendon sheath:* Hydrocortisone acetate 5–12.5 mg. *Perioperative steroid coverage:* Hydrocortisone 100 mg IV night before surgery, 1 h preop, intraop, and 4, 8, and 12 h postop; pod #1 100 mg IV q6h; pod #2 100 mg IV q8h; pod #3 100 mg IV q12h; pod #4 50 mg IV q12h; pod #5 25 mg IV q12h; then resume prior oral dosing if chronic use or DC if only perioperative coverage required. *Cerebral edema:* Dexamethasone 10 mg IV; then 4 mg IV q4–6h **Caution/Contra:** [C, ?/–] **Supplied:** Table 4, Page 248. **Notes/SE:** Hydrocortisone succinate administered systemically, acetate form intraarticular; all can cause ↑ appetite, hyperglycemia, hypokalemia, osteoporosis, nervousness, insomnia, "steroid psychosis," adrenal suppression **NIPE:** Never abruptly d/c steroids, especially in chronic treatment; taper dose

Steroids, Topical (See also Table 5, page 249)

Uses: Relief of inflammatory and pruritic manifestations of corticosteroid-responsive dermatoses **Action:** Corticosteroid, antiinflammatory **Dose:** Varies widely with indication and formulation. Table 5 (page 249) for frequency of application of various agents **Caution/Contra:** [?, ?] Contra in viral, fungal, or tubercular skin lesions **Supplied:** Table 5, page 249 **Notes/SE:** Topical use should be short term

Streptokinase (Streptase, Kabikinase)

Uses: Coronary artery thrombosis, acute massive PE, DVT, and some occluded vascular grafts **Action:** Activates plasminogen to plasmin that degrades fibrin **Dose:** *Adults. PE:* Loading dose of 250,000 IU IV through a peripheral vein over 30 min, then 100,000 IU/h IV for 24–72 h. *Coronary artery thrombosis:* 1.5 MU IV over 60 min. *DVT or arterial embolism:* Load with PE, then 100,000 IU/h for 72 h. *Peds.* 3500–4000 U/kg over 30 min, followed by 1000–1500 U/kg/h **Caution/Contra:** [C, +] Streptococcal infection or streptokinase use in last 6 mon, active bleeding, CVA, TIA, spinal surgery, or trauma in last month, vascular anomalies, severe hepatic or renal disease, endocarditis, pericarditis, severe uncontrolled HTN **Supplied:** Powder for inj 250,000, 600,000, 750,000, 1,500,000 IU **Notes/SE:** If manit inf inadequate to maintain thrombin clotting time 2–5× control, refer to the package insert, *PDR*, or the AHFS Drug Information service for adjustments. Antibodies remain 3–6 mon following dose; bleeding, hypotension, fever, bruising, rash, GI upset, hemorrhage, anaphylaxis **Interactions:** ↑ risk of bleeding with anticoagulants, ASA, heparin, indomethacin, NSAIDs, dong quai, feverfew, garlic, ginger, horse chestnut, red clover; ↓ effects with aminocaproic acid **Labs:** ↑ PT, PTT

Streptomycin **Uses:** TB **Action:** Aminoglycoside; interferes with protein synthesis **Dose:** 1–4 g/d IM in 1–2 ÷ doses (endocarditis); TB 15 mg/kg/d; ↓ dose in renal failure **Caution/Contra:** [D, +] **Supplied:** Inj 400 mg/mL **Notes/SE:** ↑ Incidence of vestibular and auditory toxicity, neurotoxicity, nephrotoxicity **Interactions:** ↑ risk of nephrotoxicity with amphotericin B, cephalosporins, cisplatin, methoxyflurane, polymyxin B, vancomycin; ↑ risk of ototoxicity with carboplatin, furosemide, mannitol, urea; ↑ effects of anticoagulants **Labs:** False + urine glucose, false ↑ urine protein **NIPE:** ↑ fluid intake

Streptozocin (Zanosar) **Uses:** Pancreatic islet cell tumors and carcinoid tumors **Action:** DNA–DNA (interstrand) cross-linking; DNA, RNA, and protein synthesis inhibitor **Dose:** 1–1.5 g/m² q4wk (single agent); 500 mg/m²/d for 5 d or 100 mg/m²/wk for 1st 2 wk q6wk (combination regimens); ↓ dose in renal failure **Caution/Contra:** [D, ?/–] Caution in renal failure. **Supplied:** Inj 1 g **Notes/SE:** N/V, duodenal ulcers; myelosuppression rare (20%) and mild; nephrotoxicity (proteinuria and azotemia often heralded by hypophosphatemia) dose limiting. Hypo-/hyperglycemia may occur; phlebitis and pain at the site of inj **Interactions:** ↑ risk of nephrotoxicity with aminoglycosides, amphotericin B, cisplatin, vancomycin; ↑ effects of doxorubicin; ↓ effects with phenytoin **NIPE:** ⊘ PRG, breastfeeding; ↑ fluid intake to 2–3 L/d

Succimer (Chemet) **Uses:** Lead poisoning **Action:** Heavy-metal-chelating agent **Dose:** *Adults & Peds.* *8–15 kg:* 100 mg PO. *16–23 kg:* 200 mg PO. *24–34 kg:* 300 mg PO. *35–44 kg:* 400 mg PO. *>45 kg:* 500 mg PO; give dose noted q8h for 5 d, q12h for 14 d; drink fluids liberally **Caution/Contra:** [C, ?] **Supplied:** Caps 100 mg **Notes/SE:** Rash, fever, GI upset, hemorrhoids, metallic taste, drowsiness, ↑ LFTs **Labs:** False + urinary ketones, false ↑ serum CPK, false ↑ uric acid **NIPE:** ⊘ take with other chelating agents; ↑ fluid intake to 2–3 L/d

Succinylcholine (Anectine, Quelicin, Sucostrin) **Uses:** Adjunct to general anesthesia to facilitate ET intubation and to induce skeletal muscle relaxation during surgery or mechanically supported ventilation **Action:** Depolarizing neuromuscular blocking agent **Dose:** *Adults.* 0.6 mg/kg IV over 10–30 s, followed by 0.04–0.07 mg/kg as needed to maintain muscle relaxation. *Peds.* 1–2 mg/kg/dose IV, followed by 0.3–0.6 mg/kg/dose at intervals of 10–20 min; ↓ in severe liver disease **Caution/Contra:** [C, M] At risk for malignant hyperthermia; myopathy; recent major burn, multiple trauma, extensive skeletal muscle denervation **Supplied:** Inj 20, 50, 100 mg/mL; powder for inj 100, 500 mg, 1 g/vial **Notes/SE:** May precipitate malignant hyperthermia, respiratory depression, or prolonged apnea; many drug interactions potentiate succinylcholine; observe for cardiovascular effects (arrhythmias, hypotension, brady/tachycardia); ↑ intraocular pressure, postoperative stiffness, salivation, myoglobinuria; in children, acute rhabdomyolysis, hyperkalemia, arrhythmia, and death **Interactions:** ↑ effects with amphotericin B, aprotinin, BBs, clindamycin, lidocaine, lithium, metoclopramide, oral contraceptives, oxytocin, phenothiazines, procainamide, procaine, quinidine, quinine, trimethaphan; ↓ effect with diazepam **Labs:** ↑ serum K+

Sucralfate (Carafate)   **Uses:** Duodenal and gastric ulcers **Action:** Forms ulcer-adherent complex that protects against acid, pepsin, and bile acid **Dose:** *Adults.* 1 g PO qid, 1 h prior to meals and hs. *Peds.* 40–80 mg/kg/d ÷ q6h; continue 4–8 wk unless healing demonstrated by x-ray or endoscopy; separate from other drugs by 2 h (can inhibit absorption); take on empty stomach (before meals acceptable) **Caution/Contra:** [B, +] **Supplied:** Tabs 1 g; susp 1 g/10 mL **Notes/SE:** Constipation frequent; diarrhea, dizziness, xerostomia; aluminum may accumulate in renal failure **Interactions:** ↓ effects of cimetidine, digoxin, levothyroxine, phenytoin, quinolones, quinidine, ranitidine, tetracyclines, theophylline, warfarin **NIPE:** Take w/o food

Sufentanil (Sufenta) [C-II]   **Uses:** Analgesic adjunct to maintain balanced general anesthesia **Action:** Potent synthetic opioid **Dose:** *Adjunctive:* 1–8 µg/kg with nitrous oxide/oxygen; maint of 10–50 µg PRN. *General anesthesia:* 8–30 µg/kg with oxygen and a skeletal muscle relaxant. *Maint:* 25–50 µg PRN. Give over 3–5 min **Caution/Contra:** [C, ?] **Supplied:** Inj 50 µg/mL **Notes/SE:** Respiratory depressant effects last longer than analgesia; bradycardia, hypotension, drowsiness, GI upset, arrhythmias, biliary tract spasm, blurred vision, pruritus **Interactions:** ↑ effects with BBs, CCBs, cimetidine, CNS depressants, alcohol **NIPE:** ↑ risk of post-op resp depression

Sulfacetamide (Bleph-10, Cetamide, Sodium Sulamyd)   **Uses:** Conjunctival infections **Action:** Sulfonamide antibiotic **Dose:** 10% oint apply qid and hs; soln for keratitis apply q2–3h depending on severity **Caution/Contra:** [C, M] Sulfonamide sensitivity; age <2 mon **Supplied:** Oint 10%; soln 10, 15, 30% **Notes/SE:** Irritation, burning; blurred vision, brow ache, Stevens–Johnson syndrome, photosensitivity **Interactions:** ↓ effects with tetracyclines **NIPE:** Not compatable with silver-containing preparations; purulent exudate inactivates drug; ↑ risk of sensitivity to light

Sulfacetamide and Prednisolone (Blephamide, others)   **Uses:** Steroid-responsive inflammatory ocular conditions with infection or a risk of infection **Action:** Antibiotic and antiinflammatory **Dose:** *Adults and Peds >2 y.* Apply oint to lower conjunctival sac qd–qid; soln 1–3 gtt 2–3 h while awake **Caution/Contra:** [C, ?/–] Sulfonamide sensitivity; age <2 mon **Supplied:** Oint sulfacetamide 10%/prednisolone 0.5%, sulfacetamide 10%/prednisolone 0.2%, sulfacetamide 10%/prednisolone 0.25%; susp sulfacetamide 10%/prednisolone 0.25%, sulfacetamide 10%/prednisolone 0.5%, sulfacetamide 10%/prednisolone 0.2% **Notes/SE:** Ophth susp can be used as an otic agent; irritation, burning, blurred vision, brow ache, Stevens–Johnson syndrome, photosensitivity **Interactions:** ↓ effects with tetracyclines **NIPE:** Not compatable with silver-containing preparations; purulent exudate inactivates drug; ↑ risk of sensitivity to light; ⊘ d/c abruptly

Sulfasalazine (Azulfidine, Azulfidine EN)   **Uses:** Ulcerative colitis, active Crohn's, juvenile RA **Action:** Sulfonamide; actions not clear **Dose: Adults.** Initially, 1 g tid–qid; ↑ to a max of 8 g/d in 3–4 ÷ doses; maint 500 mg PO qid. **Peds.** Initially, 40–60 mg/kg/24 h PO ÷ q4–6h; maint 20–30 mg/kg/24 h PO ÷ q6h; RA >6 y 30–50 mg/kg/d (%) in 2 doses, start with 1/4–1/3 described maint dose, ↑ weekly until dose reached at 1 mon, 2 g/d max; ↓ dose in renal failure **Caution/Contra:** [B (D if near term), M] Sulfonamide or salicylate sensitivity, porphyria, GI or GU obstruction; avoid in hepatic impairment **Supplied:** Tabs 500 mg; EC tabs 500 mg; oral susp 250 mg/5 mL **Notes/SE:** Can cause severe GI upset; discolors urine; dizziness, HA, photosensitivity, oligospermia, anemias, Stevens–Johnson syndrome **Interactions:** ↑ effects of anticoagulants, hypoglycemics, methotrexate, phenytoin, zidovudine; ↓ effects with antibiotics; ↓ effects of digoxin, folic acid, iron, procaine, proparacaine, sulfonylureas, tetracaine **Labs:** False + urinary glucose; false ↑ serum conjugated bilirubin, creatinine; false ↓ serum unconjugated bilirubin, K+ **NIPE:** Take >meals; ↑ fluids to 2–3 L/d; ↑ risk of photosensitivity; skin & urine may become yellow-orange

Sulfinpyrazone (Anturane)   **Uses:** Acute and chronic gout **Action:** Inhibits renal tubular absorption of uric acid **Dose:** 100–200 mg PO bid for 1 wk, then ↑ as needed to maint of 200–400 mg bid; take with food or antacids, take with plenty of fluids; avoid salicylates **Caution/Contra:** [C (per manufacturer; D per expert analysis if near term), ?/–] Avoid in renal impairment, avoid salicylates; peptic ulcer; blood dyscrasias **Supplied:** Tabs 100 mg; caps 200 mg **Notes/SE:** N/V, stomach pain, urolithiasis, leucopenia **Interactions:** ↑ effects of anticoagulants, hypoglycemics, methotrexate; ↓ effects with ASA, cholestyramine, niacin, salicylates, alcohol; ↓ effects of acetaminophen, BBs, nitrofurantoin, theophylline, verapamil **Labs:** ↓ serum uric acid **NIPE:** Take with food, ↑ fluids to 2–3 L/d

Sulindac (Clinoril)   **Uses:** Arthritis and pain **Action:** NSAID; inhibits prostaglandin synthesis **Dose:** 150–200 mg bid with food **Caution/Contra:** [B (D if 3rd trimester or near term), ?] NSAID or ASA sensitivity, peptic ulcer, GI bleeding **Supplied:** Tabs 150, 200 mg **Notes/SE:** Dizziness, rash, GI upset, pruritus, edema, ↓ renal blood flow, renal failure (may have fewer renal effects than other NSAIDs), peptic ulcer, GI bleeding **Interactions:** ↑ effects with NSAIDS, probenecid; ↑ effects of aminoglycosides, anticoagulants, cyclosporine, digoxin, lithium, methotrexate, K+-sparing diuretics; ↑ risk of bleeding with ASA, NSAIDs, alcohol, dong quai, feverfew, garlic, ginger, horse chestnut, red clover; ↓ effects with antacids, ASA; ↓ effects of BBs, captopril, diuretics, hydralazine **Labs:** ↑ serum chloride, sodium, glucose, LFTs, PT **NIPE:** Take with food; ↑ risk of photosensitivity; may take several weeks for full drug effect

Sumatriptan (Imitrex)   **Uses:** Acute treatment of migraine attacks **Action:** Vascular serotonin receptor agonist **Dose:** *SC:* 6 mg SC as a single dose PRN;

can repeat in 1 h to a max of 12 mg/24 h. *Oral:* 25 mg, repeat into 2 h, PRN, 100 mg/d max oral dose; max 300 mg/d. *Nasal spray:* 1 single spray into 1 nostril, may repeat in 2 h to a max of 40 mg/24 h **Caution/Contra:** [C, M] Avoid in patients with angina, ischemic heart disease, uncontrolled HTN, ergot use, MAOI use w/n 14 d **Supplied:** Inj 6 mg/mL; tabs 25, 50 mg; nasal spray 5, 20 mg **Notes/SE:** Pain and bruising at the inj site; dizziness, hot flashes, paresthesias, chest pain, weakness, numbness, coronary vasospasm, HTN **Interactions:** ↑ effects of weakness, incoordination and hyper-reflexia with ergots, MAOIs, and SSRIs, horehound, St. John's Wort **NIPE:** Admin drug as soon as possible >onset of migraine

Tacrine (Cognex) Uses: Mild–moderate dementia **Action:** Cholinesterase inhibitor **Dose:** 10–40 mg PO qid to 160 mg/d; separate doses from food **Caution/Contra:** [C, ?] **Supplied:** Caps 10, 20, 30, 40 mg **Notes/SE:** May ↑ LFT, HA, dizziness, GI upset, flushing, confusion, ataxia, myalgia, bradycardia **Interactions:** ↑ effects with cimetidine, quinolones, SSRIs, ↑ effects of BBs, cholinergics, cholinesterase inhibitors, succinylcholine, theophylline; ↓ effects with tobacco, food; ↓ effects of anticholinergics, levodopa **Labs:** ↑ ALT **NIPE:** If taken with food ↓ drug plasma levels by 30%; may take up to 6 wk for ALT elevations

Tacrolimus [FK-506] (Prograf, Protopic) Uses: Prophylaxis of organ rejection, eczema **Action:** Macrolide immunosuppressant **Dose:** *IV:* 0.05–0.1 mg/kg/d as cont inf. *PO:* 0.15–0.3 mg/kg/d ÷ into 2 doses. *Eczema:* Apply bid, continue 1 wk after clearing; ↓ dose in hepatic/renal impairment **Caution/Contra:** [C, –] Do not use with cyclosporine **Supplied:** Caps 1, 5 mg; inj 5 mg/mL; ointment 0.03, 0.1% **Notes/SE:** Neurotoxicity and nephrotoxicity, HTN, edema, HA, insomnia, fever, pruritus, hypo-/hyperkalemia, hyperglycemia, GI upset, anemia, leukocytosis, tremors, paresthesias, pleural effusion, seizures, lymphoma

Tadalafil (Cialis) Uses: Erectile dysfunction **Action:** Phosphodiesterase 5 inhibitor **Dose:** *Adults.* 10 mg PO before sexual activity w/o regard to meals (20 mg Max); 5 mg (10 mg max) in renal and mild hepatic insufficiency **Caution:** [B, –] **Contra:** Nitrates, α-blockers (except tamsulosin), severe hepatic insufficiency **Supplied:** 5, 10, 20 mg tabs **SE:** HA, flushing, dyspepsia, rhinitis, back pain, myalgia **Notes:** Longest acting of class (36 h) **Interactions:** ↑ effects with ketoconazole, ritonavir, and other cytochrome P450 CYP3A4 inhibitors; ↑ hypotension with antihypertensives, alcohol; ↓ effects with P450 CYP3A4 inducers such as rifampin, antacids **NIPE:** ↑ risk of priapism; use barrier contraception to prevent STDs

Tamoxifen (Nolvadex) Uses: Breast CA (postmenopausal, estrogen receptor positive), endometrial CA, melanoma, reduction of breast CA risk in high-risk women **Action:** Nonsteroidal antiestrogen; mixed agonist–antagonist effect **Dose:** 20–40 mg (typically 10 mg bid or 20 mg/d) **Caution/Contra:** [D, –] Caution in leukopenia, thrombocytopenia, hyperlipidemia **Supplied:** Tabs 10, 20 mg **Notes/SE:** Uterine malignancy and thrombotic events noted when administered to reduce risk of breast CA; menopausal symptoms (hot flashes, N/V) in pre-menopausal patients; vaginal bleeding and menstrual irregularities; skin rash, pruritus vulvae, dizziness, HA, peripheral edema; acute flare of bone metastasis pain and hypercalcemia; retinopathy reported (high dose); ↑ risk of PRG in pre-menopausal women by inducing ovulation **Interactions:** ↑ effects with bromocriptine, grapefruit juice; ↑ effects of coumadin, cyclosporine, warfarin; ↓ effects with antacids, aminoglutethimide, letrozole, medroxyprogesterone, rifamycins **Labs:** ↑ calcium , T4, BUN, creatinine, LFTs **NIPE:** ⊘ PRG or breast-feeding; use barrier contraception; ↑ risk of photosensitivity

Tamsulosin (Flomax) **Uses:** BPH **Action:** Antagonist of prostatic α-receptors **Dose:** 0.4 mg/d; do not crush, chew, or open caps **Caution/Contra:** [NA/NA (not for use in women)] **Supplied:** Caps 0.4, 0.8 mg **Notes/SE:** HA, dizziness, syncope, somnolence, decreased libido, GI upset, retrograde ejaculation, rhinitis, rash, angioedema **Interactions:** ↑ effects with cimetidine; ↓ hypotension with doxazosin, prazosin, terazosin **NIPE:** Ensure neg test results for prostate CA <drug administration

Tazarotene (Tazorac) **Uses:** Facial acne vulgaris; stable plaque psoriasis up to 20% body surface area **Action:** Keratolytic **Dose:** *Adults & Peds >12 y. Acne:* Cleanse face, dry, and apply thin film qd hs on acne lesions. *Psoriasis:* Apply hs **Caution/Contra:** [X, ?/–] Retinoid sensitivity **Supplied:** Gel 0.05, 0.1% **Notes/SE:** Burning, erythema, irritation, rash, photosensitivity, desquamation, bleeding, skin discoloration **Interactions:** ↑ risk of photosensitivity with quinolones, phenothiazines, sulfonamides, tetracyclines, thiazide diuretics **NIPE:** ⊘ PRG or breast-feeding; use contraception; use sunscreen for ↑ photosensitivity risk

Tegaserod maleate (Zelnorm) **Uses:** Short-term treatment of constipation-predominant IBS in women **Action:** 5HT$_4$ serotonin agonist **Dose:** 6 mg PO bid pc for 4–6 wk; may continue for 2nd course **Caution/Contra:** [B, ?/–] Contra in severe renal, moderate–severe hepatic impairment, Hx of bowel obstruction, gallbladder disease, sphincter of Oddi dysfunction, abdominal adhesions **Supplied:** Tabs 2, 6 mg **Notes/SE:** Do not administer if diarrhea present, as ↑ GI motility; DC if abdominal pain worsens **NIPE:** Take before meals

Telmisartan (Micardis) **Uses:** HTN, CHF, DN **Action:** Angiotensin II receptor antagonist **Dose:** 40–80 mg/d **Caution/Contra:** [C (1st trimester; D 2nd and 3rd trimesters), ?/–] Angiotensin II receptor antagonist sensitivity **Supplied:** Tabs 40, 80 mg **Notes/SE:** Edema, GI upset, HA, angioedema, renal impairment, orthostatic hypotension **Interactions:** ↑ effects with alcohol; ↑ effects of digoxin; ↓ effects of warfarin **Labs:** ↑ creatinine, ↓ HMG **NIPE:** Take w/o regard to food; ⊘ PRG; use barrier contraception

Temazepam (Restoril) [C-IV] **Uses:** Insomnia **Action:** Benzodiazepine **Dose:** 15–30 mg PO hs PRN; ↓ dose in elderly **Caution/Contra:** [X; ?/–] Narrow-angle glaucoma **Supplied:** Caps 7.5, 15, 30 mg **Notes/SE:** Confusion, dizziness, drowsiness, hangover **Interactions:** ↑ effects with cimetidine, disulfiram, kava kava, valerian; ↑ CNS depression with anticonvulsants, CNS depressants, alcohol; ↑ effects of haloperidol, phenytoin; ↓ effects with aminophylline, dyphylline, oral contraceptives, oxitriphylline, rifampin, theophylline, tobacco; ↓ effects of levodopa **NIPE:** ⊘ d/c abruptly after prolonged use, use in PRG or breast-feed

Tenecteplase (TNKase)   **Uses:** Reduction of mortality associated with AMI **Action:** Thrombolytic; TPA **Dose:** 30–50 mg; see following table: **Caution/Contra:** [C, ?] Bleeding, CVA, major surgery (intracranial, intraspinal) or trauma w/n 2 mon **Supplied:** Inj 50 mg, reconstitute with 10 mL sterile water **Notes/SE:** Bleeding, hypersensitivity **Interactions:** ↑ risk of bleeding with anticoagulants, ASA, clopidogrel, dipyridamole, ticlopidine, vitamin K antagonists; ↓ effects with aminocaproic acid **NIPE:** Eval for s/s bleeding

Tenecteplase Dosing

Weight (kg)	TNKase (mg)	TNKase^a Volume (mL)
<60	30	6
≥60–70	35	7
≥70–80	40	8
≥80–90	45	9
≥90	50	10

^{a}From one vial of reconstituted TNKase.

Tenofovir (Viread)   **Uses:** HIV infection **Action:** Nucleotide reverse transcriptase inhibitor **Dose:** 300 mg PO qd with a meal **Caution/Contra:** [B, ?/–] CrCl <60 mL/min; caution with known risk factors for liver disease **Supplied:** Tabs 300 mg **Notes/SE:** GI upset, metabolic syndrome, hepatotoxicity; separate didanosine doses by 2 h **Interactions:** ↑ effects with acyclovir, cidofovir, ganciclovir, indinavir, lopinavir, ritonavir, valacyclovir, food; ↓ effects of didanosine, lamivudine, ritonavir **Labs:** ↑ LFTs, triglycerides, serum and urine glucose **NIPE:** Take with food, take 2 h < or 1 h >didanosine, lopinavir/ritonavir

Terazosin (Hytrin)   **Uses:** BPH and HTN **Action:** α_1-Blocker (blood vessel and bladder neck/prostate) **Dose:** Initially, 1 mg PO hs; ↑ 20 mg/d max **Caution/Contra:** [C, ?] α-Antagonist sensitivity **Supplied:** Tabs 1, 2, 5, 10 mg; caps 1, 2, 5, 10 mg **Notes/SE:** Hypotension and syncope following 1st dose; dizziness, weakness, nasal congestion, peripheral edema common, palpitations, GI upset **Interactions:** ↑ effects with antihypertensives, diuretics; ↑ effects of finasteride; ↓ effects with NSAIDs, α-blockers, ephedra, garlic, ginseng, saw palmetto, yohimbe; ↓ effects of clonidine **Labs:** ↓ albumin, HMG, HCT, WBCs **NIPE:** Take w/o regard to food, ⊘ d/c abruptly

Terbinafine (Lamisil) **Uses:** Onychomycosis, athlete's foot **Action:** Inhibits squalene epoxidase resulting in fungal death **Dose:** *Oral:* 250 mg/d PO for 6–12 wk. *Topical:* Apply to affected area; ↓ dose in renal/hepatic impairment **Caution/Contra:** [B, –] Liver disease or kidney impairment **Supplied:** Tabs 250 mg; cream 1% **Notes/SE:** Effect may take months due to need for new nail growth; do not use occlusive dressings; HA, dizziness, rash, pruritus, alopecia, GI upset, taste perversion, neutropenia, retinal damage, Stevens–Johnson syndrome **Interactions:** ↑ effects with cimetidine; ↑ effects of dextromethorphan, theophylline, caffeine; ↓ effects with rifampin; ↓ effects of cyclosporine **Labs:** LFT abnormalities

Terbutaline (Brethine, Bricanyl) **Uses:** Reversible bronchospasm (asthma, COPD); inhibition of labor **Action:** Sympathomimetic **Dose:** *Adults. Bronchodilator:* 2.5–5 mg PO qid or 0.25 mg/0.25 mg SC; may repeat in 15 min (max 0.5 mg in 4 h). *Met-dose inhaler:* 2 inhal q4–6h. *Premature labor:* Acutely 2.5–10 mg/min/IV, gradually ↑ as tolerated q10–20min; maint 2.5–5 mg PO q4–6h until term. *Peds. Oral:* 0.05–0.15 mg/kg/dose PO tid; max 5 mg/24 h; ↓ dose in renal failure **Caution/Contra:** [B, +] Caution with diabetes, HTN, hyperthyroidism; tachycardia **Supplied:** Tabs 2.5, 5 mg; inj 1 mg/mL; met-dose inhaler **Notes/SE:** Caution with diabetes, HTN, hyperthyroidism; high doses may precipitate β₁-adrenergic effects; nervousness, trembling, tachycardia, HTN, dizziness **Interactions:** ↑ effects with MAOIs, TCAs; ↓ effects with BBs **Labs:** ↑ LFTs, serum glucose **NIPE:** Take oral dose with food

Terconazole (Terazol 7) **Uses:** Vaginal fungal infections **Action:** Topical antifungal **Dose:** 1 applicatorful or 1 supp intravaginally hs for 7 d **Caution/Contra:** [C, ?] **Supplied:** Vaginal cream 0.4%, vaginal supp 80 mg **Notes/SE:** Vulvar or vaginal burning **NIPE:** insert cream or supp high into vagina, complete full course of treatment, ⊘ intercourse during drug treatment, ↑ risk of breakdown of latex condoms & diaphragms with drug

Teriparatide (Forteo) **WARNING:** Do not use if ? baseline risk for osteosarcoma; ? incidence of osteosarcoma in rats **Uses:** Rx osteoporosis in postmenopausal women and men with idiopathic/hypogonadal osteoporosis **Action:** Human PTH; stimulates bone formation **Dose:** 20 mcg sq QD, 2 y max **Caution:** [C,–] **Contra:** N/A **Supplied:** 750 mcg (3 mL pre-filled pen injector) **SE:** Nausea, dizziness, leg cramps, HA, orthostatic hypotension (first few doses) **Notes:** Admin into thigh or abdominal wall; keep pen refrigerated **Labs:** ↑ serum calcium, uric acid, urine calcium **NIPE:** ⊘ Take if h/o Paget's Disease; bone metastases or malignancy, or h/o radiation therapy; take w/o regard to food; not used to prevent osteoporosis

Tetanus Immune Globulin Uses: Passive immunization against tetanus for a suspected contaminated wound and unknown immunization status Action: Passive immunization Dose: *Adults & Peds.* 250–500 U IM (higher doses if delayed therapy); Table 9, page 257 Caution/Contra: [C, ?] Thimerosal sensitivity Supplied: Inj 250-U vial or syringe Notes/SE: May begin active immunization series at different inj site if required; pain, tenderness, erythema at inj site; fever, angioedema, muscle stiffness, anaphylaxis Interactions: ↓ immune response when admin with Td NIPE: Drug does not cause AIDs or hepatitis

Tetanus Toxoid Uses: Protection against tetanus Action: Active immunization Dose: Based on previous immunization status (Table 9, page 257) Caution/Contra: [C, ?] Chloramphenicol use, neurologic symptoms with previous use, active infection (for routine primary immunization) Supplied: Inj tetanus toxoid, fluid, measured in limes flocculation (Lf) units of toxoid: 4–5 Lf units/0.5 mL; tetanus toxoid, adsorbed, 5, 10 Lf units/0.5 mL Notes/SE: Local erythema, induration, sterile abscess; chills, fever, neurologic disturbances Interactions: Delay of active immunity if given with tetanus immune globulin; ↓ immune response if given to pts taking corticosteroids or immunosuppressive drugs NIPE: Stress the need for timely completion of immunization series

Tetracycline (Achromycin V, Sumycin) Uses: Broad-spectrum antibiotic treatment against *Staphylococcus, Streptococcus, Chlamydia, Rickettsia,* and *Mycoplasma* Action: Bacteriostatic; inhibits protein synthesis Dose: *Adults.* 250–500 mg PO bid–qid. *Peds >8 y.* 25–50 mg/kg/24 h PO q6–12h; ↓ dose in renal/hepatic impairment Caution/Contra: [D, +] Do not use with antacids; children <8 y Supplied: Caps 100, 250, 500 mg; tabs 250, 500 mg; oral susp 250 mg/5 mL Notes/SE: Can stain tooth enamel and depress bone formation in children; photosensitivity, GI upset, renal failure, pseudotumor cerebri, hepatic impairment Interactions: ↑ effects of anticoagulants, digoxin; ↓ effects with antacids, cimetidine, laxatives, penicillin, iron suppl, dairy products; ↓ effects of oral contraceptives Labs: False neg of urinary glucose, serum folate; false ↑ serum glucose; NIPE: ⊘ take with dairy products, take w/o food; use barrier contraception

Theophylline (Theolair, Somophyllin, others) Uses: Asthma, bronchospasm Action: Relaxes smooth muscle of the bronchi and pulmonary blood vessels Dose: *Adults.* 900 mg PO ÷ q6h; SR products may be ÷ q8–12h × (maint). *Peds.* 16–22 mg/kg/24 h PO ÷ q6h; SR products may be ÷ q8–12h × (maint); ↓ dose in hepatic failure Caution/Contra: [C, +] Arrhythmia, hyperthyroidism, uncontrolled seizures Supplied: Elixir 80, 150 mg/15 mL; liq 80, 160 mg/15 mL; caps 100, 200, 250 mg; tabs 100, 125, 200, 225, 250, 300 mg; SR caps 50, 75, 100, 125, 200, 250, 260, 300 mg; SR tabs 100, 200, 250, 300, 400, 450, 500 mg Notes/SE: See drug levels in Table 2 (page 244); many drug interactions; N/V, tachycardia, and seizures; nervousness, arrhythmias Interactions: ↑ effects with allopurinol, BBs, CCBs, cimetidine, corticosteroids, macrolide antibiotics, oral contraceptives, quinolones, rifampin, tacrine, tetracyclines, verapamil, zileuton; ↑ effects of digitalis; ↓ effects with barbiturates, loop diuretics, thyroid hormones, tobacco, St John's Wort; ↓ effects of benzodiazepines, lithium, phenytoin **Labs:** False + ↑ uric acid, ↑ bilirubin, ESR **NIPE:** Use barrier contraception; take with food if GI upset; caffeine foods ↑ drug effects; smoking ↓ drug effects

Thiamine [Vitamin B₁]

Thiamine [Vitamin B_1] **Uses:** Thiamine deficiency (beriberi), alcoholic neuritis, Wernicke's encephalopathy **Action:** Dietary supplementation **Dose:** *Adults. Deficiency:* 100 mg/d IM for 2 wk, then 5–10 mg/d PO for 1 mon. *Wernicke's encephalopathy:* 100 mg IV in single dose, then 100 mg/d IM for 2 wk. *Peds.* 10–25 mg/d IM for 2 wk, then 5–10 mg/24 h PO for 1 mon **Caution/Contra:** [A (C if doses exceed RDA), +] **Supplied:** Tabs 5, 10, 25, 50, 100, 500 mg; inj 100, 200 mg/mL **Notes/SE:** IV thiamine use associated with anaphylactoid reaction; give IV slowly; angioedema, paresthesias, rash **Interactions:** ↑ effects of neuromuscular blocking drugs; **Labs:** False + uric acid; interference with theophylline levels

Thiethylperazine (Torecan)

Thiethylperazine (Torecan) **Uses:** N/V **Action:** Antidopaminergic antiemetic **Dose:** 10 mg PO, PR, or IM qd–tid; ↓ dose in hepatic failure **Caution/Contra:** [X, ?] Phenothiazine and sulfite sensitivity **Supplied:** Tabs 10 mg; supp 10 mg; inj 5 mg/mL **Notes/SE:** Extrapyramidal reactions may occur; xerostomia, drowsiness, orthostatic hypotension, tachycardia, confusion **Interactions:** ↑ effects with atropine, CNS depressants, epinephrine, lithium, MAOIs, TCAs, alcohol; ↑ effects of antihypertensives, phenytoin; ↓ effects of bromocriptine, cabergoline, levodopa **Labs:** ↑ serum prolactin level, interferes with PRG test **NIPE:** May cause tardive dyskinesia; ↑ risk of photosensitivity

6-Thioguanine [6-TG] (Tabloid)

6-Thioguanine [6-TG] (Tabloid) **Uses:** AML, ALL, CML **Action:** Purine-based antimetabolite (substitutes for natural purines interfering with nucleotide synthesis) **Dose:** 2–3 mg/kg/d; ↓ dose in severe renal/hepatic impairment **Caution/Contra:** [D, –] Resistance to mercaptopurine **Supplied:** Tabs 40 mg **Notes/SE:** Myelosuppression (especially leukopenia and thrombocytopenia), N/V/D, anorexia, stomatitis, rash, hyperuricemia; hepatotoxicity occurs rarely **Interactions:** ↑ bleeding with anticoagulants, NSAIDs, salicylates, thrombolytics **Labs:** ↑ serum and urine uric acid **NIPE:** Take w/o food; ↑ fluids to 2–3 L/d; ⊘ exposure to infection

Thioridazine (Mellaril)

Thioridazine (Mellaril) **WARNING:** Dose-related QT prolongation **Uses:** Psychotic disorders; short-term treatment of depression, agitation, organic brain syndrome **Action:** Phenothiazine antipsychotic **Dose:** *Adults.* Initially, 50–100 mg PO tid; maint 200–800 mg/24 h PO in 2–4 ÷ doses. *Peds >2 y.* 0.5–3 mg/kg/24 h PO in 2–3 ÷ doses **Caution/Contra:** [C, ?] Phenothiazine sensitivity **Supplied:** Tabs 10, 15, 25, 50, 100, 150, 200 mg; oral conc 30, 100 mg/mL; oral susp 25, 100 mg/5 mL **Notes/SE:** Low incidence of extrapyramidal effects; ventricular arrhythmias; hypotension, dizziness, drowsiness, neuroleptic malignant syndrome, seizures, skin discoloration, photosensitivity, constipation, sexual dysfunction, blood dyscrasias, pigmentary retinopathy, hepatic impairment **Interactions: ↑ effects with BBs; ↑ effects of anticholinergics, antihypertensives, antihistamines, CNS depressants, nitrates, alcohol; ↓ effects with barbiturates, lithium, tobacco; ↓ effects of levodopa **Labs:** False + and neg urinary PRG test; false + urine bilirubin and amylase; ↑ serum LFTs; **NIPE:** ↑ risk of photosensitivity – use sunscreen, take with food; ⊘ d/c abruptly; disturbance of temperature regulation; urine color change to reddish brown

Thiothixene (Navane)   **Uses:** Psychotic disorders **Action:** Antipsychotic **Dose:** *Adults & Peds >12 y. Mild–moderate psychosis:* 2 mg PO tid, up to 20–30 mg/d. *Severe psychosis:* 5 mg PO bid; ↑ to a max of 60 mg/24 h PRN. *IM use:* 16–20 mg/24 h ÷ bid–qid; max 30 mg/d. *Peds <12 y.* 0.25 mg/kg/24 h PO ÷ q6–12h **Caution/Contra:** [C, ?] Phenothiazine sensitivity **Supplied:** Caps 1, 2, 5, 10, 20 mg; oral conc 5 mg/mL; inj 2, 5 mg/mL **Notes/SE:** Drowsiness and extrapyramidal side effects most common; hypotension, dizziness, drowsiness, neuroleptic malignant syndrome, seizures, skin discoloration, photosensitivity, constipation, sexual dysfunction, blood dyscrasias, pigmentary retinopathy, hepatic impairment **Interactions:** ↑ effects with BBs; ↑ effects of anticholinergics, antihistamines, BBs, CNS depressants, nitrates, alcohol; ↓ effects with barbiturates, lithium, tobacco, caffeine; ↓ effects of levodopa **Labs:** ↑ serum glucose, cholesterol; ↓ serum uric acid; false + urinary PRG test **NIPE:** ↑ risk of photosensitivity – use sunscreen; take with food; ⊘ d/c abruptly; disturbance of temperature regulation; darkens urine color

Tiagabine (Gabitril)   **Uses:** Adjunctive therapy in treatment of partial seizures **Action:** Inhibition of GABA **Dose:** Initial 4 mg/d, ↑ by 4 mg during 2nd wk; ↑ PRN by 4–8 mg/d based on response, 56 mg/d/max **Caution/Contra:** [C, M] **Supplied:** Tabs 4, 12, 16, 20 mg **Notes/SE:** Use gradual withdrawal; used in combination with other anticonvulsants; dizziness, HA, somnolence, memory impairment, tremors **Interactions:** ↑ effects with valproate; ↑ effects of CNS depressants, alcohol; ↓ effects with barbiturates, carbamazepine, phenobarbital, phenytoin, primidone, rifampin, ginkgo biloba **NIPE:** Take with food; ⊘ d/c abruptly

Ticarcillin (Ticar)   **Uses:** Infections due to gram– bacteria (*Klebsiella, Proteus, E. coli, Enterobacter, P. aeruginosa,* and *Serratia*) involving the skin, bone, respiratory tract, urinary tract, and abdomen and septicemia **Action:** Bactericidal; inhibits cell wall synthesis **Dose:** *Adults.* 3 g IV q4–6h. *Peds.* 200–300 mg/kg/d IV ÷ q4–6h; ↓ dose in renal failure **Caution/Contra:** [B, +] Penicillin sensitivity **Supplied:** Inj **Notes/SE:** Often used in combination with aminoglycosides; interstitial nephritis, anaphylaxis, bleeding, rash, hemolytic anemia **Interactions:** ↑ effects with probenecid; ↑ effects of anticoagulants, methotrexate; ↓ effects with tetracyclines, ↓ effects of aminoglycosides **Labs:** False ↑ urine glucose, ↑ serum AST, ALT, alkaline phosphatase **NIPE:** Monitor for s/s superinfection; frequent loose stools may be due to pseudomembranous colitis

Ticarcillin/Potassium Clavulanate (Timentin)   **Uses:** Infections caused by gram– bacteria (*Klebsiella, Proteus, E. coli, Enterobacter, P. aeruginosa,*

cisplatin, other neoplastic drugs, radiation therapy; ↑ in duration of neutropenia with filgrastim **Labs:** ↑ AST, ALT, bilirubin **NIPE:** Monitor CBC; ⊘ PRG, breast-feeding, immunizations; avoid exposure to infection; use barrier contraception

Torsemide (Demadex)   **Uses:** Edema, HTN, CHF, and hepatic cirrhosis **Action:** Loop diuretic; inhibits reabsorption of Na and Cl in ascending loop of Henle and distal tubule **Dose:** 5–20 mg/d PO or IV **Caution/Contra:** [B, ?] Sulfonylurea sensitivity **Supplied:** Tabs 5, 10, 20, 100 mg; inj 10 mg/mL **Notes/ SE:** Orthostatic hypotension, HA, dizziness, photosensitivity, electrolyte imbalance, blurred vision, renal impairment **Interactions:** ↑ risk of ototoxicity with aminoglycosides, cisplatin; ↑ effects with thiazides; ↑ effects of anticoagulants, antihypertensives, lithium, salicylates; ↓ effects with barbiturates, carbamazepine, cholestyramine, NSAIDs, phenytoin, phenobarbital, probenecid, dandelion **NIPE:** Monitor electrolytes, BUN, creatinine, glucose, uric acid; take w/o regard to food Monitor for s/s tinnitus

Tramadol (Ultram)   **Uses:** Moderate–severe pain **Action:** Centrally acting analgesic **Dose:** 50–100 mg PO q4–6h PRN, not to exceed 400 mg/d **Caution/Contra:** [C, ?/–] Opioid dependency; MAOIs **Supplied:** Tabs 50 mg **Notes/SE:** Lowers seizure threshold, tolerance or dependence may develop; dizziness, HA, somnolence, GI upset, respiratory depression, anaphylaxis (sensitivity to codeine) **Interactions:** ↑ effects with cimetidine, CNS depressants, MAOIs, phenothiazines, quinidine, TCAs, alcohol, St. John's Wort; ↑ effects of digoxin, warfarin; ↓ effects with carbamazepine **Labs:** ↑ creatinine, LFTs, ↓ HMG **NIPE:** Take w/o regard to food

Tramadol/Acetaminophen (Ultracet)   **Uses:** Short-term management of acute pain (<5 d) **Action:** Centrally acting analgesic; nonnarcotic analgesic **Dose:** 2 tab PO q4–6h PRN; 8 tab/d max; *Elderly/renal impairment:* Use lowest possible dose; 2 tab q12h max if CrCl <30 **Caution/Contra:** [C, –] Contra in allergy to either drug, in acutely intoxicated patients; caution in seizures, hepatic/renal impairment, or Hx addictive tendencies **Supplied:** Tab 37.5 mg tramadol/325 mg APAP **Notes/SE:** Avoid alcohol use; SSRIs, TCAs, opioids, MAOIs increase risk of seizures; dizziness, somnolence, tremor, HA, risk of seizures, N/V/D, constipation, xerostomia, liver toxicity, rash, pruritus, ↑ sweating, physical dependence **Interactions:** ↑ effects with cimetidine, CNS depressants, MAOIs, phenothiazines, quinidine, TCAs, alcohol, St. John's Wort; ↑ effects of digoxin, warfarin; ↓ effects with carbamazepine **Labs:** ↑ creatinine, LFTs, ↓ HMG **NIPE:** Take w/o regard to food; ⊘ take other acetaminophen-containing drugs

Trandolapril (Mavik)   **WARNING:** Use in PRG in 2nd/3rd trimester can result in fetal death **Uses:** HTN, CHF, LVD, post-AMI **Action:** ACE inhibitor **Dose:** *HTN:* 2–4 mg/d. *CHF/LVD:* 4 mg/d; ↓ dose in severe renal/hepatic impairment **Caution/Contra:** [D, +] ACE inhibitor sensitivity, angioedema with ACE inhibitors **Supplied:** Tabs 1, 2, 4 mg **Notes/SE:** Hypotension, bradycardia, dizziness, hyperkalemia, GI upset, renal impairment, cough, angioedema **Interactions:** ↑ effects with diuretics; ↑ effects of insulin, lithium; ↓ effects with ASA, NSAIDs; **NIPE:** ⊘ take if pregnant or breast-feeding; ⊘ K⁺-containing salt substitutes

Trazodone (Desyrel) **Uses:** Depression and insomnia associated with anxiety and depression **Action:** Antidepressant; inhibits reuptake of serotonin and norepinephrine **Dose:** *Adults & Adolescents.* 50–150 mg PO qd–qid; max 600 mg/d. *Sleep:* 50 mg PO, qhs, PRN **Caution/Contra:** [C, ?/–] **Supplied:** Tabs 50, 100, 150, 300 mg **Notes/SE:** May take 1–2 wk for symptomatic improvement; anticholinergic side effects; dizziness, HA, sedation, nausea, xerostomia, syncope, confusion, tremor, hepatitis, extrapyramidal reactions **Interactions:** ↑ effects with fluoxetine, phenothiazines; ↑ risk of serotonin syndrome with MAOIs, SSRIs, venlafaxine, St. John's Wort; ↑ CNS depression with barbiturates, CNS depressants, opioids, sedatives, alcohol; ↑ hypotension with antihypertensives, neuroleptics; nitrates, alcohol; ↑ effects of clonidine, digoxin, phenytoin; ↓ effects with carbamazepine **NIPE:** Take with food; ↑ fluids to 2–3 L/d; ⊘ d/c abruptly; ↑ risk of priapism

Treprostinil Sodium (Remodulin) **Uses:** NYHA Class II–IV pulmonary arterial hypertension **Action:** Vasodilation, inhibition of platelet aggregation **Dose:** 0.625–1.25 ng/kg/min cont inf **Caution/Contra:** [B, ?/–] Initiate in monitored setting; do not DC or reduce dose abruptly **Supplied:** 1, 2.5, 5, 10 mg/mL inj **Notes/SE:** inf site reactions **Interactions:** ↑ effects with antihypertensives; ↑ effects of anticoagulants **NIPE:** Teach care of inf site and pump; use barrier contraception; once med vial used discard >14 d

Tretinoin, Systemic [Retinoic Acid] (Vesanoid) **Uses:** APL induction therapy **Action:** Differentiating agent; all-*trans* retinoic acid **Dose:** 45 mg/m²/d in ÷ doses for approximately 40 d; with food **Caution/Contra:** [D, ?] Retinoid sensitivity **Supplied:** Caps 10 mg **Notes/SE:** Cutaneous (dryness, chafing), neurologic (HA), hypertriglyceridemia, and treatment-related leukocytosis is reported in APL, as well as "retinoic acid syndrome" **Interactions:** ↑ effects with ketoconazole; ↑ skin irritation with topical acne drugs such as those containing sulfur, resorcinol, benzoyl peroxide, salicylic acid **Labs:** Monitor cholesterol, triglycerides, LFTs, CBC, platelets **NIPE:** Take with food; low-fat diet; ↑ fluids to 2–3 L/d; ⊘ PRG or breast-feeding; use two forms of contraception; neg PRG test <starting drug; ↑ risk of suicidal ideation; ↑ risk of photosensitivity

Tretinoin, Topical [Retinoic Acid] (Retin-A, Avita, Renova) **Uses:** Acne vulgaris, sun-damaged skin, wrinkles (aka photo aging), some skin CAs **Action:** Exfoliant retinoic acid derivative **Dose:** *Adults & Peds >12 y.* Apply qd hs; if irritation develops, ↓ frequency; photoaging, start 0.025%, increase to 0.1% over several months; apply only every 3 d if on neck area; dark skin may require bid application **Caution/Contra:** [C, ?] Retinoid sensitivity **Supplied:** Cream 0.025, 0.05, 0.1%; gel 0.01, 0.025, 0.1%; microformulation gel 0.1%; liq 0.05% **Notes/SE:** Avoid sunlight; edema; skin dryness, erythema, scaling, changes in pigmentation, stinging, photosensitivity **Interactions:** ↑ photosensitivity with quinolones, phenothiazines, sulfonamides, tetracyclines, thiazides, dong quai, St. John's Wort; ↑ skin irritation with topical sulfur, resorcinol, benzoyl peroxide, salicylic acid; ↑ effects with vit A suppl and foods with excess vit A such as fish oils **NIPE:** ⊘ Apply to mucous membranes, wash skin and apply med >30 min, wash hands >application; avoid breast-feeding, PRG use contraception

Triamcinolone and Nystatin (Mycolog-II) Uses: Cutaneous candidiasis **Action:** Antifungal and antiinflammatory **Dose:** Apply lightly to area bid; max 25 d **Caution/Contra:** [C, ?] Varicella; systemic fungal infections **Supplied:** Cream and oint 15, 30, 60, 120 mg **Notes/SE:** Local irritation, hypertrichosis, changes in pigmentation **Interactions:** ↓ effects with barbiturates, phenytoin, rifampin; ↓ effects of salicylates, vaccines **NIPE:** Avoid eyes; ⊘ apply to open skin/wounds, eyes, mucous membranes

Triamterene (Dyrenium) Uses: Edema associated with CHF, cirrhosis **Action:** K⁺-sparing diuretic **Dose:** *Adults.* 100–300 mg/24 h PO ÷ qd–bid. *Peds.* 2–4 mg/kg/d in 1–2 ÷ doses; ↓ dose in renal/hepatic impairment **Caution/Contra:** [B (manufacturer; D expert opinion), ?/–] Hyperkalemia, renal impairment, diabetes; caution with other K⁺-sparing diuretics **Supplied:** Caps 50, 100 mg **Notes/SE:** Hyperkalemia, blood dyscrasias, liver damage, and other reactions **Interactions:** ↑ risk of hyperkalemia with ACEIs, K⁺ supplements, K⁺-sparing drugs, K⁺-containing drugs, K⁺ salt substitutes; ↑ effects with cimetidine, indomethacin; ↑ effects of amantadine, antihypertensives, lithium; ↓ effects of digitalis **Labs:** False ↑ serum digoxin **NIPE:** Take with food, blue discoloration of urine, ↑ risk of photosensitivity - use sunscreen

Triazolam (Halcion) [C-IV] Uses: Short-term management of insomnia **Action:** Benzodiazepine **Dose:** 0.125–0.25 mg/d PO hs PRN; additive CNS depression with alcohol and other CNS depressants; ↓ dose in elderly **Caution/Contra:** [X, ?/–] Narrow-angle glaucoma; cirrhosis, amprenavir, ritonavir, nelfinavir **Supplied:** Tabs 0.125, 0.25 mg **Notes/SE:** Tachycardia, chest pain, drowsiness, fatigue, memory impairment, GI upset **Interactions:** ↑ effects with azole antifungals, cimetidine, clarithromycin, ciprofloxin, CNS depressants, disulfiram, digoxin, erythromycin, fluvoxamine, isoniazid, protease inhibitors, troleandomycin, verapamil, alcohol, grapefruit juice, kava kava, valerian; ↓ effects of levodopa; ↓ effects with carbamazepine, phenytoin, rifampin, theophylline **NIPE:** ⊘ PRG or breast-feeding; ⊘ d/c abruptly >long-term use

Triethanolamine (Cerumenex) Uses: Cerumen removal **Action:** Ceruminolytic agent **Dose:** Fill the ear canal and insert the cotton plug; irrigate with water after 15 min; repeat PRN **Caution/Contra:** [C, ?] Perforated tympanic membrane, otitis media **Supplied:** Soln 6, 12 mL **Notes/SE:** Local dermatitis, pain, erythema, pruritus **NIPE:** Warm solution to body temp <use for better effect

Triethylene-Triphosphamide (Thio-Tepa, Tespa, TSPA) Uses: Hodgkin's and NHLs; leukemia; breast, ovarian, and bladder CAs (IV and intravesical therapy), preparative regimens for allogeneic and autologous BMT in high

doses **Action:** Polyfunctional alkylating agent **Dose:** 0.5 mg/kg q1–4wk, 6 mg/m^2 IM or IV ×4 d q2–4wk, 15–35 mg/m^2 by cont IV inf over 48 h; 60 mg into the bladder and retained 2 h q1–4wk; 900–125 mg/m^2 in ABMT regimens (the highest dose that can be administered w/o ABMT is 180 mg/m^2); 1–10 mg/m^2 (typically 15 mg) IT once or twice a wk; 0.8 mg/kg in 1–2 L of soln may be instilled intraperitoneally; ↓ dose in renal failure **Caution/Contra:** [D, –] **Supplied:** Inj 15 mg **Notes/SE:** Myelosuppression, N/V, dizziness, HA, allergy, paresthesias, alopecia

Trifluoperazine (Stelazine)   **Uses:** Psychotic disorders **Action:** Phenothiazine; blocks postsynaptic CNS dopaminergic receptors in the brain **Dose:** *Adults.* 2–10 mg PO bid. *Peds 6–12 y.* 1 mg PO qd–bid initially, gradually ↑ to 15 mg/d; ↓ dose in elderly/debilitated patients **Caution/Contra:** [C, ?/–] Hx blood dyscrasias; phenothiazine sensitivity **Supplied:** Tabs 1, 2, 5, 10 mg; oral conc 10 mg/mL; inj 2 mg/mL **Notes/SE:** Oral conc must be diluted to 60 mL or more prior to administration; requires several wks for onset of effects; orthostatic hypotension, EPS, dizziness, neuroleptic malignant syndrome, skin discoloration, lowered seizure threshold, photosensitivity, blood dyscrasias **Interactions:** ↑ hypotensive effects with antihypertensives, nitrates, sulfadoxine-pyrimethamine, alcohol; ↑ effects of anticholinergics; ↑ CNS depression with antihistamines, CNS depressants, narcotics, alcohol; ↓ effects with barbiturates, lithium, caffeine, tobacco; ↓ effects of guanadrel, guanethidine, levodopa **Labs:** ↑ LFTs, serum prolactin levels, ↓ HMG, HCT, platelets, false PRG test results + or neg **NIPE:** Use sunscreen due to photosensitivity; affects body temperature regulation; reddish brown urine color change; ⊘ d/c abruptly > long-term use

Trifluridine (Viroptic)   **Uses:** Herpes simplex keratitis and conjunctivitis **Action:** Antiviral **Dose:** 1 gt q2h (max 9 gt/d); ↓ to 1 gt q4h after healing begins; treat up to 14 d **Caution/Contra:** [C, M] **Supplied:** Soln 1% **Notes/SE:** Local burning, stinging **NIPE:** Store in refrigerator; ⊘ use if soln discolored; >admin exert pressure on lacrimal sac for 1 min

Trihexyphenidyl (Artane)   **Uses:** Parkinson's disease **Action:** Blocks excess acetylcholine at cerebral synapses **Dose:** 2–5 mg PO qd–qid **Caution/Contra:** [C, +] Narrow-angle glaucoma, GI obstruction, MyG, bladder obstructions **Supplied:** Tabs 2, 5 mg; SR caps 5 mg; elixir 2 mg/5 mL **Notes/SE:** Dry skin, constipation, xerostomia, photosensitivity, tachycardia, arrhythmias **Interactions:** ↑ effects with MAOIs, phenothiazines, quinidine, TCAs; ↑ effects of amantadine, anticholinergics, digoxin; ↓ effects with antacids, tacrine; ↓ effects of chlorpromazine, haloperidol, tacrine **Labs:** False ↑ T3, T4 **NIPE:** Take with food; monitor for urinary hesitancy or retention; ⊘ d/c abruptly; ↑ risk of heat stroke

Trimethobenzamide (Tigan)   **Uses:** N/V **Action:** Inhibits medullary chemoreceptor trigger zone **Dose:** *Adults.* 250 mg PO or 200 mg PR or IM tid–qid PRN. *Peds.* 20 mg/kg/24 h PO or 15 mg/kg/24 h PR or IM in 3–4 ÷ doses (not recommended for infants) **Caution/Contra:** [C, ?] Benzocaine sensitivity; inj in children; suppositories in premature infants or neonates **Supplied:** Caps 100, 250 mg;

supp 100, 200 mg; inj 100 mg/mL **Notes/SE:** In the presence of viral infections, may mask emesis or mimic CNS effects of Reye's syndrome; may cause parkinsonian-like syndrome; drowsiness, hypotension, dizziness; hepatic impairment, blood dyscrasias, seizures **Interactions:** ↑ CNS depression with antidepressants, antihistamines, opioids, sedatives, alcohol; ↑ risk of extrapyramidal effects

Trimethoprim (Trimpex, Proloprim)
Uses: UTI due to susceptible gram+ and gram– organisms; suppression of UTI **Action:** Inhibits dihydrofolate reductase **Dose:** *Adults.* 100 mg/d PO bid or 200 mg/d PO. *Peds.* 4 mg/kg/d in 2 ÷ doses; ↓ dose in renal failure **Caution/Contra:** [C, +] Megaloblastic anemia due to folate deficiency **Supplied:** Tabs 100, 200 mg; oral soln 50 mg/5 mL **Notes/SE:** Rash, pruritus, megaloblastic anemia, hepatic impairment, blood dyscrasias **Interactions:** ↑ effects with dapsone; ↑ effects of dapsone, phenytoin, procainamide; ↓ efficacy with rifampin **Labs:** ↑ LFTs, BUN, creatinine **NIPE:** ↑ fluids to 2–3 L/d; ↑ risk of folic acid deficiency

Trimethoprim-Sulfamethoxazole [Co-Trimoxazole] (Bactrim, Septra)
Uses: UTI treatment and prophylaxis, otitis media, sinusitis, bronchitis, and *Shigella, P. carinii,* and *Nocardia* infections **Action:** SMX-inhibiting synthesis of dihydrofolic acid; TMP-inhibiting dihydrofolate reductase to impair protein synthesis **Dose:** *Adults.* 1 DS tab PO bid or 5–20 mg/kg/24 h (based on TMP) IV in 3–4 ÷ doses. *P. carinii:* 15–20 mg/kg/d IV or PO (TMP) in 4 ÷ doses. *Nocardia:* 10–15 mg/kg/d IV or PO (TMP) in 4 ÷ doses. *UTI prophylaxis:* 1 PO qd. *Peds.* 8–10 mg/kg/24 h (TMP) PO ÷ into 2 doses or 3–4 doses IV; do not use in newborns; ↓ dose in renal failure; maintain hydration **Caution/Contra:** [B (D if near term), +] Sulfonamide sensitivity, porphyria, megaloblastic anemia with folate deficiency, significant hepatic impairment, age <2 mon; interacts with warfarin **Supplied:** Regular tabs 80 mg TMP/400 mg SMX; DS tabs 160 mg TMP/800 mg SMX; oral susp 40 mg TMP/200 mg SMX/5 mL; inj 80 mg TMP/ 400 mg SMX/5 mL **Notes/SE:** Synergistic combination; allergic skin reactions, photosensitivity, GI upset, Stevens–Johnson syndrome, blood dyscrasias, hepatitis **Interactions:** ↑ effect of dapsone, methotrexate, phenytoin, sulfonylureas, warfarin, zivoudine; ↓ effects with rifampin; ↓ effect of cyclosporine **Labs:** ↑ serum bilirubin, alkaline phosphatase, creatinine **NIPE:** ↑ risk of photosensitivity – use sunscreen; ↑ fluids to 2–3 L/d

Trimetrexate (Neutrexin)
WARNING: Must be used with leucovorin to avoid toxicity **Uses:** Moderate–severe PCP **Action:** Inhibits dihydrofolate reductase **Dose:** 45 mg/m² IV q24h for 21 d; ↓ in hepatic impairment **Caution/Contra:** [D, ?/–] Methotrexate sensitivity **Supplied:** Inj **Notes/SE:** Administer with leucovorin 20 mg/m² IV q6h for 24 d; use cytotoxic cautions; infuse over 60 min; seizure, fever, rash, GI upset, anemias, and ↑ LFTs, peripheral neuropathy, renal impairment **Interactions:** ↑ effects with azole antifungals, cimetidine, erythromycin; ↓ effects with rifabutin, rifampin; ↓ effects of pneumococcal immunization **Labs:** ↑ LFTs, serum creatinine **NIPE:** ⊘ PRG, breast-feeding use contraception; avoid exposure to infection

Trimipramine (Surmontil)   **Uses:** Depression **Action:** TCA; increases synaptic conc of serotonin and/or norepinephrine in CNS **Dose:** 50–300 mg/d PO hs; avoid grapefruit juice **Caution/Contra:** [C, ?] Narrow-angle glaucoma **Supplied:** Caps 25, 50, 100 mg **Notes/SE:** Arrhythmias, hypotension, tachycardia, confusion, photosensitivity, sexual dysfunction, xerostomia, constipation, urinary retention, EPS, hepatic damage, blood dyscrasias; do not DC abruptly in hyperthyroid patients **Interactions:** ↑ risks of arrhythmias with quinolones, procainamide, pimozide, quinidine, thyroid drugs; ↑ effects with BBs, cimetidine, CNS depressants, fluoxetine, oral contraceptives, propoxyphene, quinidine, SSRIs, alcohol, St. John's Wort; ↑ effects of anticoagulants; ↓ effects of barbiturates, carbamazepine, clonidine, guanabenz, guanethidine; ↓ effects with tobacco use **Labs:** ↑ serum glucose **NIPE:** Take with food; ↑ risk of photosensitivity—use sunscreen; ◌ d/c abruptly, may take 2–4 wk for full effects

Triptorelin (Trelstar Depot, Trelstar LA)   **Uses:** Palliation of advanced prostate CA **Action:** ↓ Gonadotropin secretion when given continuously; following 1st administration, there is a transient surge in LH, FSH, testosterone, and estradiol. After chronic/continuous administration (usually 2–4 wk), a sustained decrease in LH and FSH secretion and marked reduction of testicular and ovarian steroidogenesis is observed. A reduction of serum testosterone similar to surgical castration. **Dose:** 3.75 mg IM monthly or 11.25 mg IM q3mon **Caution/Contra:** [X, NA] Not indicated in females **Supplied:** Inj depot 3.75 mg; LA 11.25 mg **Notes/SE:** Dizziness, emotional lability, fatigue, HA, insomnia, HTN, diarrhea, vomiting, impotence, urinary retention, UTI, pruritus, anemia, inj site pain, musculoskeletal pain, allergic reactions **Interactions:** ↑ risk of severe hyperprolactinemia with antipsychotics, metoclopramide **Labs:** Suppression of pituitary-gonadal function **NIPE:** ◌ PRG or breast-feeding; may cause hot flashes; initial ↑ bone pain

Urokinase (Abbokinase)   **Uses:** PE, DVT, restore patency to IV catheters **Action:** Converts plasminogen to plasmin that causes clot lysis **Dose:** **Adults & Peds.** *Systemic effect:* 4400 IU/kg IV over 10 min, followed by 4400–6000 IU/kg/h for 12 h. *Restore catheter patency:* Inject 5000 IU into catheter and gently aspirate **Caution/Contra:** [B, +] Do not use w/n 10 d of surgery, delivery, or organ biopsy; bleeding, CVA, vascular malformation **Supplied:** Powder for inj 5000 IU/mL, 250,000-IU vial **Notes/SE:** Bleeding, hypotension, dyspnea, bronchospasm, anaphylaxis, cholesterol embolism **Interactions:** ↑ risk of bleeding with anticoagulants, ASA, heparin, indomethacin, NSAIDs, phenylbutazone, feverfew, garlic, ginger, ginkgo biloba; ↓ effects with aminocaproic acid **Labs:** ↑ PT, PTT; ↓ fibrinogen, plasminogen

Valacyclovir (Valtrex)   **Uses:** Herpes zoster; genital herpes **Action:** Prodrug of acyclovir; inhibits viral DNA replication **Dose:** 1 g PO tid. *Genital herpes:* 500 mg bid ×7 d. *Herpes prophylaxis:* 500–1000 mg/d; ↓ dose in renal failure **Caution/Contra:** [B, +] **Supplied:** Caplets 500 mg **Notes/SE:** HA, GI upset, dizziness, pruritus, photophobia **Interactions:** ↑ effects with cimetidine, probenecid **Labs:** ↑ LFTs, creatinine **NIPE:** Take w/o regard to food; ↑ fluids to 2–3 L/d; begin drug at first sign of s/s

Valdecoxib (Bextra) **Uses:** RA, osteoarthritis, primary dysmenorrhea **Action:** COX-2 inhibition **Dose:** *Arthritis:* 10 mg PO bid, PRN *Dysmenorrhea:* 20 mg PO bid Caution/Contra: [C, ?] Asthma, urticaria, allergic-type reactions after ASA or NSAIDs, sulfonamide hypersensitivity **Supplied:** Tabs 10, 20 mg **Notes/SE:** ↑ LFT, GI ulceration or bleeding; dizziness, edema, HTN, HA, peptic ulcer, renal failure; serious hypersensitivity reactions have occurred, including Stevens–Johnson syndrome **Interactions:** ↑ effects with azole antifungals; ↑ effects of dextromethorphan, lithium, warfarin; ↓ effects of ACEIs, diuretics **Labs:** ↑ LFTs, BUN, creatinine **NIPE:** Take with food if GI upset; ↑ fluids to 2–3 L/d

Valganciclovir (Valcyte) **Uses:** Treatment of CMV **Action:** Ganciclovir prodrug; inhibits viral DNA synthesis **Dose:** Induction, 900 mg PO bid with food ×21 days, then 900 mg/d PO **Caution/Contra:** Caution in renal impairment [C, ?/–] **Supplied:** Tabs 450 mg **Notes/SE:** Dose adjustment in renal dysfunction; bone marrow suppression, requires frequent CBCs; renal function monitoring required; caution with imipenem/cilastatin, nephrotoxic drugs **Interactions:** ↑ effects with cytotoxic drugs, immunosuppressive drugs, probenecid; ↑ risks of nephrotoxicity with amphotericin B, cyclosporine; ↑ effects with didanosine **Labs:** ↑ serum creatinine **NIPE:** Take with food; ⊘ PRG, breast-feeding, alcohol, NSAIDs; use contraception for at least 3 mon >drug treatment

Valproic Acid (Depakene, Depakote) **Uses:** Rx epilepsy, mania; prophylaxis of migraines **Action:** Anticonvulsant; increases the synthesis of GABA **Dose:** *Adults & Peds.* Seizures: 30–60 mg/kg/24 h PO ÷ tid (after initiation of 10–15 mg/kg/24 h). *Mania:* 750 mg in 3 ÷ doses, ↑ 60 mg/kg/d max. *Migraines:* 250 mg bid, ↑ 1000 mg/d max; ↓ dose in hepatic impairment **Caution/Contra:** [D, +] Hepatic impairment **Supplied:** Caps 250 mg; syrup 250 mg/5 mL **Notes/SE:** Monitor LFTs and serum levels (Table 2, page 243); phenobarbital and phenytoin may alter levels; somnolence, dizziness, GI upset, diplopia, ataxia, rash, thrombocytopenia, hepatitis, pancreatitis, prolonged bleeding times, alopecia, weight gain; hyperammonemic encephalopathy reported in patients with urea cycle disorders **Interactions:** ↑ effects with clarithromycin, erythromycin, felbamate, isoniazid, salicylates, troleandomycine; ↑ effects of anticoagulants, lamotrigine, nimodipine, phenobarbital, primidone, zidovudine; ↑ CNS depression with CNS depressants, haloperidol, loxapine, maprotiline, MAOIs, phenothiazines, thioxanthenes, TCAs, alcohol; ↓ effects with cholestyramine, colestipol; ↓ effects of clozapine, rifampin **Labs:** ↑ LFTs; altered TFTs, false + urinary ketones **NIPE:** Take with food for GI upset; ⊘ PRG, breast-feeding; d/c abruptly

Valsartan (Diovan) **WARNING:** Use during 2nd/3rd trimester of PRG can cause fetal harm **Uses:** HTN, CHF, DN **Action:** Angiotensin II receptor antagonist **Dose:** 80–160 mg/d; caution with K⁺-sparing diuretics or K⁺ supplements

Caution/Contra: [C (1st trimester; D 2nd and 3rd trimesters), ?/–] Severe hepatic impairment, biliary cirrhosis, biliary obstruction, primary hyperaldosteronism, bilateral renal artery stenosis **Supplied:** Caps 80, 160 mg **Notes/SE:** Hypotension, dizziness **Interactions:** ↑ effects with diuretics, lithium; ↑ risk of hyperkalemia with K⁺ sparing diuretics, K⁺ supplements, trimethoprim **Labs:** ↑ LFTs, K⁺, ↓ HMG, HCT **NIPE:** Take w/o regard to food; ⊘ PRG, breastfeeding; use contraception

Vancomycin (Vancocin, Vancoled) **Uses:** Serious MRSA infections; enterococcal infections; oral Rx of *C. difficile* pseudomembranous colitis **Action:** Inhibits cell wall synthesis **Dose:** *Adults.* 1 g IV q12h; for colitis 125–500 mg PO q6h. *Peds (NOT neonates).* 40 mg/kg/24 h IV in ÷ doses q6–12h; ↓ in renal insufficiency **Caution/Contra:** [C, M] **Supplied:** Caps 125, 250 mg; powder for oral soln; powder for inj 500 mg, 1000 mg, 10 g/vial **Notes/SE:** Not absorbed PO, local effect in gut only; give IV dose slowly (over 1 h) to prevent "red-neck syndrome"; ↓ in renal insufficiency (for drug levels, Table 2, page 242). Ototoxic and nephrotoxic; GI upset (oral), neutropenia **Interactions:** ↑ ototoxicity and nephrotoxicity with ASA, aminoglycosides, cyclosporine, clisplatin, loop diuretics; ↓ effects of methotrexate **Labs:** ↑ BUN, **NIPE:** Take with food, ↑ fluid to 2–3 L/d

Vardenafil (Levitra) **WARNING:** May prolong QTc interval **Uses:** Erectile dysfunction **Action:** Phosphodiesterase 5 inhibitor **Dose:** *Adults.* 10 mg PO 60 min <sexual activity; 2.5 mg with CYP3A4 inhibitors; no more than once daily or >20 mg; ⊘ fatty meals **Caution:** [B, –] **Contra:** Nitrates **Supplied:** 2.5, 5,10, 20 mg tabs **SE:** Hypotension, HA, dyspepsia, priapism **Notes:** Concomitant α-blockers may cause hypotension; caution in pts with cardiovascular, hepatic, or renal disease **Interactions:** ↑ effects with erythromycin, keotconazole, indinavir, ritonavir; ↑ effects of α blockers, nitrates; ↓ effects of indinavir, ritonavir **NIPE:** Take w/o regard to food; ↑ risk of priapism

Varicella Virus Vaccine (Varivax) **Uses:** Prevention of varicella (chickenpox) infection **Action:** Active immunization **Dose:** *Adults & Peds.* 0.5 mL SC, repeated in 4–8 wk **Caution/Contra:** [C, M] Contra in immunocompromised patients; neomycin-anaphylactoid reaction, blood dyscrasias; immunosuppressive drugs; avoid PRG for 3 mon after inj **Supplied:** Powder for inj **Notes/SE:** Live attenuated virus; may cause mild varicella infection; fever, local reactions, irritability, GI upset **Interactions:** ↓ effects with acyclovir, immunosuppressant drugs **NIPE:** ⊘ salicylates for 6 wk >immunization; N PRG for 3 mon >immunization

Vasopressin [Antidiuretic Hormone, ADH] (Pitressin) **Uses:** Diabetes insipidus; relieves gaseous GI tract distention; severe GI bleeding **Action:** Posterior pituitary hormone, potent GI vasoconstrictor **Dose:** *Adults & Peds. Diabetes insipidus:* 2.5–10 U SC or IM tid–qid or 1.5–5.0 U IM q1–3d of the tannate. *GI hemorrhage:* 0.2–0.4 U/min; ↓ dose in cirrhosis; caution in vascular disease **Caution/Contra:** [B, +] **Supplied:** Inj 20 U/mL **Notes/SE:** HTN, arrhythmias, fever, vertigo, GI upset, tremor **Interactions:** ↑ vasopressor effects with guanethidine, neostigmine; ↑ antidiuretic effects with carbamazepine, chlorpropamide, clofibrate, fludricortisone, phenformin urea, TCAs; ↓ antidiuretic effects with demeclocycline, lithium, heparin, phenytoin, alcohol **Labs:** ↑ cortisol level **NIPE:** Take 1–2 glasses H_2O with drug

Vecuronium (Norcuron) Uses: Skeletal muscle relaxation during surgery or mechanical ventilation **Action:** Nondepolarizing neuromuscular blocker **Dose:** *Adults & Peds.* 0.08–0.1 mg/kg IV bolus; maint 0.010–0.015 mg/kg after 25–40 min; additional doses q12–15min PRN; ↓ dose in severe renal/hepatic impairment **Caution/Contra:** [C, ?] **Supplied:** Powder for inj 10 mg **Notes/SE:** Drug interactions causing ↑ effect of vecuronium (eg, aminoglycosides, tetracycline, succinylcholine); fewer cardiac effects than with pancuronium; bradycardia, hypotension, rash **Interactions:** ↑ neuromuscular blockade with aminoglycosides, BBs, CCBs, clindamycin, furosemide, lincomycin, quinidine, tetracyclines, thiazide diuretics, verapamil; ↑ respiratory depression with opioids; ↓ effects with phenytoin **NIPE:** Will not provide pain relief or sedation

Venlafaxine (Effexor) Uses: Depression, generalized anxiety, social anxiety disorder **Action:** Potentiation of CNS neurotransmitter activity **Dose:** 75–375 mg/d ÷ into 2–3 equal doses; ↓ dose in renal/hepatic impairment **Caution/Contra:** [C, ?/–] MAOIs **Supplied:** Tabs 25, 37.5, 50, 75, 100 mg; ER caps 37.5, 75, 150 mg **Notes/SE:** HTN, HA, somnolence, GI upset, sexual dysfunction; actuates mania or seizures **Interactions:** ↑ effects with cimetidine, desipramine, haloperidol, MAOIs; ↑ risk of serotonin syndrome with buspirone, lithium, meperidine, sibutramine, sumatriptan, SSRIs, TCAs, trazodone, St. John's Wort **Labs:** ↑ LFTs, creatinine **NIPE:** Take with food; ⊘ d/c abruptly; d/c MAOI 14 days <start of this drug; ↑ fluids to 2–3 L/d; may take 2–3 wk for full effects

Verapamil (Calan, Isoptin) Uses: Angina, essential HTN, arrhythmias; migraine prophylaxis **Action:** Ca^{2+} channel blocker **Dose:** *Adults. Arrhythmias:* 2nd line for PSVT with narrow QRS complex and adequate BP 2.5–5.0 mg IV over 1–2 min; repeat 5–10 mg in 15–30 min PRN (30 mg max). *Angina:* 80–120 mg PO tid, ↑ 480 mg/24 h max. *HTN:* 80–180 mg PO tid or SR tabs 120–240 mg PO qd to 240 mg bid. *Peds.* <1 y: 0.1–0.2 mg/kg IV over 2 min (may repeat in 30 min). *1–16 y:* 0.1–0.3 mg/kg IV over 2 min (may repeat in 30 min); 5 mg max. *Oral: 1–5 y:* 4–8 mg/kg/d in 3 ÷ doses. *>5 y:* 80 mg q6–8h; ↓ dose in renal/hepatic impairment **Caution/Contra:** [C, +] Conduction disorders, cardiogenic shock; caution with elderly patients **Supplied:** Tabs 40, 80, 120 mg; SR tabs 120, 180, 240 mg; SR caps 120, 180, 240, 360 mg; inj 5 mg/2 mL **Notes/SE:** Gingival hyperplasia, constipation, hypotension, bronchospasm, heart rate or conduction disturbances **Interactions:** ↑ effects with antihypertensives, nitrates, quinidine, alcohol, grapefruit juice; ↑ effects of buspirone, carbamazepine, cyclosporine, digoxin, prazosin, quinidine, theophylline, warfarin; ↓ effects with antineoplastics, barbiturates, NSAIDs, ↓ effects of lithium, rifampin **Labs:** ↑ ALT,

AST, alkaline phosphatase **NIPE:** Take with food; ↑ fluids and bulk foods to prevent constipation

Vinblastine (Velban, Velbe) WARNING: Chemotherapeutic agent; handle with caution

Uses: Hodgkin's and NHLs, mycosis fungoides, CAs (testis, renal cell, breast, small-cell lung, AIDS-related Kaposi's sarcoma, choriocarcinoma), histiocytosis X **Action:** Inhibits microtubule assembly through binding to tubulin **Dose:** 0.1–0.5 mg/kg/wk (4–20 mg/m²); ↓ dose in hepatic failure **Caution/Contra:** [D, ?] IT use **Supplied:** Inj 1 mg/mL **Notes/SE:** Myelosuppression (especially leukopenia), N/V (rare), constipation, neurotoxicity (like vincristine but less frequent), alopecia, rash; myalgia tumor pain **Interactions:** ↑ effects with erythromycin, itraconazole; ↓ effects with glutamic acid, tryptophan; ↑ effects of phenytoin **Labs:** ↑ uric acid **NIPE:** ↑ fluids to 2–3 L/d; ⊘ PRG or breastfeeding; use contraception for at least 2 mon >drug; photosensitivity – use sunscreen; ⊘ admin immunizations

Vincristine (Oncovin, Vincasar PFS) WARNING: Chemotherapeutic agent; handle with caution

Uses: ALL, breast and small-cell lung carcinoma, sarcoma (eg, Ewing's, rhabdomyosarcoma), Wilms' tumor, Hodgkin's and NHLs, neuroblastoma, multiple myeloma **Action:** Promotes disassembly of mitotic spindle, causing metaphase arrest **Dose:** 0.4–1.4 mg/m² (single doses 2 mg/max); ↓ dose in hepatic failure **Caution/Contra:** [D, ?] IT use **Supplied:** Inj 1 mg/mL **Notes/SE:** Neurotoxicity commonly dose limiting, jaw pain (trigeminal neuralgia), fever, fatigue, anorexia, constipation and paralytic ileus, bladder atony; no significant myelosuppression with standard doses; soft-tissue necrosis possible with extravasation **Interactions:** ↑ effects with CCBs; ↑ effects of methotrexate; ↑ risk of bronchospasm with mitomycin; ↓ effects of digoxin, phenytoin **NIPE:** ↑ fluids to 2–3 L/d; reversible hair loss; avoid exposure to infection; ⊘ admin immunizations

Vinorelbine (Navelbine) WARNING: Chemotherapeutic agent; handle with caution

Uses: Breast and non-small-cell lung CA (alone or with cisplatin) **Action:** Inhibits polymerization of microtubules, impairing mitotic spindle formation; semisynthetic vinca alkaloid **Dose:** 30 mg/m²/wk; ↓ dose in hepatic failure **Caution/Contra:** [D, ?] IT use **Supplied:** Inj 10 mg **Notes/SE:** Myelosuppression (especially leukopenia), mild GI effects, and infrequent neurotoxicity (6–29%); constipation and paresthesias (rare); tissue damage can result from extravasation **Interactions:** ↑ risk of granulocytopenia with cisplatin; ↑ pulmonary effects with mitomycin, paclitaxel **Labs:** ↑ LFTs **NIPE:** ⊘ PRG or breast-feeding; use contraception; ⊘ infectious environment; ↑ fluids to 2–3 L/d

Vitamin B₁, See Thiamine (page 219)
Vitamin B₆, See Pyridoxine (page 196)
Vitamin B₁₂, See Cyanocobalamin (page 76)
Vitamin K, See Phytonadione (page 186)
Voriconazole (VFEND) Uses: Invasive aspergillosis, serious infections caused by *Scedosporium* or *Fusarium* spp **Action:** Inhibits ergosterol synthesis

Dose: *IV:* 6 mg/kg q12h × 2, then 4 mg/kg bid; may reduce to 3 mg/kg/dose. *PO:* <40 kg–100 mg q12h, up to 150 mg; >40 kg–200 mg q12 h, up to 300 mg. ↓ dose in mild/moderate hepatic impairment **Caution/Contra:** [D,?/–] Severe hepatic impairment **Supplied:** Tabs 50, 200 mg; 200 mg inj **Notes/SE:** Must screen for multiple drug interactions (eg, increase dose when given with phenytoin); maintain oral doses on empty stomach; visual changes, fever, rash, GI upset, ↑ LFTs **Interactions:** ↑ effects with delavirdine, efavirenz; ↑ effects of benzodiazepines, buspirone, CCBs, cisapride, cyclosporine, ergots, pimozide, quinidine, sirolimus, sulfonylureas, tacrolimus, terfenidine; ↓ effects with carbamazepin, mephobarbital, phenobarbital, rifampin, ribabutin **NIPE:** Take w/o food; ↑ risk of photosensitivity; ⊗ PRG or breast-feeding;

Warfarin (Coumadin) Uses: Prophylaxis and Rx of PE and DVT, AF with embolization, other postoperative indications **Action:** Inhibits vitamin K-dependent production of clotting factors in the order VII-IX-X-II **Dose:** Table 10 (page 258) for anticoagulation guidelines. *Adults.* Adjust to keep INR 2.0–3.0 for most; mechanical valves' INR is 2.5–3.5. *ACCP guidelines:* 5 mg initially (unless rapid therapeutic INR needed), use 7.5–10 mg or patient elderly or has other bleeding risk factors ↓. *Alternative:* 10–15 mg PO, IM, or IV qd for 1–3 d; maint 2–10 mg/d PO, IV, or IM; follow daily INR initially to adjust dosage. *Peds.* 0.05–0.34 mg/kg/24 h PO, IM, or IV; follow PT/INR to adjust dosage; monitor vitamin K intake; consider ↓ doses in hepatic impairment or elderly **Caution/Contra:** [X, +] Severe hepatic or renal disease, bleeding, peptic ulcer **Supplied:** Tabs 1, 2, 2.5, 3, 4, 5, 6, 7.5, 10 mg; inj **Notes/SE:** INR preferred test rather than PT; follow INR; bleeding caused by excessive anticoagulation (PT >3× control or INR >5.0–6.0); to rapidly correct excessive anticoagulation, use vitamin K, FFP, or both; highly teratogenic; do not use in PRG. Caution patient on taking warfarin with other meds, especially ASA. *Common warfarin interactions*: Potentiated by APAP, alcohol (with liver disease), amiodarone, cimetidine, ciprofloxacin, co-trimoxazole, erythromycin, fluconazole, flu vaccine, isoniazid, itraconazole, metronidazole, omeprazole, phenytoin, propranolol, quinidine, tetracycline. Inhibited by barbiturates, carbamazepine, chlordiazepoxide, cholestyramine, dicloxacillin, nafcillin, rifampin, sucralfate, high vitamin K foods; bleeding, alopecia, skin necrosis, purple toe syndrome **Labs:** ↑ PTT; false ↓ serum theophylline levels **NIPE:** Reddish discoloration of urine; ⊗ PRG or breast-feeding; use Barrier contraception; monitor for bleeding

Witch Hazel (Tucks Pads, others) Uses: After bowel movement cleansing to decrease local irritation or relieve hemorrhoids; after anorectal surgery, episiotomy **Dose:** Apply PRN **Caution/Contra:** [?, ?] **Supplied:** Presoaked pads, liq **Notes/SE:** Mild itching or burning

Zafirlukast (Accolate) Uses: Prophylaxis and chronic Rx of asthma **Action:** Selective and competitive inhibitor of leukotrienes **Dose:** 20 mg bid; empty stomach **Caution/Contra:** [B, –] Interacts with warfarin, can ↑ PT **Supplied:** Tabs

20 mg **Notes/SE:** Not for acute asthma; hepatic dysfunction, usually reversible on discontinuation; HA, dizziness, GI upset; Churg–Strauss syndrome;\ **Interactions:** ↑ effects with ASA; ↑ effects of CCBs, cyclosporine; ↑ risk of bleeding with warfarin; ↓ effects with erythromycin, theophylline, food **Labs:** ↑ ALT **NIPE:** Take w/o food; ⊘ use for acute asthma attack

Zalcitabine (Hivid)   **WARNING:** Use with caution in patients with neuropathy, pancreatitis, lactic acidosis, hepatitis **Uses:** HIV **Action:** Antiretroviral agent **Dose:** 0.75 mg PO tid; ↓ dose in renal failure **Caution/Contra:** [C, +] **Supplied:** Tabs 0.375, 0.75 mg **Notes/SE:** May be used in combination with zidovudine; peripheral neuropathy, pancreatitis, fever, malaise, anemia, hypo-/hyperglycemia, hepatic impairment **Interactions:** ↑ risk of peripheral neuropathy with amphotericin B, aminoglycosides, cisplatin, didanosine, disulfiram, foscarnet, isoniazid, phenytoin, ribavirin, vincristine; ↑ effects with cimetidine, metoclopramide; probenecid; ↓ effects with antacids **Labs:** ↑ LFTs, lipase, triglycerides **NIPE:** Use barrier contraception; take w/o regard to food

Zaleplon (Sonata)   **Uses:** Insomnia **Action:** A nonbenzodiazepine sedative hypnotic, a pyrazolopyrimidine **Dose:** 5–20 mg hs PRN; ↓ dose in renal/hepatic insufficiency, elderly **Caution/Contra:** [C, ?/–] Caution in mental/psychologic conditions **Supplied:** Caps 5, 10 mg **Notes/SE:** HA, edema, amnesia, somnolence, photosensitivity **Interactions:** ↑ CNS depression with cimetidine, CNS depressants, imipramine, thioridazine, alcohol; ↓ effects with carbamazepine, phenobarbital, phenytoin, rifampin **NIPE:** Rapid effects of drug; take w/o food ⊘ d/c abruptly

Zanamivir (Relenza)   **Uses:** Influenza A and B **Action:** Inhibits viral neuraminidase **Dose:** *Adults & Peds >7 y.* 2 inhal (10 mg) bid for 5 d; initiate w/n 48 h of symptoms **Caution/Contra:** [C, M] Pulmonary disease **Supplied:** Powder for inhal 5 mg **Notes/SE:** Uses a Diskhaler for administration; bronchospasm, HA, GI upset **Labs:** ↑?LFTS, CPK **NIPE:** Does not reduce risk of transmitting virus

Zidovudine (Retrovir)   **WARNING:** Neutropenia, anemia, lactic acidosis, and hepatomegaly with steatosis **Uses:** HIV infection **Action:** Inhibits reverse transcriptase **Dose:** *Adults.* 200 mg PO tid or 300 mg PO bid or 1–2 mg/kg/dose IV q4h. *Pregnancy:* 100 mg PO 5x/d until the start of labor, then during labor 2 mg/kg over 1 h followed by 1 mg/kg/h until clamping of the umbilical cord. *Peds.* 160 mg/m^2/dose q8h; ↓ dose in renal failure **Caution/Contra:** [C, ?/–] **Supplied:** Caps 100 mg; tabs 300 mg; syrup 50 mg/5 mL; inj 10 mg/mL **Notes/SE:** Hematologic toxicity, HA, fever, rash, GI upset, malaise **Interactions:** ↑ effects with fluconazole, phenytoin, probenecid, trimethoprim, valporoic acid, vinblastine, vincristine; ↑ hematologic toxicity with adriamycin, dapsone, ganciclovir, interferon-α; ↓ effects with rifampin, ribavirin, stavudine **NIPE:** Take w/o food monitor for s/s opportunistic infection; monitor for anemia

Zidovudine and Lamivudine (Combivir)   **WARNING:** Neutropenia, anemia, lactic acidosis, and hepatomegaly with steatosis **Uses:** HIV infections

Action: Combination inhibitors of reverse transcriptase **Dose:** *Adults & Peds >12 y.* 1 tab bid; ↓?dose in renal failure **Caution/Contra:** [C, ?/–] **Supplied:** Caps zidovudine 300 mg/lamivudine 150 mg **Notes/SE:** An alternative to ↓ number of caps for combination therapy with the two agents; hematologic toxicity, HA, fever, rash, GI upset, malaise, pancreatitis **Interactions:** ↑ effects with fluconazole, phenytoin, probenecid, trimethoprim, valporoic acid, vinblastine, vincristine; ↑ hematologic toxicity with adriamycin, dapsone, ganciclovir, interferon-α; ↓ effects with rifampin, ribavirin, stavudine **NIPE:** Take w/o food; monitor for s/s opportunistic infection; monitor for anemia

Zileuton (Zyflo) **Uses:** Prophylaxis and chronic treatment of asthma **Action:** Inhibitor of 5-lipoxygenase **Dose:** 600 mg qid **Caution/Contra:** [C, ?/–] Hepatic impairment **Supplied:** Tabs 600 mg **Notes/SE:** Must take on a regular basis; not for acute asthma; hepatic damage, HA, GI upset, leucopenia **Interactions:** ↑ effects of propranolol, terfenadine, theophylline, warfarin **Labs:** ↑ LFTs, ↓ WBCs; **NIPE:** Take w/o regard to food

Ziprasidone (Geodon) **Uses:** Schizophrenia, acute agitation **Action:** Atypical antipsychotic **Dose:** 20 mg PO bid with food, may increase in 2-day intervals up to 80 mg bid; agitation 10–20 mg IM PRN up to 40 mg/d. Separate 10-mg doses by 2h and 20-mg doses by 4 h **Caution/Contra:** [C, –] QT prolongation, recent MI, uncompensated heart failure, meds that prolong QT interval **Supplied:** Caps 20, 40, 60, 80 mg; Inj 20 mg/mL **Notes/SE:** Caution in hypokalemia/hypomagnesemia, bradycardia; monitor electrolytes; rash, somnolence, respiratory disorder, EPS, weight gain, orthostatic hypotension **Interactions:** ↑ effects with ketoconazole; ↑ effects of antihypertensives; ↑ CNS depression with anxiolytics, sedatives, opioids, alcohol; TCAs, thioridazine, risk of prolonged QT with cisapride, chlorpromazine, clarithromycin, diltiazem, erythromycin, levofloxacin, mefloquine, pentamidine, TCAs, thioridazine; ↓ effects with amphetamines, carbamazepine; ↓ effects of levodopa **Labs:** ↑ prolactin, cholesterol, triglycerides **NIPE:** May take wks before full effects, take with food, ↑ risk of tardive dyskinesia

Zoledronic acid (Zometa) **Uses:** Hypercalcemia of malignancy (HCM), ↓ skeletal-related events in prostate CA, multiple myeloma, and metastatic bone lesions **Action:** Bisphosphonate: inhibits osteoclastic bone resorption **Dose:** *HCM:* 4 mg IV over at least 15 min; may retreat in 7 days if adequate renal function. *Bone lesions/myeloma:* 4 mg IV over at least 15 min repeat q3–4wk PRN; prolonged with Cr ↑ **Caution/Contra:** [C, ?/–] Contra if bisphosphonate hypersensitive; caution with loop diuretics and aminoglycosides; adverse effects ↑ with renal dysfunction; caution in ASA-sensitive asthmatics **Supplied:** Vial 4 mg **Notes/SE:** Requires vigorous prehydration; do not exceed recommended doses/inf duration to minimize dose-related renal dysfunction; follow Cr; fever, flu-like syndrome, GI upset, insomnia, anemia, electrolyte abnormalities **Interactions:** ↑ risk of hypocalcemia with diuretics; ↑ risk of nephrotoxicity with aminoglycosides, thalidomide **NIPE:** ↑ fluids to 2–3 L/d

Zolmitriptan (Zomig) **Uses:** Rx acute migraine **Action:** Selective serotonin agonist; causes vasoconstriction **Dose:** Initial 2.5 mg, may repeat after 2 h to 10 mg max in 24 h **Caution/Contra:** [C, ?/–] Ischemic heart disease, Prinzmetal's angina, uncontrolled HTN, accessory conduction pathway disorders, ergots, MAOIs **Supplied:** Tabs 2.5, 5 mg **Notes/SE:** Dizziness, hot flashes, paresthesias, chest tightness, myalgia, diaphoresis **Interactions:** ↑ effects with cimetidine, MAOIs, oral contraceptives, propranolol; ↑ risk of prolonged vasospasms with ergots; ↑ risk of serotonin syndrome with sibutramine, SSRIs **NIPE:** Admin to relieve migraines; not for prophylaxis

Zolpidem (Ambien) **Uses:** Short-term treatment of insomnia **Action:** Hypnotic agent **Dose:** 5–10 mg PO hs PRN; ↓ dose in elderly, hepatic insufficiency **Caution/Contra:** [B, +] **Supplied:** Tabs 5, 10 mg **Notes/SE:** HA, dizziness, drowsiness, nausea, myalgia **Interactions:** ↑ CNS depression with CNS depressants, sertraline, alcohol ↑ effects of ketoconazole; ↓ effects of rifampin; **NIPE:** Take w/o food; ⊘ d/c abruptly if long-term use; may develop tolerance to drug

Zonisamide (Zonegran) **Uses:** Partial seizures **Action:** Anticonvulsant **Dose:** Initial 100 mg/d; may ↑ to 400 mg/d **Caution/Contra:** [C, –] Hypersensitivity to sulfonamides, oligohidrosis and hypothermia in peds **Supplied:** Caps 100 mg **Notes/SE:** Dizziness, drowsiness, confusion, ataxia, memory impairment, paresthesias, psychosis, nystagmus, diplopia, tremor; anemia, leukopenia; GI upset, nephrolithiasis, Stevens–Johnson syndrome; monitor for ↓ sweating and ↑ body temperature **Interactions:** ↓ effects with carbamazepine, phenobarbital, phenytoin, valproic acid **Labs:** ↑ serum alkaline phosphatase, ALT, AST, creatinine, BUN, ↓ glucose, sodium **NIPE:** ⊘ d/c abruptly, ↑ fluids to 2–3 L/d; take w/o regard to food

TABLES

TABLE 1
Quick Guide to Dosing of Acetaminophen Based on the Tylenol Product Line

	Suspension^a Drops and Original Drops 80 mg/0.8 mL Dropperful	Chewable^a Tablets 80-mg tabs	Suspension^a Liquid and Original Elixir 160 mg/5 mL	Junior^a Strength 160-mg Caplets/Chewables	Regular^b Strength 325-mg Caplets/Tablets	Extra Strength^b 500-mg Caplets/Gelcaps
Birth–3 mo/ 6–11 lb/ 2.5–5.4 kg	½ dppr^c (0.4 mL)					
4–11 mo/ 12–17 lb/ 5.5–7.9 kg	1 dppr^c (0.8 mL)		½ tsp			
12–23 mo/ 18–23 lb/ 8.0–10.9 kg	1½ dppr^c (1.2 mL)		¾ tsp			
2–3 y/24–35 lb/ 11.0–15.9 kg	2 dppr^c (1.6 mL)	2 tab	1 tsp			
4–5 y/36–47 lb/ 16.0–21.9 kg		3 tab	1½ tsp			

240

6–8 y/48–59 lb/ 22.0–26.9 kg	4 tab	2 tsp	2 cap/tab		
9–10 y/60–71 lb/ 27.0–31.9 kg	5 tab	2½ tsp	2½ cap/ tab		
11 y/72–95 lb/ 32.0–43.9 kg	6 tab	4 tsp	3 cap/tab		
Adults & children 12 y and over/ 96 lb and over/ 44.0 kg and over			4 cap/tab	1 or 2 caps/ tabs	2 caps/ gel

241

TABLE 2
Common Drug Levels[a]

Drug	When to Sample	Therapeutic Levels	Usual Half-Life	Potentially Toxic Levels
Antibiotics				
Gentamicin	Peak: 30 min after 30-min infusion (peak level not necessary if extended-interval dosing: 6 mg/kg/dose) Trough: <0.5 h before next dose	Peak: 5–8 µg/mL Trough: <2 µg/mL <1.0 µg/mL for extended intervals (6 mg/kg/dose) (peak levels not needed with extended-interval dosing)	2 h	Peak: >12 µg/mL
Tobramycin	Same as above	Same as above	Same as above	Same as above
Amikacin	Same as above	Peak: 20–30 µg/mL	2 h	Peak: >35 µg/mL
Vancomycin	Peak: 1 h after 1-h infusion Trough: <0.5 h before next dose	Peak: 30–40 µg/mL	6–8 h	Peak: >50 µg/mL Trough: >15 µg/mL

242

Anticonvulsants

Carbamazepine	Trough: just before next oral dose	8–12 µg/mL (monotherapy) 4–8 µg/mL (polytherapy)	15–20 h	Trough: >12 µg/mL
Ethosuximide	Trough: just before next oral dose	40–100 µg/mL	30–60 h	Trough: >100 µg/mL
Phenobarbital	Trough: just before next dose	15–40 µg/mL	40–120 h	Trough: >40 µg/mL
Phenytoin	May use free phenytoin to monitor[b] Trough: just before next dose	10–20 µg/mL	Concentration-dependent	>20 µg/mL
Primidone	Trough: just before next dose [primidone is metabolized to phenobarb; order levels separately]	5–12 µg/mL	10–12 h	>12 µg/mL
Valproic acid	Trough: just before next dose	50–100 µg/mL	5–20 h	>100 µg/mL

243

TABLE 2
(Continued)

Drug	When to Sample	Therapeutic Levels	Usual Half-Life	Potentially Toxic Levels
Bronchodilators				
Caffeine	Trough: just before next dose	Adults 5–15 µg/mL Neonates 6–11 µg/mL	Adults 3–4 h Neonates 30–140 h	20 µg/mL
Theophylline (IV)	IV: 12–24 h after infusion started	5–15 µg/mL	Nonsmoking adults 8 h Children and smoking adults 4 h	>20 µg/mL
Theophylline (PO)	Peak levels: not recommended Trough level: just before next dose	5–15 µg/mL		
Cardiovascular Agents				
Amiodarone	Trough: just before next dose	1–2.5 µg/mL	30–100 days	>2.5 µg/mL

244

	Sampling Time	Therapeutic Range	Half-Life	Toxic Level
Digoxin	Trough: just before next dose (levels drawn earlier than 6 h after a dose will be artificially elevated)	0.8–2.0 ng/mL	36 h	>2 ng/mL
Disopyramide	Trough: just before next dose	2–5 µg/mL	4–10 h	>5 µg/mL
Flecainide	Trough: just before next dose	0.2–1.0 µg/mL	11–14 h	>1.0 µg/mL
Lidocaine	Steady-state levels are usually achieved after 6–12 h	1.2–5.0 µg/mL	1.5 h	>6.0 µg/mL
Procainamide	Trough: just before next oral dose	4–10 µg/mL NAPA + Procaine: 5–30 µg/mL	Procaine: 3–5 h NAPA: 6–10 h	>10 µg/mL >30 µg/mL NAPA + Procaine: 0.5 µg/mL
Quinidine	Trough: just before next oral dose	2–5 µg/mL	6 h	
Other Agents				
Amitriptyline plus nortriptyline	Trough: just before next dose	120–250 ng/mL		
Nortriptyline	Trough: just before next dose	50–140 ng/mL		
Lithium	Trough: just before next dose	0.5–1.5 mEq/mL	18–20 h	>1.5 mEq/mL

245

TABLE 2
(Continued)

Drug	When to Sample	Therapeutic Levels	Usual Half-life	Potentially Toxic Levels
Imipramine plus desipramine	Trough: just before next dose	150–300 ng/mL		
Desipramine	Trough: just before next dose	50–300 ng/mL		
Methotrexate	By protocol	<0.5 μmol/L after 48 h		
Cyclosporine	Trough: just before next dose	Highly variable Renal: 150–300 ng/mL (RIA) Hepatic: 150–300 ng/mL	Highly variable	
Doxepin	Trough: just before next dose	100–300 ng/mL		
Trazodone	Trough: just before next dose	900–2100 ng/mL		

Results of therapeutic drug monitoring *must* be interpreted in light of the complete clinical situation. For information on dosing or interpretation of drug levels contact the pharmacist or an order for a pharmacokinetic consult may be written in the patient's chart. Modified and reproduced with permission from the *Pharmacy and Therapeutics Committee Formulary*, 41st ed., Thomas Jefferson University Hospital, Philadelphia, PA.
bMore reliable in cases of uremia and hypoalbuminemia.

246

TABLE 3
Local Anesthetic Comparison Chart for Commonly Used Injectable Agents

Agent	Proprietary Names	Onset	Duration	mg/kg	Volume in 70-kg Adult[a]
					Maximum Dose
Bupivacaine	Marcaine, Sensoricaine	7–30 min	5–7 h	3	70 mL of 0.25% solution
Lidocaine	Xylocaine, Anestacon	5–30 min	2 h	4	28 mL of 1% solution
Lidocaine with epinephrine (1:200,000)		5–30 min	2–3 h	7	50 mL of 1% solution
Mepivacaine	Carbocaine	5–30 min	2–3 h	7	50 mL of 1% solution
Procaine	Novocaine	Rapid	30 min–1 h	10–15	70–105 mL of 1% solution

[a]To calculate the maximum dose if not a 70-kg adult, use the fact that a 1% solution has 10 mg of drug per milliliter.

247

TABLE 4
Comparison of Systemic Steroids

Drug	Relative Equivalent Dose (mg)	Mineralo-corticoid Activity	Duration (h)	Route
Betamethasone	0.75	0	36–72	PO, IM
Cortisone (Cortone)	25.00	2	8–12	PO, IM
Dexamethasone (Decadron)	0.75	0	36–72	PO, IV
Hydrocortisone (Solu-Cortef, Hydrocortone)	20.00	2	8–12	PO, IM, IV
Methylprednisolone acetate (Depo-Medrol)	4.00	0	36–72	PO, IM, IV
Methylprednisolone succinate (Solu-Medrol)	4.00	0	8–12	PO, IM, IV
Prednisone (Deltasone)	5.00	1	12–36	PO
Prednisolone (Delta-Cortef)	5.00	1	12–36	PO, IM, IV

TABLE 5
Topical Steroid Preparations

Agent	Common Trade Names	Potency	Apply
Alclometasone dipropionate	Aclovate, cream, oint 0.05%	Low	bid/tid
Amcinonide	Cyclocort, cream, lotion, oint 0.1%	High	bid/tid
Betamethasone			
Betamethasone valerate	Valisone cream, lotion 0.01%	Low	qd/bid
Betamethasone valerate	Valisone cream 0.01, 0.1%, oint, lotion 0.1%	Intermediate	qd/bid
Betamethasone dipropionate	Diprosone cream 0.05%	High	qd/bid
Betamethasone dipropionate	Diprosone aerosol 0.1%		
Betamethasone dipropionate, augmented	Diprolene oint, gel 0.05%	Ultrahigh	qd/bid
Clobetasol propionate	Temovate cream, gel, oint, scalp, soln 0.05%	Ultrahigh	bid (2 wk max)
Clocortolone pivalate	Cloderm cream 0.1%	Intermediate	qd-qid
Desonide	DesOwen, cream, oint, lotion 0.05%	Low	bid-qid
Desoximetasone			
Desoximetasone 0.05%	Topicort LP cream, gel 0.05%	Intermediate	
Desoximetasone 0.25%	Topicort cream, oint	High	
Dexamethasone base	Aeroseb-Dex aerosol 0.01%	Low	bid-qid
	Decadron cream 0.1%		
Diflorasone diacetate	Psorcon cream, oint 0.05%	Ultrahigh	bid/qid
Fluocinolone			
Fluocinolone acetonide 0.01%	Synalar cream, soln 0.01%	Low	bid/tid
Fluocinolone acetonide 0.025%	Synalar oint, cream 0.025%	Intermediate	bid/tid

TABLE 5
(Continued)

Agent	Common Trade Names	Potency	Apply
Fluocinolone acetonide 0.2%	Synalar-HP cream 0.2%	High	bid/tid
Fluocinonide 0.05%	Lidex, anhydrous cream, gel, soln 0.05%	High	bid/tid oint
	Lidex-E aqueous cream 0.05%		
Flurandrenolide	Cordran cream, oint 0.025%	Intermediate	bid/tid
	cream, lotion, oint 0.05%	Intermediate	bid/tid
	tape, 4 μg/cm²	Intermediate	qd
Fluticasone propionate	Cutivate cream 0.05%, oint 0.005%	Intermediate	bid
Halobetasol	Ultravate cream, oint 0.05%	Very High	bid
Halcinonide	Halog cream 0.025%, emollient base 0.1% cream, oint, solution 0.1%	High	qd/tid
Hydrocortisone			
Hydrocortisone	Cortizone, Caldecort, Hycort, Hytone, etc.	Low	tid/qid
	aerosol 1%, cream: 0.5, 1, 2.5%, gel 0.5%, oint 0.5, 1, 2.5%, lotion 0.5, 1, 2.5%, paste 0.5%, soln 1%		
Hydrocortisone acetate	Corticaine cream, oint 0.5, 1%	Low	tid/qid
Hydrocortisone butyrate	Locoid oint, soln 0.1%	Intermediate	bid/tid
Hydrocortisone valerate	Westcort cream, oint 0.2%	Intermediate	bid/tid

250

Mometasone furoate	Elocon 0.1% cream, oint, lotion	Intermediate	qd
Prednicarbate	Dermatop 0.1% cream	Intermediate	bid
Triamcinolone			
Triamcinolone acetonide 0.025%	Aristocort, Kenalog cream, oint, lotion 0.025%	Low	tid/qid
Triamcinolone acetonide 0.1%	Aristocort, Kenalog cream, oint, lotion 0.1% Aerosol 0.2 mg/2-sec spray	Intermediate	tid/qid
Triamcinolone acetonide 0.5%	Aristocort, Kenalog cream, oint 0.5%	High	tid/qid

TABLE 6
Comparison of Insulins

Type of Insulin	Onset (h)	Peak (h)	Duration (h)
Ultra Rapid			
Humalog (lispro)	Immediate	0.5–1.5	3–5
NovoLog (insulin aspart)	Immediate	0.5–1.5	3–5
Rapid			
Regular Iletin II	0.25–0.5	2.0–4.0	5–7
Humulin R	0.5	2.0–4.0	6–8
Novolin R	0.5	2.5–5.0	5–8
Velosulin	0.5	2.0–5.0	6–8
Intermediate			
NPH Iletin II	1.0–2.0	6–12	18–24
Lente Iletin II	1.0–2.0	6–12	18–24
Humulin N	1.0–2.0	6–12	14–24
Novolin L	2.5–5.0	7–15	18–24
Novulin 70/30	0.5	7–12	24
Prolonged			
Ultralente	4.0–6.0	14–24	28–36
Humulin U	4.0–6.0	8–20	24–28
Lantus (insulin glargine)	4.0–6.0	No peak	24
Combination Insulins			
Humalog Mix (lispro protamine/ lispro)	0.25–0.5	1–4	24

TABLE 7
Some Oral Contraceptives (see page 174 for dosing information)

Drug (Manufacturer)	Estrogen (μg)[a]	Progestin (mg)[b]
Monophasics		
Alesse 21, 28 (Wyeth)	Ethinyl estradiol (20)	Desogestrel (0.15)
Brevicon 21, 28 (Watson)[c]	Ethinyl estradiol (35)	Norethindrone (0.5)
Demulen 1/35 21 (Searle)[c]	Ethinyl estradiol (35)	Ethynodiol diacetate (1)
Demulen 1/50 21 (Searle)[c]	Ethinyl estradiol (50)	Ethynodiol diacetate (1)
Desogen 28 (Organon)	Ethinyl estradiol (30)	Desogestrel (0.15)
Genora 1/50 28 (Physicians total care)	Mestranol (50)	Norethindrone (1)
Genora 1/35 21, 28 (Physicians total care)	Ethinyl estradiol (35)	Norethindrone (1)
Levlen 21, 28 (Berlex)	Ethinyl estradiol (30)	Levonorgestrel (0.15)
Levlite 21, 28 (Berlex)	Ethinyl estradiol (20)	Levonorgestrel (0.1)
Levora 21, 28 (Watson)	Ethinyl estradiol (30)	Levonorgestrel (0.15)
Loestrin 1.5/30 21, 28 (Parke-Davis)	Ethinyl estradiol (30)	Norethindrone acetate (1, 5)
Loestrin 1/20 21, 28 (Parke-Davis)	Ethinyl estradiol (20)	Norethindrone acetate (1)
Lo/Ovral (Wyeth)[c]	Ethinyl estradiol (30)	Norgestrel (0.3)
Low-Ogestrel (Watson)	Ethinyl estradiol (30)	Norgestrel (0.3)
Modicon 28 (Ortho-McNeil)	Ethinyl estradiol (35)	Norethindrone (0.5)
Necon 1/50 21, 28 (Watson)	Mestranol (50)	Norethindrone (1)
Necon 0.5/35E 21, 28 (Watson)	Ethinyl estradiol (35)	Norethindrone (0.5)
Necon 1/35 21, 28 (Watson)	Ethinyl estradiol (35)	Norethindrone (1)
Nelova 0.5/35E 21 (Warner-Chilcott)[c]	Ethinyl estradiol (35)	Norethindrone (0.5)
Nelova 1/35 21 (Warner-Chilcott)	Ethinyl estradiol (35)	Norethindrone (1)
Nelova 1/50 21 (Warner-Chilcott)[c]	Mestranol (50)	Norethindrone (1)
Nordette 21 (Wyeth)[c]	Ethinyl estradiol (30)	Levonorgestrel (0.15)

253

TABLE 7
(Continued)

Drug (Manufacturer)	Estrogen (μg)[a]	Progestin (mg)[b]
Norinyl 1/35 21, 28 (Watson)	Ethinyl estradiol (35)	Norethindrone (1)
Norinyl 1/50 21, 28 (Watson)	Mestranol (50)	Norethindrone (1)
Ogestrel-28 (Watson)	Ethinyl estradiol (50)	Norgestrel (0.5)
Ortho-Cept 21 (Ortho-McNeil)[c]	Ethinyl estradiol (30)	Desogestrel (0.15)
Ortho-Cyclen 21 (Ortho-McNeil)[c]	Ethinyl estradiol (35)	Norgestimate (0.25)
Ortho-Novum 1/35 21 (Ortho-McNeil)[c]	Ethinyl estradiol (35)	Norethindrone (1)
Ortho-Novum 1/50 21 (Ortho-McNeil)[c]	Mestranol (50)	Norethindrone (1)
Ovcon 35 21, 28 (Warner Chilcott)	Ethinyl estradiol (35)	Norethindrone (0.4)
Ovcon 50 21, 28 (Warner Chilcott)	Ethinyl estradiol (50)	Norethindrone (1)
Ovral (Wyeth-Ayerst)[c]	Ethinyl estradiol (50)	Norgestrel (0.5)
Zovia 1/50E 21, 28 (Watson)	Ethinyl estradiol (50)	Ethynodiol diacetate (1)
Zovia 1/35E 21, 28 (Watson)	Ethinyl estradiol (35)	Ethynodiol diacetate (1)

Biphasics

Jenest-28 (Organon)	Ethinyl estradiol (35)	Norethindrone (0.5, 1)
Necon 10/11 21, 28 (Watson)[c]	Ethinyl estradiol (35)	Norethindrone (0.5, 1)
Nelova 10/11 21 (Warner-Chilcott-McNeil)	Ethinyl estradiol (35)	Norethindrone (0.5, 1)
Ortho-Novum 10/11 21 (Ortho)[c]	Ethinyl estradiol (35, 35)	Norethindrone (0.5, 1.0)

Triphasics[d]

Estrostep 28 (Parke-Davis)	Ethinyl estradiol (20, 30, 35)	Norethindrone acetate (1)
Mircette 28 (Organon)	Ethinyl estradiol (20, 0, 10),	Desogestrel (0.15)
Ortho Tri-Cyclen (Ortho-McNeil)[c]	Ethinyl estradiol (35, 35, 35)	Norgestimate (0.18, 0.215, 0.25)

254

Ortho-Novum 7/7/7 21 (Ortho-McNeil)[c]	Ethinyl estradiol (35, 35, 35)	Norethindrone (0.5, 0.75, 1.0)
Tri-Levlen 21, 28 (Berlex)	Ethinyl estradiol (30, 40, 30)	Levonorgestrel (0.05, 0.075, 0.125)
Tri-Norinyl 21, 28 (Watson)	Ethinyl estradiol (35, 35, 35)	Norethindrone (0.5, 1.0, 0.5)
Triphasil-21 (Wyeth)[c]	Ethinyl estradiol (30, 40, 30)	Levonorgestrel (0.05, 0.075, 0.125)
Trivora-28 (Watson)	Ethinyl estradiol (30, 40, 30)	Levonorgestrel (0.05, 0.075, 0.125)

Progestin Only

Micronor (Ortho-McNeil)	None	Norethindrone (0.35)
Nor-QD (Watson)	None	Norethindrone (0.35)
Ovrette (Wyeth-Ayerst)	None	Norgestrel (0.075)

[a] Ethinyl estradiol and mestranol are not equivalent microgram for microgram; the results of some studies indicate that 35 μg of ethinyl estradiol is equivalent to 50 μg of mestranol.

[b] Different progestins are not equivalent milligram for milligram.

[c] Also available in a 28-d regimen at slightly different cost.

[d] Estrogen/progesterone dose varies based on time of cycle (ie, day 1–7, 8–14, 15–21).

TABLE 8
Some Common Oral Potassium Supplements

Brand Name	Salt	Form	mEq Potassium/ Dosing Unit
Glu-K	Gluconate	Tablet	2 mEq/tablet
Kaochlor 10%	KCl	Liquid	20 mEq/15 mL
Kaochlor S-F 10% (sugar-free)	KCl	Liquid	20 mEq/15 mL
Kaochlor Eff	Bicarbonate/ KCl/citrate	Effervescent tablet	20 mEq/tablet
Kaon elixir	Gluconate	Liquid	20 mEq/15 mL
Kaon	Gluconate	Tablets	5 mEq/tablet
Kaon-Cl	KCl	Tablet, SR	6.67 mEq/tablet
Kaon-Cl 20%	KCl	Liquid	40 mEq/15 mL
KayCiel	KCl	Liquid	20 mEq/15 mL
K-Lor	KCl	Powder	15 or 20 mEq/packet
Klorvess	Bicarbonate/ KCl	Liquid	20 mEq/15 mL
Klotrix	KCl	Tablet, SR	10 mEq/tablet
K-Lyte	Bicarbonate/ citrate	Effervescent tablet	25 mEq/tablet
K-Tab	KCl	Tablet, SR	10 mEq/tablet
Micro-K	KCl	Capsules, SR	8 mEq/capsule
Slow-K	KCl	Tablet, SR	8 mEq/tablet
Tri-K	Acetate/bicarbonate and citrate	Liquid	45 mEq/15 mL
Twin-K	Citrate/gluconate	Liquid	20 mEq/5 mL

SR = sustained release.

TABLE 9
Tetanus Prophylaxis

History of Absorbed Tetanus Toxoid Immunization	Clean, Minor Wounds		All Other Wounds[a]	
	Td[b]	TIG[c]	Td[d]	TIG[c]
Unknown or <3 doses	Yes	No	Yes	Yes
<3 doses	No[e]	No	No[f]	No

[a] Such as, but not limited to, wounds contaminated with dirt, feces, soil, saliva, etc; puncture wounds; avulsions; and wounds resulting from missiles, crushing, burns, and frostbite.

[b] Td = tetanus-diphtheria toxoid (adult type), 0.5 mL IM.
- For children <7 y, DPT (DT, if pertussis vaccine is contraindicated) is preferred to tetanus toxoid alone.
- For persons >7 y, Td is preferred to tetanus toxoid alone.
- DT = diphtheria-tetanus toxoid (pediatric), used for those who cannot receive pertussis.

[c] TIG = tetanus immune globulin, 250 U IM.

[d] If only 3 doses of fluid toxoid have been received, then a fourth dose of toxoid, preferably an adsorbed toxoid, should be given.

[e] Yes, if >10 y since last dose.

[f] Yes, if >5 y since last dose.

Source: Based on guidelines from the Centers for Disease Control and Prevention and reported in *MMWR*.

TABLE 10
Oral Anticoagulant Standards of Practice

Thromboembolic Disorder	INR	Duration
Deep Venous Thrombosis		
High-risk surgery (prophylaxis)	10 mg night before surgery 5 mg night of surgery	Short term only
Treatment: single episode	2–3	3–6 mo
Recurrent systemic embolism	2–3	Indefinite
Prevention of Systemic Embolism		
Atrial fibrillation (AF)[a]	2–3	Indefinite
AF: cardioversion	2–3	3 wk prior; 4 wk post sinus rhythm
Valvular heart disease	2–3	Indefinite
Cardiomyopathy	2–3	Indefinite
Acute Myocardial Infarction		
Prevention of systemic embolization	2–3	<3 mo
Prevention of recurrence	2.5–3.5	Indefinite
Prosthetic Valves		
Tissue heart valves	2–3	3 mo
Bileaflet mechanical valves in aortic position	2–3	2–3 mo Indefinite
Other mechanical prosthetic valves[b]	2.5–3.5	Indefinite

[a]With high-risk factors or multiple moderate risk factors.

[b]May add aspirin 81 mg to warfarin in patients with ball–cage valves or with additional risk factors.

INR = international normalized ratio.

Source: Based on data published in *Chest* 2001;119 Supplement 1S–307S.

TABLE 11
Serotonin 5-HT₁ Receptor Agonists

Drug	Initial Dose	Repeat Dose	Max. Dose/24h	Supplied
Almotriptan (Axert)	6.25 or 12.5 mg PO	× 1 in 2 h	25 mg	Tabs 6.25, 12.5 mg
Frovatriptan (Frova)	2.5 mg PO	in 2 h	7.5 mg	Tabs 2.5 mg
Naratriptan (Amerge)	1 or 2.5 mg PO[a]	in 4 h	5 mg	Tabs 1, 2.5 mg
Rizatriptan (Maxalt)	5 to 10 mg PO[b]	in 2 h	30 mg	Tabs 5,10 mg Disintegrating tabs 5, 10 mg
Sumatriptan (Imitrex)	25, 50, or 100 mg PO 5–20 mg intranasally 6 mg SC	in 2 h in 2 h in 1 h	200 mg 40 mg 12 mg	Tabs 25,50 mg Nasal spray 5, 20 mg Inj 12 mg/mL
Zolmitriptan (Zomig)	2.5 or 5 mg PO	in 2 h	10 mg	Tabs 2.5,5 mg

Precautions/contraindications: [C, M]; ischemic heart disease, coronary artery vasospasm, Prinzmetal's angina, uncontrolled HTN, hemiplegic or basilar migraine, ergots, use of another serotonin agonist within 24 h, use with MAOI. Side effects: dizziness, somnolence, paresthesias, nausea, flushing, dry mouth, coronary vasospasm, chest tightness, HTN, GI upset.

[a]Reduce dose in mild renal and hepatic insufficiency (2.5 mg/d MAX); contraindicated with severe renal (CrCl <15 mL/min) or hepatic impairment.

[b]Initiate therapy at 5 mg PO (15 mg/d max) in patients receiving propranolol.

259

INDEX

NOTE: Page numbers followed by t indicate tables.